协和百年纪念文集

The Legacy of PUMC：Centennial Essays

主　编　蒋育红
〔美〕玛丽·布朗·布洛克（Mary Brown Bullock）

 中国协和医科大学出版社

图书在版编目（CIP）数据

协和百年纪念文集 / 蒋育红，（美）玛丽·布朗·布洛克（Mary Brown Bullock）主编 . —北京：中国协和医科大学出版社，2017. 9
ISBN 978 - 7 - 5679 - 0897 - 0

Ⅰ.①协…　Ⅱ.①蒋…　②玛…　Ⅲ.①北京协和医学院 – 纪念文集 – 汉、英　Ⅳ.①R199. 2 – 53

中国版本图书馆 CIP 数据核字（2017）第 179534 号

协和百年纪念文集
The Legacy of PUMC：Centennial Essays

主　　编：	蒋育红　[美] 玛丽·布朗·布洛克（Mary Brown Bullock）	
责任编辑：	顾良军	

出版发行：中国协和医科大学出版社
（北京东单三条九号　邮编 100730　电话 65260431）

网　　址：www. pumcp. com
经　　销：新华书店总店北京发行所
印　　刷：中煤（北京）印务有限公司

开　　本：710×1000　1/16 开
印　　张：34. 5
字　　数：480 千字
版　　次：2017 年 9 月第 1 版
印　　次：2017 年 9 月第 1 次印刷
定　　价：58. 00 元

ISBN 978 - 7 - 5679 - 0897 - 0

（凡购本书，如有缺页、倒页、脱页及其他质量问题，由本社发行部调换）

序 言

1917 年 9 月，在中国北京紫禁城一公里开外的豫王府中，举办了隆重的北京协和医学院（Peking Union Medical College，PUMC）奠基典礼。在中美双方的见证下，一座承载着崇高使命的建筑群庄严地落下奠基石。从此，在东单三条胡同矗立起中国现代医学教育史上的丰碑，在这个中西合璧的宫殿式建筑群里，孕育了中国现代医学的跨越发展和巨大进步。过去一百年中，从这个殿堂走出了众多在中国现代医学史上叱咤风云、做出杰出贡献的医学大师、医学教育家、公共卫生及护理先驱、卓越的医师们，在中国各地乃至世界的医学大舞台上为我国的医学发展和世界人民健康做出了不可磨灭的贡献。

百年来，协和坚守初心。协和建立之初即确立了"建立远东乃至世界最好的医学院，与欧美最好的医学院媲美"的愿景（vision）。一个世纪以来，协和人坚守"科学济人道"的理念，秉承"严谨、博精、勤奋、奉献"的精神，不断谱写出辉煌的篇章，在中国创建并发展了医学领域众多分支学科，被称为中国医学科学的圣殿、中国现代医学教育的摇篮。大量国内外历史研究者把目光聚焦到了这里。而随着中国医学科学院与中国协和医学院（协和 1952 - 1959 年间的名字）合并，到 1959 年协和历史上第二次复校及以后的历史也逐渐成为中外学者关注的焦点。本书之所以不同于以往其他关于协和历史书籍，就在于它给读者提供了这个独特医学机构在更长的历史节点中的发展轨迹，给予人们更多的深度思考和想象空间。

百年来，协和科教并进。医学科学研究与教育是百年协和立足之本。对北京猿人头盖骨的研究，对麻黄素的研究，中国公共卫生城市社区医疗与农村三级卫生体系的创建，众多基础医学学科——解剖、生化、生理、药学等研究在中国的创建及发展，享有盛誉的、典范式的住院医师培训制度的建立与发展，护理高等教育的开办等等，一个又一个成绩的取得都是协和人奋斗的结果。在建国后，特别是与中国医学科学院合并以后，新的协和继续为我国人民的健康福祉做出了巨大贡献。本书中原院校长刘德培院士所撰写文章中所述，就是院校所做出的众多成就中的代表。协和今天的辉煌，是所有"协和人"共同努力的结果。今天的协和传承历史优秀传统，在创新中寻求更大的发展，为全球医学及人类健康做出更大贡献。正如原院校长巴德年院士在本书中热情洋溢地概括了"协和的创造力"、协和为中国医学事业培养了领导力，这是协和的历史传承、也是协和的发展动力。

百年来，协和包容合作。协和的历史和今天是在国际合作的大背景下书写的。犹如本书一样，是中外学者精诚合作的结果。主编之一玛丽·布洛克（Mary Bullock）发表过多部关于协和历史及洛克菲勒基金会的专著，是国际上此领域著名学者。她长期致力于促进中美学术及人文交往，对协和一直非常关注并充满深厚的情谊和热爱。本书的几位其他国外学者，也都从其不同的角度对协和历史上的人物及事件开展了深入的研究，提供了多个视角。他们只是众多研究者中的代表。同时，来协和的国外客座教授，研究和教学工作完成返回后，其职业生涯有了新的飞跃，如协和第一任校长麦可林（Franklin C. Mclean）回美国后担任了美国芝加哥大学医学院院长；再有协和前几任护理学院院长，包括来自约翰·霍普金斯的沃安娜（Anna Wolfe）、胡志敏（E. Hodgman）等回美国后的职业生涯都有很大发展；世界知名的公共卫生专家、协和第一任公共卫生系主任兰安生（John Grant）把协和及中国经验推向世界。虽然一段时间里，协和由于各种原因中断了同国外的交往，但到了改革开放初期，在首批访美的科学代表团就有协和医学大师吴阶平、林巧稚、黄家驷，协和再次成为中美间乃至全球医学合作交流的纽带与桥梁。

传播知识、培养人才、科学研究和服务社会是现代大学的四大功能，大学的核心使命是通过培养造就有价值观的一流人才去探索未知、传播知识以及开拓创新。伟大的时代造就了协和的今天和明天。今天的协和人在医学科学上的努力与探索，是建立在协和深厚的底蕴与当今协和人对新知识不懈追求之上的。本书是协和百年历史的一个缩影。面对下一个百年，协和人将继续励精图治，开拓创新，将北京协和医学院全面建成世界一流医学院校，为国民健康作出新的贡献！

曹雪涛
中国医学科学院院长
北京协和医学院校长
2017 年 8 月

Preface

The grand cornerstone laying ceremony of Peking Union Medical College (PUMC) was held in September 1917, at the former Prince Yu's Mansion, a kilometer away from the Forbidden City – the heart of China. Representatives from China and the United States presented witnessed the grand ceremony and the embarking of an institution bearing the lofty mission in China's modern medicine. What was to be built in Dongdan Santiao would be a landmark of modern Chinese medical education. This palace-like complex, combining Chinese and Western architecture has fostered the dramatic improvement and the great advancement of modern medicine in China. Over the past one hundred years, the medical masters, educators, public health and nursing pioneers, and distinguished physicians in the history of China's modern medicine coming out of the College and marching to the medical arenas in China, advancing medicine, making indelible contributions to the health and well-being of the Chinese people and the people of the world.

Over the past hundred years, PUMC adheres to its original ambition. The cornerstone embodied the founders' visions ever since its beginning-establishing the best medical school in the Far East and in the world, comparable to the top ones in Europe and North America. The stone recorded PUMC's glory and splendid past. Upholding the belief in "science for humanity" and motto of "rigorousness, excellence, diligence, dedication", PUMC has written brilliant chapters in its history, establishing and developing disciplines in modern medicine in China, making itself a sacred altar of medical sciences and the cradle of modern medical education in China. In the past, a large number of domestic and foreign researchers of history devoted themselves to the researches into PUMC history. The history of the founding of Chinese Academy of Medical

Sciences (CAMS) and its consolidation with China Union Medical College (the name of PUMC from 1952 to 1959) until the second resumption of PUMC in 1959 and thereafter gradually attracts attention from Chinese and foreign scholars. The reason why this book is different from other books on PUMC history is that it covers a longer historical period and readers can track the trajectory of this unique institution, therefore inviting deeper thinking into the history and the institution itself.

Over the past a hundred years, PUMC has always been the institution simultaneously advancing medical research and education. Medical research and education are the bedrocks of PUMC. Out of hardworking and unyielding effort, PUMC people made such tremendous progress in the research of the Peking Man, ephedrine, the creation of China's public health care system both community-based health care in cities and the three-tiered health system in rural areas, the establishment and development of disciplines in basic medicine, such as in anatomy, biochemistry, physiology and pharmacy, and others in China, as well as the establishment and development of the prestigious exemplary residency training program and the nursing higher education. After the founding of the People's Republic of China, especially after the consolidation with CAMS, "the New PUMC" made great contribution to the wellbeing of the Chinese people. In this book, the article written by Academician Liu Depei, former President of CAMS, presents some of the achievements of CAMS. The brilliant achievements of PUMC today are the results of the concerted efforts made by generations of the PUMC family. The PUMC will continue its great heritage and tradition, seeking further advancement from innovation and making greater contribution to medicine and wellbeing of the whole world. As the former President Ba Denian enthusiastically summarizes "PUMC' s Creativity" in this book-PUMC has created the leadership for the Chinese medical causes. This is the historical heritage of PUMC and also the momentum for its future development.

Over the past hundred years, PUMC has emphasized oncooperation and inclusiveness. PUMC's history is brimmed with stories of international cooperation. As exemplified by this book, PUMC is the result of cooperation between Chinese and foreign scholars. Mary Bullock, one of the editors of this book, has published a number of monographs on the history of PUMC and the Rockefeller Foundation. She, as an internationally renowned scholar in this field, has long devoted herself to the promotion of academic and cultural exchanges between China and the United States. Other China and foreign scholars-the authors of this book, have carried out in-depth research into the history of PUMC from different perspectives, providing multiple points of view. And they are just examples among many researchers in this field. In history, PUMC was a model for international medical exchanges. Historically, PUMC is the base for international medical talents. Foreign visiting professors, after completing their research and teaching tasks, returned home and made new leaps in their careers. For example, Franklin C. Mclean who was the first President of PUMC, assumed office of Dean for the Medical School of University of Chicago after returning to the United States. Former deans of the School of Nursing-Anna Wolfe and E. Hodgman, among others, from John Hopkins, had found their career development and advancement back in America. John Grant, the world's leading public health experts, was the first dean of PUMC's Public Health Department and brought his experience of PUMC and China to the world. Although the Cold War and the Cultural Revolution interrupted China's exchanges with foreign countries, yet in the early years of China's reform and opening-up, among the first scientific delegations to the US, one was led by medical masters Wu Jieping and Lin Qiaozhi as well as former President of CAMS/PUMC Huang Jiasi who not only contributed every effort to restore PUMC twice, but also played an important role, together with Wu Jieping in restoring the medical exchanges between China and the United States, making PUMC once again an irreplaceable link in Sino-US medical cooperation and exchanges and with other countries in the world.

For a modern university, disseminating Knowledge, educating, researching, and serving the society are the four functions. The core mission of a university is to explore the unknown, disseminate knowledge, and innovate through cultivating the talents of high caliber. The great era has shaped PUMC's present and lead to its future. Today, PUMC, embedded in rich heritage will pursuit unyieldingly and continue its effort in new discoveries in medical sciences. This book is only a microcosm of history. Marching into the next a hundred years, the PUMC people will continue the great tradition, its effort, vision and ambition, taking the challenges and pushing the boundaries in knowledge, forging the college into a top medical school in the world and serving the wellbeing globally.

Xuetao Cao

President

Chinese Academy of Medical Sciences &

Peking Union Medical College

August 2017

前　言

玛丽·布朗·布洛克（Mary Brown Bullock）

玛丽·布朗·布洛克（Mary Brown Bullock），杜克昆山大学第一任美国执行副校长，曾担任美国中华医学基金会（CMB）董事会主席。她的出版物包括：《洛克菲勒基金会与协和模式》（An American Transplant：The Rockefeller Foundation and Peking Union Medical College）（1980）及《油王：洛克菲勒在中国》（The Oil Prince's Legacy：Rockefeller Philanthropy in China）（2011）。她也曾经担任过艾格尼丝·斯科特学院（Agnes Scott College）的前校长以及埃莫瑞大学（Emory University）的杰出客座教授。

对于任何机构来说，百年纪念日都是一个里程碑，对于北京协和医学院（简称"协和"）可能更是如此。构思于 20 世纪初期，按照约翰·霍普金斯医学院为原型，由美国人资助的三十多年里，协和经历了多重变迁和转向。在国民政府时代从西方教员过渡到中国教师；（新中国成立后）从美国帝国主义的标志性象征，过渡到中国军事医学的主要贡献者；从几次闭校，以及十几个不同校名的变更，到与中国医学科学院合并，直至成为当今中国优秀高等医学学府。

1917 年 9 月 24 日，在豫王府依稀可见的大殿建筑的衬托下，协和落下了奠基石。洛克菲勒基金会为协和购买了清廷王府的院落，王府的建筑成为新式的现代医疗中心的建筑模型。参加仪式的贵宾体现了其国际性，其中有中国教育总长范源濂，同时美国海军陆战队乐队则演奏了得体的音乐。协和第一任校长麦可林（Franklin McLean）博士总结了该机构的宗旨：

> ……在这里建立一个机构，即致力于医学教学、研究和救治病患，在各方面都力求完美，具有同国外最好的同类医学院所具有的高标准……一旦给予这个国家学习和研究的机会。她将能培养出引以为豪的医疗专业人士，也可以在世界领导者中迅速地占据一席之地……[1]

本书的文章追溯了从这个中美混合的仪式开始，一直到世纪更替之时协和师生发挥的作用。文章建立在以往中国国内和国际的研究基础上，这些研究描绘了这段历史的不同方面。虽然协和历史大多人都耳熟能详，但几个关键问题尚需要进一步阐述：这个来自美国的移植体如何在现代中国的历史沧桑中存活下来？它如何影响中国现代医学的发展和方向？本书的作者们通过更全面的目光看待协和的国际特征，尤其是其对中国现代医学和医学教育的贡献，同时首次深入探讨该机构是如何超越20世纪50年代、60年代高度政治化等问题。回答这些问题，需要通过访谈、调查和出版物，同时也揭示了一代代的杰出协和教师及校友领导力。通过查阅存储于北京和纽约的塔里镇（Tarrytown）的关于美国中华医学基金会（China Medical Board）和协和的档案，作者们获得了丰富的新资料。

本书作者包括中外学者、医学史学家及在协和担任过多年领导职位的人士。不同的文章风格有助于对这一历史更多样化、更细微和更国际化的理解。本书作为一个整体，既有赞美也有反思，以呈献给协和百年。

本书中有两篇文章述及协和历史的国际化，当然在其他文章中也曾提到这个主题。从达尔文·斯塔普顿撰写的《"对医学教育的国际贡献"：北京协和医学院的全球化背景》一文中，我们可以更清晰地了解到洛克菲勒基金会创建的协和并非自成一体，而是其更广推动力的一部分，同时也是在全球不同地区推进医学教育的一个特殊模式。因此，从这个理念出发，协和与美国、加拿大、德国、英国、法国甚至日本的机构都联系起来。在民国时期，几乎所有协和毕业生都会在国外学习一两年后返回中国。通常他们要去不同国家或不同机构，巩固了机构之间的长期联系。虽然参照了约翰·霍普金斯的办学模式，协和仍为公共卫生事业做出了自己独特的贡献，并被国际公共卫生专家（特别是国际联盟）的公共卫生专家所熟知。而协和的全球影响力也扩展到其科学出版物。到20世纪20年代中期，在每年出版的几十个专业出版物上，协和发表的文章超过百篇。

阿瑞尔·波尔格浩特（Arie Berghout）关于斯乃博（Isadore Snapper）的文章，提供了在中日战争（即抗日战争。——译者注）期间协和的国际关系之研究案例。斯乃博是来自荷兰的犹太科学家，国际知名度很高，纳粹占领荷兰后逃离到北京避难。1938年，他被任命为内科教授和主任。在日本占领北京的艰难岁月中，斯乃博给协和带来了其对医学的求知欲和独特的授课风格。阿瑞尔·波尔格浩特的研究利用了斯乃博的信件和文章，详细描述了那个时期协和的境况——患者、疾病、工作人员和文化。尤其能够说明问题的是斯乃博与中医之相遇。鉴于斯乃博的生物化学和整体医学的欧洲思想，他能够赏识中医医师的工作。望、闻、问、切的顺序，对于中医师的诊断是非常重要的。斯乃博堪称这些技艺的大师。此外，他不仅切脉，也彻底地检查人体的其他部分、乃至全身。重要的是，斯乃博还把患者家属告诉他的信息非常认真地记录下来。[2]1941年，斯乃博虽被日本逮捕并软禁，却还是发表了在当时对协和最重要的记录——题为《中国给西医的教材：北京协和医学院对地域医学的贡献》的著作。这本书成为国际畅销书，向世界各地的医生介绍了中国的疾病模式和协和。

本书有其他三篇文章与协和国际化有关，分别是关于林巧稚、杨崇瑞[3]、刘士豪的传记性文章。作为从协和开办之初的十几年里毕业的学生，这三位医生的一生跨越民国时期和中华人民共和国的最初几十年。这个轨迹可以深入洞察"老协和"毕业生所经历的复杂的时代变迁，以及他（她）们在人民共和国时期怎样以不同方式继续领导现代医学。杨崇瑞和林巧稚无可争议地成为孕产妇和儿童健康的领导者，在中国创造了现代助产专业和产科。作为精英，她们是受过教育的基督徒女性，所做工作触及社会敏感问题——如转变生产的操作方式和计划生育。像许多其他协和毕业生一样，她们在 20 世纪 20 年代和 30 年代在伦敦、维也纳、芝加哥和巴尔的摩留学。她们把欧洲和美国的经验带回到自己创办的机构中。这两位女性的传记作家蒋菲婷（Tina Johnson）观察到：

> 杨崇瑞和林巧稚的传记提醒我们，医药和公共卫生、政治、妇女的生活及社会对女性的期望的转变。与中国历史上传统的封闭与父权制并行下，这两位女性打破了妇女的传统模式。由协和领导的医学专业为妇女打开了职业发展和个人成长的通道，而商业或法律或其他专业在当时都没有能够做到。[1]

虽然杨崇瑞的工作与国民党的公共卫生项目紧密相连，但她在新中国时期，直到反"右"运动中失去领导职位之前，都在卫生部的妇幼工作中发挥了重要的领导作用。相比之下，林巧稚与中国领导层关系更好。从 20 世纪 50 年代开始，直到 20 世纪 80 年代初去世，她一直是"妇女解放、全民医疗保健、医疗与科学研究之星"的全国榜样。与其他医生相比，林巧稚的偶像形象 —— 体现在电影、邮票和纪念雕像中 —— 既是协和医学卓越传统的持续，也是在政治上及公众心目中的证明。

李乃适的文章介绍了协和在内分泌学上的两代领导人 —— 刘士豪及其学生史轶蘩。刘士豪与史轶蘩的成就体现着协和的一大优势 —— 基础和临床研究的整合。在李乃适对刘士豪的研究中，我们看到了协和毕业生的不同原型 —— 从 20 世纪 20 年代中期一直持续到 70 年代初期在生物化学领域的杰出研究生涯。1924 年，作为协和第二届毕业生的刘士豪，在学生时代已经在科学研究方面取得优异成绩，毕业后不久在《中华医学杂志》上就发表了两篇关于"鱼肝油对搐搦症钙磷代谢的影响"的文章。住院医阶段结束之后，他去了美国洛克菲勒医学研究所，在美国领先的生物化学家范斯莱克（Donald D. van Slyke）指导下学习，发表了关于骨软化症和其他代谢疾病的开创性研究。抗美援朝战争结束后，他成为协和生物化学系主任。他撰写的教科书《生物化学与临床医学的联系》

"是当时中国内科医生和外科医生最有影响力的医书"。李乃适认为，刘士豪是转化医学早期践行者：刘士豪在其书中的序言指出，"如果能引起生物化学工作者深入临床，临床工作者深入生化，使二者更密切地结合起来，向医学进军，则本书的抛砖引玉之目的即已达到。"虽然刘士豪的研究在那个时代由于政治运动中断了，但他的不懈努力继续推动着临床内分泌学的新发展。

史轶蘩比刘士豪年轻三十岁。作为刘士豪的学生，她于 1949 年正式加入协和。她的职业生涯所跨越的 20 世纪 50 年代和 60 代，正是协和最动荡的年代。然而，在刘士豪的指导下，她的研究与临床技能不断增强。"文革"后，她领导了协和内分泌部门重建工作，并于 80 年代初在美国国立卫生研究院（NIH）进修。在 NIH 她主要关注的是脑垂体研究，并在回国后继续从事这方面的研究。1996 年，史轶蘩当选中国工程院院士。

在对内分泌学这两位"大师"经历的研究基础之上，李乃适反思了"老协和"的整体教育情况。他比较了刘士豪与史轶蘩的教育和经验，强调了几代协和人的教育经历和价值观的连续性。他赞扬了"老协和"标志性的基础研究与临床医学的整合方法，也肯定当前"将基础医学研究和临床医学研究结合"的教学，但对就业市场以及重视发表文章与短期医疗培养的变化表示遗憾。他在文章的结尾中写道："在当前的评价体系下，如何提高协和毕业生的竞争力？能否培养出当代的刘士豪和史轶蘩？这将是协和医学教育所面临的严峻挑战。"

"林巧稚等协和著名毕业生的领导生涯及其令人叹服的医学实践，影响了公众对协和的看法及协和的命运。"《"老协和"的回忆》提升了人们对协和教育核心特征的认识。玛丽·布洛克（Mary Bullock）撰写的《"老协和"的回忆》一章，展示了她在 1984 年至 2008 年期间对五十名协和毕业生的访谈中采集到的信息。访谈许多年长的受访者时，这些记忆不可避免地铭记着协和的科学和道德标准、必不可少的 8 年制教育以及以病人为中心的文化。而这些 20 世纪 30 年代、50 年代和 60 年代的毕业生们的人生经历说明，指责协和是"象牙塔的精英教育"与事实不符。虽然在教育上条件优越，但协和毕业生没有游离于抗日战争和国内战争的沧桑磨难，也未摆脱 20 世纪 50 和 60 年代的政治运动以及多次闭校的影响。事实上，大部分受访者的大段职业生涯，都是在协和的医学圣殿的校园围墙之外度过。他们为天津、上海、广州和成都的机构提供了大量的医疗专业知识，并去了宁夏、甘肃和西藏的农村地区。他们的医疗专业精神经受住了考验，并固守强劲的、有些理想化的协和记忆，他们成了二十世纪末协和复兴的关键参照点。

张大庆撰写的《北京协和医学院早期的中药研究：从 1910 年到 1941 年》则在几个不同的方面有新突破。他指出虽然许多传教士拒绝中医，但还有些传教士对中药的科学价值表示了兴趣，力图研究和运用不同的传统治病草药，部分原因是中国腹地缺少西医西药。他还指出，协和药学系的研究人员是中国最早将中药最为重要的经典文献翻译成英文的，并运用现代科学方法研究传统药材的药理和药化。最重要的人物当属伊博恩博士（Bernard Read）。1909 年，伦敦会派伊博恩到协和医学堂——北京协和医学院的前身任教。多年之后，洛克菲勒基金会派他在约翰·霍普金斯大学、哈佛大学、芝加哥大学，最终到耶鲁大学接受高级博士生培训。他的《本草新注》评估了中国经典《本草纲目》，并介绍了欧洲和日本的研究成果，成为中医药的经典参考书目。伊博恩还发表了关于动物药物、禽类药物、中国药用植物等方面的广泛研究成果。

最重要的是协和为年轻中国学者创造了良好的研究氛围，其中最著名的是陈克恢。此人研究了中药材麻黄，最终以发现了麻黄碱而闻名遐迩。在英国和瑞士受过教育的赵承嘏，先在法国制药公司担任研究部主任，后到协和。在协和的实验室里，赵承嘏研究分析了 30 多种中药的化学成分。正如张大庆对协和科学群体所做出的总结："……他们建立了系统研究整理祖国医药学的一套科学方法"。张大庆枚列协和药学系对中医药研究的出版物的清单，发现从 1927 年至 1948 年刊发在《中国生理学杂志》上的 88 篇关于中医药的论文中，有 33 篇来自协和。在 20 世纪 30 年代中期，协和药学系的主要领导被邀请组建专门研究中国药物的机构。

赵承嘏创办了国立北平研究院药物研究所，后来成为中国科学院的一部分。伊博恩应上海雷氏德医学研究院之邀，离开了协和。

我们把目光从集中展示协和历史优秀传承，转向关注 20 世纪 50 年代和 60 年代的协和。本书有三个章节涉及这个时期：胡成撰写的《"新协和"的医学专业化（1951－1966）》、白玛丽撰写的《收归国有之后的北京协和医学院（1949－1985）年》以及蒋育红撰写的《中国医学科学院的成立及其早期运作（1956－1966）》。这三篇文章以各自不同的角度发掘了许多细节，包括新政府对由美国人资助的协和及其影响进行更符合新时代的大众卫生政策的改革。每篇的侧重点也都有所不同。协和虽然看起来经历了很大的变化，但其作为现代西方医学的中心坚持了下来。胡成对此时医学专业化的观点是：

> 协和国有化之后，曾大力铲除"崇美、亲美、恐美"的情绪。当中共宣布"向科学进军"时，着眼于推进高端医学科学研究和恢复顶尖高等医学教育，则必须要继承"老协和"所建立的医学专业化。[5]

白玛丽的观点是，协和从 1952 年至 1956 年军管之后，超出多数人的预期，即"协和作为中国西方科学的生物医学研究中心而坚持下来，重要原因是取决于军队在协和的改革。军队领导下的政治运动公开谴责了美国对协和的影响，却没有对西方医学本身进行直接的批评。"[6] 蒋育红则认为，尽管 1956 年按照苏联模式所建立的中国医学科学院及其研究机构最初影响到了协和的教育力量，然而这两个机构的整合实际上又扩大了协和教师研究的平台，使中国医学科学院/北京协和医学院（CAMS／PUMC）成为中国的国家医学科学中心。而且，从 1957 年至 1984 年，黄家驷（协和 1933 届）作为中国医学科学院院长和协和校长，坚持不懈地努力重新恢复协和 8 年制教育。他终于在 1959 年取得了短暂成功。经过文革的漫长间隔，协和于 1979 年再次复校。[7]

胡成和蒋育红都有意避免对"反美主义"的大框架描述，重点关注协和内部的不同群体——激进派和温和派，以及他们如何应对那个时代的激烈政治运动。胡成提供了相当多的细节，展现不同的协和人如何应对铲除美国影响的压力以及在那个时期为医治更多病人而进行的医疗改革等。坚持"协和标准"是当时协和领导者拒绝极"左"做法的一个方法，特别是 20 世纪 50 年代初及"大跃进"时期。支持改革的激进人士认为，协和的标准应该放在"解决人民生产的实际问题"。胡成阐述了中国政治领导人一次又一次地转向协和的医疗专业化，以满足这个国家的卫生需求。

白玛丽虽也描绘了 20 世纪 50 年代的政治运动，给出的解释却有所不同。解放军"将学校融入国家军事医疗基础设施，让所有师生入伍"[9]。协和成为解放军培训基地，并为著名的 301 医院提供了教员。20 世纪 50 年代初，轰轰烈烈的思想改造和"三反"运动，重点是批判协和的西方出身，而不是西医本身。即使所实施的改革更具平等主义，解放军仍尽全力"维护中国协和医学院（当时协和的名称）作为国家的西方生物医学之象征"。白玛丽确信，西方生物医学的核心合法性被保留下来，在军队领导之下，同时也被中国化了。协和成为"中国新医学的最初标志之一，在这种新医学的框架之下，中国的国家政权，特别是军队在其范围内对西医进行监管"[10]。

蒋育红撰写的章节是关于 1956 年创建的中国医学科学院（医科院）案例及其与协和的关系。受苏联影响和对科技进步的渴望，致使中国领导人认识到要建立一个高水平的医学研究中心。1956 年，以（国民党时代）的中央卫生研究院的八个研究所为主干成立了中国医学科学院。1957 年，协和被纳入医科院，医科院院部当时（现在）设在协和校园之中，研究工作继续进行，教学则被中止（直到 1959 年复校）。协和的教授要学习俄语，许多人与苏联的生物医学科学有过交往。蒋育红详细介绍协和适应苏联模式面临的困难。苏联模式更加分散，研究人员和教授有更多的自主权。她强调了黄家驷在基础研究和精英教育方面的政治需求之领导作用。她重点展现了黄家驷的领导作用，及其更加关注基础研究与精英教育。

综合这三章内容，我们可以认为是讲述协和在 20 世纪 50 年代和 60 年代经历的政治风暴，并揭示了存续协和核心身份的不同方式：医疗专业人士公认的临床功效、意想不到与解放军的联盟以及其调整自身认同身份，终于成为中国医学科学院的一部分。

最后一部分"新生"，这三章是由协和的学术带头人、现任教务长马超以及两位前院校长巴德年和刘德培撰写。他们概述了解放后协和的校友、教师和研究状况。

马超撰写的《协和学子：百年回顾》，着重论及了协和的医学教育及其校友。他详细描述了八年制医学教育的历史，展示八年制在过去六十多年来是如何继续和没有间断的调试。从 1954 届毕业生张志南教授的回忆中，马超描述了许多著名协和教授的教学法，阐述了他们的技艺和对病人的重视。他由此大量谈及了"老协和"课程的连续性。

这篇文章特别有价值的部分，是提供了从 1956 ～ 2008 年间协和的校友调查结果。虽然只有 26.4% 的受访者寄回了问卷，但协和校友们还是提供了宝贵的信息。调查图标显示，女毕业生人数从 1950 年代的约 30%，增加到最近的 2000 ～ 2008 年的 50% 以上，以及可预期的专业职称水平的提高。最有意义的是 1979 ～ 1989 年毕业生的职业生涯，与之前和之后的毕业生都不同。"文革"后的毕业的最初一届学生倾向于在国外或中国其他地方学习和生活而很少回到协和。这些数字与在此期间出国留学的其他专业的人数相一致。1990 年后，部分由于在中国提供了更好的居住、实习和研究机会，毕业生更多转向在国内就职，包括在协和的工作。

2001 ～ 2012 年间担任医科院和协和主要领导的刘德培，把医学研究作为自己讲述协和工作的重点，这反映在他撰写的中国医学科学院和协和重大科技成果的一章。通过突出展示最重要的研究成果，刘德培提醒我们，医科院/协和的研究人员在 1956 年至 1980 年期间的中国独立自主的医学突破中起到了关键作用。就流行病和传染病方面来看，这包括开发脊髓灰质炎疫苗、进行麻风病防治和以后的艾滋病的创新治疗。医科院肿瘤医院开展的食道癌研究和阜外医院开展的心血管疾病研究都大大提高了这些疾病治疗效果。医科院/协和的研究者还在细胞遗传学、人类基因组研究和基因治疗多个领域取得了进展。刘德培也谈及常被忽视的药物研究部分，指出此时研究成功开发了很多新药，包括中药。

1992～2001年间担任医科院和校长的巴德年，通过改进科研设施，鼓励更多协和毕业生留在中国。他负责修建的教学楼是自20世纪20年代以来协和首个主要新的建筑工程。他撰写的章节详尽介绍了协和教师和毕业生对协和/医科院的贡献，同时也讲述了他们对许多其他医疗机构和政府部门及研究机构做出的巨大贡献。他列举了很多人的名单，具体展示了自1950年以来协和在中国各地的影响，还概述了一些主要的科研成果。

本书最后一章《让我们共同迎接挑战——写在协和百年之际》，是由北京大学医学部前任主任、著名的肿瘤专家柯杨撰写。她提到协和诸多贡献，同时也利用协和纪念其成立百年之际，引起人们注意中国医学教育面临的持续挑战。她提及医学教育需要向更全面发展，包括培育许多不同的卫生专业人员。人民生活的变化——技术更新和全球化——为重新建立病人和医生之间的信任提供了大背景，需要满足培训当今的医生的多维度要求。她写道：

> 与此同时，年轻人经历了信仰危机，社会诚信危机，职业多元性选择，物质利益的诱惑……当今的医学生正经历前所未有的焦虑。这些都要求我们对医学生加强"全人教育"和职业精神的引导，做出全面努力，助其综合能力的提高。唯有这样才能让医学生更加坚定、自信与成熟。总之，今日的医学生再也不是当年选择了学医就坚定不移、就两耳不闻窗外事、一心只读"圣贤书"了。医学教育再也不能像过去那样单纯地传授医学知识与技能而不关心医学生的心灵成长。我们不能等待社会的进步和体制的完善，我们必须做出教育的改变和应对。[11]

柯杨呼吁继续进行教育改革，提醒所有庆祝协和百年之人戒骄戒躁，在协和第二个百年以新的活力和领导力打造未来。

参考书目

1. 引自 Mary Ferguson. *China Medical Board and Peking Union Medical College*（China Medical Board：New York，1970），40.

2. 见阿瑞尔·波尔格浩特文章，本书 P107。

3. 杨崇瑞毕业于协和前身。

4. 见蒋菲婷文章，本书 P37。

5. 见胡成文章，本书 P231。

6. 见白玛丽文章，本书 P326。

7. 见蒋育红文章，本书 P287。

8. 同上。

9. 见白玛丽文章，本书 P326。

10. 同上。

11. 见柯杨文章，本书 P496。

Introduction

Mary Brown Bullock

Mary Brown Bullock was the first executive Vice Chancellor of Duke Kunshan University and was chair of the China Medical Board from 2005 to 2014. Her publications include An American Transplant: The Rockefeller Foundation and Peking Union Medical College (1980) and The Oil Prince's Legacy: Rockefeller Philanthropy in China (2011). She was the former president of Agnes Scott College and visiting distinguished professor of Chinese history at Emory University.

To arrive at a centennial anniversary is a milestone for any institution, but perhaps even more so for Peking Union Medical College (PUMC). Conceived in the early 20th century in the image of Johns Hopkins Medical School and funded by Americans for more than three decades, PUMC weathered multiple transitions-from a western to a Chinese faculty during the Republican era, from an iconic symbol of American imperialism to a major contributor to China's military medicine, from years of closure and more than a dozen different names, from an appendage of the Chinese Academy of Medical Sciences to a revitalized pre-eminent Chinese medical university today.

PUMC's cornerstone was laid on September 24, 1917 in full view of the still-standing Ceremonial Hall of Prince Yu's palace. The Manchu prince's property had been bought by the Rockefeller Foundation for PUMC and its Qing palace became the architectural model for the new modern medical complex. The assembled dignitaries were an international cast including Fan Yuanlien,

Minister of Education and the U. S. Marine Band played appropriate music. Dr. Franklin McLean, the first director summarized the purpose of the institution:

> *...to establish here an institution devoted to medical teaching and research and the care of the sick, complete in every respect, and with the high standards of work that are already existent in the best of similar institutions abroad ... Given the opportunity for study and research, this country should develop a medical professional to be proud of, and one that may easily take its place among the leaders of the world.* [1]...

The essays in this volume trace the role of PUMC and its students and faculty from this hybrid Sino-American ceremonial beginning across the subsequent century. They build on previous studies, both Chinese and international, which have portrayed different aspects of this history. While the basic PUMC story is thus fairly well known several key questions require further elaboration: how did this American transplant survive amid the vicissitudes of modern China? how did it influence the shape and direction of China's modern medicine? The authors here in address these questions by providing a more comprehensive look at PUMC's international character, its contributions to China's modern medicine and medical education, and the first in-depth look at how the institution traversed the highly political 1950s and 1960s. The research and institutional leadership of successive cohorts of PUMC faculty and alumni are reviewed through interviews, surveys, and their publications. Access to the China Medical Board and PUMC archives in both Beijing and Tarrytown, New York have provided rich new source material.

The authors are both Chinese and international, both historians of medicine and those who have spent years in leadership positions at PUMC. The differing essay styles contribute to a more varied, nuanced and internationalized understanding of this history. Taken as a whole, with both praise and critique, they stand as a tribute to PUMC's centennial anniversary.

The international aspects of PUMC's history are the subjects of two of the essays and are touched on in others. Darwin Stapleton's " ' An International Contribution to Medical Education ' : The Global Context of Peking Union Medical College" provides a clear understanding of the degree to which the creation of PUMC by the Rockefellers was not *sui generis* but was part of a broader thrust to advance a particular model of medical education in different parts of the globe. From its conception, therefore, PUMC was linked to institutions in the United States, Canada, Germany, the United Kingdom, France and even Japan. During the Republican period almost all of the PUMC graduates studied abroad for a year or two and returned to China. Usually they would spend time in more than one country and at more than one institution, solidifying longer term institutional ties. Even as it drew on the Johns Hopkins model, PUMC developed its own distinct contributions to public health which were well-known by international public health specialists, especially those in the League of Nations. And PUMC's global reach extended to its scientific publications as well - by the mid-1920s over 100 articles were published *each year* in "several dozen professional publications. "

Arie Berghout's essay on Isidore Snapper provides a case study of PUMC's international connections during the Sino-Japanese war. A Jewish scientist from the Netherlands with a wide international reputation Snapper sought refuge in Beijing from the Nazi occupation. Appointed Professor and Chair of Medicine in 1938 Snapper brought his medical curiosity and distinct lecturing style to PUMC during the difficult years of Japanese occupation of Beijing. Berghout's writing, which draws from Snapper's letters and articles, conveys a detailed picture of PUMC - its patients, diseases, staff and culture during this era. Snapper's encounter with traditional Chinese medicine is especially revealing. Given

Snapper's European ideas regarding bio-chemistry and holistic medicine Snapper could appreciate the role of the Chinese physician:

> *For the Chinese physician the sequence of inspection, listening, interview, and finally the investigation of the pulse, was very important to reach a diagnosis. Snapper was a master of these skills, and moreover, he not only investigated the pulse, but also and very thoroughly the other parts of the human body, the whole body. Importantly, Snapper took also the story the patient's family told him very seriously into account.* [2]

Captured and placed under house arrest by the Japanese, in 1941 Snapper nonetheless published the most important account of PUMC to that date. Titled *Chinese Lessons to Western Medicine: A Contribution to Geographical Medicine from the Clinics of Peiping Union Medical College.* This book became an international best-seller, introducing physicians the world over to Chinese disease patterns and PUMC.

Three others associated with PUMC are given biographical treatment here: Lin Qiaozhi, Yang Chongrui and Liu Shihao and Shi Yifan. Graduates of PUMC[3] from its first decade the lives of these two women and one male physician spanned both the Republican period and the first decades of the People's Republic of China. This trajectory gives insight into the complex transitions experienced by graduates of "old PUMC" and the differing ways in which they continued to lead modern medicine in the People's Republic. Yang and Lin became the undisputed leaders of maternal and child-health, creating modern midwifery and obstetrics in China. As elite, educated Christian women they tackled socially sensitive issues such as transforming birth practices and family planning. Like so many of the other PUMC graduates they studied abroad in the 1920s and 1930s - in London, Vienna, Chicago, and Baltimore. They brought the experiences of Europe as well as the United States to the institutions they created. Their biographer, Tina Johnson, observes that

> *The biographies of Yang and Lin remind us about the shifting landscape of medicine and public health, of politics, and of women's lives and society's expectations of them. These two women broke the molds for women, juxtaposed on the traditional Chinese history of seclusion and patriarchy. The medical profession led by PUMC gave women an outlet for professional development and personal growth in ways that business or law or other professions did not.* [4]

Although Yang's work had been closely tied to the public health programs of the Guomindang she played an important role as director of Women's and Infants work in the PRC's Ministry of Health until she lost her leadership role during the anti-rightist campaign. In contrast Lin, with close ties to the PRC leadership, emerged from the 1950s until her death in the early 1980s as the national model for "emancipated women, health care for all, stellar medical and scientific research." More than any other physician Lin Qiaozhi's iconic image – replicated in movies, stamps, and commemorative statues – was a continuing political and public testimony to the medical excellence of Peking Union Medical College.

Li Naishi's chapter explores two generations of PUMC leaders in endocrinology - Liu Shihao and his student, Shi Yifan. The lives of Liu and Shi reflect one of the great strengths of PUMC - the integration of basic and clinical research. In Li Naishi's portrayal of Liu Shihao we see a different prototype of the PUMC graduate - a distinguished research career in biochemistry that continued from the mid 1920s to the early 1970s. Graduating in PUMC's second class, 1924, Liu excelled in scientific research as a student, publishing two articles on "The Influence of Cod Liver Oil on the Calcium and Phosophorous metabolism in tetany" in the *Chinese Medical Journal* shortly after his graduation. After residency he went to the United States where he studied with the leading American biochemist Donald D. van Slyke at the Rockefeller Institute and published pioneering articles on osteomalacia and other metabolic diseases. He became head of PUMC's department of biochemistry after the Korean War and his textbook, *The Relationship between Biochemistry and Clinical Medicine* "was the most influential medical book for physicians and surgeons at that time in China." Li sees Liu as an early practitioner of translational medicine, citing Liu's forward: "If the book could make biochemists engage in clinical work, and the clinicians engage in biochemistry, so that the two worked closely together and march toward medical science, then the purpose of this book as the humble trailblazer has been realized." Although interrupted during the political movements of the era, Liu Shihao's research continued to break new ground for clinical endocrinology.

Almost thirty years younger, Shi Yifan was Liu's student, formally entering PUMC in 1949. Her career thus spans the 1950s and 1960s, periods of considerable turmoil at PUMC. Mentoring by Liu Shihao, however, enhanced both her research and her clinical skills. She led in the reconstitution of PUMC's endocrinology department after the Cultural Revolution and spent time in the United States at the National Institutes of Health in the early 1980s. There she was introduced to experimental animal research, honing her research on the pituitary gland which she was able to continue upon return to China. In 1996 she was elected a member of the Chinese Academy of Engineering Science.

Li Naishi draws on his portrayals of these two "masters" of endocrinology to reflect on the overall education of the "old PUMC." He illustrates the continuity of PUMC's educational experience and values across the generations in comparing the training and experience of Liu and Shi. In extolling the integration of basic research and clinical medicine which was the hallmark of "old PUMC," he also commends the current educational program "covering basic medical research and clinical medical research simultaneously," but laments changes in the job market which value publications and short-term medical training. He concludes: "How can we cultivate contemporary Liu Shihao and Shi Yifan? This will be a huge challenge to PUMC. "

The leadership careers and compelling medical practices of well-known PUMC graduates such as Lin Qiaozhi influenced public perceptions and the survival of PUMC. Memories of the "old PUMC" also heightened awareness of the core characteristics of a PUMC education. Mary Bullock's essay "Memories of Old PUMC" conveys information gleaned from interviews with fifty PUMC graduates in 1984 and 2008. Conducted when many of the interviewees were quite elderly these memories inevitably memorialized PUMC's scientific and ethical standards, the indispensable 8-year curriculum, and the patient-centered culture. But the life experiences of these cohorts who graduated in the 1930s, 1950s, and 1960s belie the charge of ivy-tower elitism. Privileged in their education the PUMC graduates were not exempt from the vicissitudes of the Sino-Japanese and Civil War, the political campaigns of the 1950s and 1960s, and the multiple closures of PUMC. In fact, most of those interviewed spent the bulk of their medical careers outside of PUMC's hallowed halls - lending their considerable medical expertise to lesser institutions in Tianjin, Shanghai, Guangzhou and Chengdu. Or in rural villages in Ningxia, Gansu and Tibet. Their medical professionalism endured and in clinging to a powerful, if idealized memory of PUMC, they became key reference points for its revival at the end of the twentieth century.

Zhang Daqing's chapter "Traditional Chinese Medical (TCM) Research in PUMC: 1910 – 1941" breaks new ground in several different ways. He demonstrates that although many missionaries rejected Chinese medicine, others were interested in the scientific value of TCM and sought to both study and use different traditional herbal remedies, in part because in China's hinterland western medicine was in short supply. He also demonstrates that researchers in

PUMC's Department of Pharmacology were among the first in China to translate the most important compendiums of Chinese medicine into English, and to use modern scientific methods to study both the pharmacology and the chemistry of traditional herbs. The key individual was Dr. Bernard Read, assigned by the London Missionary Society to the Union Medical College, PUMC's predecessor, in 1909. Over the years the Rockefeller Foundation sent him for advanced doctoral training in biochemistry at Johns Hopkins, Harvard, Chicago and eventually Yale. His "New Notes on Materia Medica" reviewed China's classic Pen Ts'ao Kang Mu but also introduced findings from European and Japanese studies and became a classic reference for TCM. Read published a wide range of studies on topics such as animal drugs, avian drugs, Chinas' medicinal plants and so on.

Most importantly he created a climate for younger Chinese scholars, best known of whom is Chen Kehui whose work on the Chinese plant *ma huang* led to the well-known discovery of ephedrine. Also T. Q. Chou, trained in England and Switzerland, was brought to PUMC from his position as director of the research department of a French pharmaceutical company. His laboratory work at PUMC led to the analysis of the chemical composition of more than 30 kinds of traditional Chinese drugs. As Zhang notes about this PUMC scientific community: "…they established a set of scientific methods for the country to assort the TCM herbal medicine in a systematic way. " Zhang includes a list of the most important publications on TCM from PUMC's Department of Pharmacology, noting that of 88 papers published on TCM in *The Chinese Journal of Physiology* from 1927 to 1948 thirty-seven came from PUMC.

In the mid-1930s the key leaders from PUMC's Department of Pharmacology were invited to lead new Chinese institutes dedicated to the study of China's *materia medica*. T. Q. Chou became the Director of the Institute of Materia Medica of the National Academy of Peiping, later the Chinese Academy of Science. Read left PUMC to lead the Henry Lester Institute of Medical

Research in Shanghai.

We turn from highlighting aspects of PUMC's historical legacy to look more closely at PUMC during the 1950s and 1960s. Three chapters address this period: Hu Cheng's "The New PUMC and Its Medical Professionalism (1951 – 1966), Mary Brazelton's "Peking Union Medical College After Nationalization, 1949 – 1985," and Jiang Yuhong: "Establishing and Strengthening the Chinese Academy of Medical Sciences 1956 – 1966".

Each provides considerable detail about the various ways in which the new Communist government sought to discredit the American origins and influences on PUMC and to enforce reforms that brought the institution more in line with the mass health policies of the new era. But each uses a different focus to illustrate that, despite what appear to be draconian changes, PUMC is able to persist as a center of modern, western medicine. For Hu Cheng the perspective is that of medical professionalism:

> "*The Chinese Communist Party (CCP) made a great effort to root out the sentiments of the 'worship-America, pro-America, or fear-America,' in the faculty and staffs after it nationalized PUMC.... However, at a time when the CCP declared "advancing toward science," aiming at promoting the research on high level medical science and attempting to resume the top medical education, it had to carry on the heritage of medical professionalism established by the 'old PUMC.'*" [5]

For Mary Brazelton, the perspective is that of the People's Liberation Army which was given control of PUMC from 1952 – 1956, contrary to what might be expected, Brazelton demonstrates that "the endurance of PUMC as an institute of scientific Western biomedicine in China was largely contingent upon the reforms that the PLA instituted there … . political campaigns under Army leadership decried American influences on the College but avoided direct criticisms of Western medical science itself. "[6] Jiang Yuhong argues that although the creation of the Soviet model Chinese Academy of Medical Sciences (CAMS) and its research institutes in 1956 initially curtailed PUMC's education program the integration of the two institutions in fact expanded the platform of PUMC's research faculty, enabling CAMS/PUMC to become a national center for scientific medicine in China. As the leader of CAMS/PUMC from 1957 until 1984 Huang Jiasi (Chia-ssu '33) was persistent in his efforts to reconstitute the PUMC 8-year education program, succeeding briefly in 1959 and, after a long Cultural Revolution hiatus, then again in 1979. [7]

Both Hu Cheng and Jiang Yuhong deliberately avoid the "grand narratives of anti-Americanism" and focus on the different groups of people within PUMC-radicals and moderates – and how they coped with the intense political campaigns of the era. Hu provides considerable detail on how different PUMC groups responded to the pressures to reject American influences and to accelerate medical reforms that treated more patients and, during the Great Leap Forward, greatly exaggerated the claims of medical research. Advocacy of "PUMC standards" was one way for PUMC leaders to resist change, especially the changes of the early 1950s and the Great Leap Forward. Proponents of radical change argued that PUMC's standards should address "solving practical problems for people's production. " Hu illustrates that time and time again China's political leaders returned to PUMC's medical professionalism to serve the health needs of the country.

Mary Brazelton also depicts the political campaigns of the 1950s but interprets their results differently. The PLA " integrated the school into the national military medical infrastructure, enlisting all faculty and students. "[9]

PUMC became a training site for the PLA and staffed the famous 301 Hospital. While the thought reform and Three-Antis campaigns of the early 1950s were fully implemented the focus was on castigating the western origins of PUMC medicine but not western medicine itself. The PLA made every effort to "preserve CUMC as a national symbol of Western biomedicine" even as it implemented reforms that were more egalitarian. Brazelton affirms that the core legitimacy of western bio-medicine was preserved even as it was simultaneously sinified under military leadership: PUMC became "one of the first symbols of a new medicine in China, one in which the Chinese state - and especially its military army asserted authority over Western medicine within its borders." [10]

Jiang Yuhong's chapter is a case study of the creation of the Chinese Academy of Medical Sciences in 1956 and its relationship to PUMC. Influenced by the Soviet Union and the desire to advance scientifically, Chinese leaders acknowledged the need to establish high level centers for medical research. In 1956, the eight institutes of the (Guomindang era) Central Institute of Health were constituted as the Chinese Academy of Medical Sciences. In 1957 PUMC was incorporated into CAMS: CAMS' headquarters were (and are) located at PUMC, its research programs continued but the education program formally ceased (until it re-opened in 1959). PUMC's faculty had studied Russian and many were engaged in exchanges with Russian biomedical sciences. Jiang details the difficulties faced in adapting the Soviet model which was more decentralized and provided more autonomy for researchers and professors than China's centralized model. She highlights the leadership role of Huang Jiasi who endeavored to bridge the political demand that "scientific research should relate to practice" with a focus on basic research and elite education.

Taken together these three chapters illuminate the political struggles faced by PUMC during the 1950s and 1960s but also the several different ways in which its core identity persisted: through the acknowledged clinical efficacy of medical professionals, through an un-expected alliance with the PLA, and in modifying its identity to become part of the Chinese Academy of Medical Science.

Three chapters in the final section, Revitalization, are written by PUMC academic leaders - Ma Chao, current PUMC Dean, and two previous presidents, Ba Denian and Liu Depei. They provide an overview of PUMC's alumni, faculty, and research since liberation.

In Ma Chao's chapter on "PUMC Alumni: A Centennial Review" the evolution of PUMC's medical education and its alumni take center stage. He provides a detailed chronology of the 8-year curriculum noting how it continued, and was sometimes modified, over six decades. Drawing from the recollections of Professor Zhang Zhinan, '54, he describes the pedagogy of many famous PUMC professors, illustrating both their techniques and also their values of patient care. In doing so he illustrates considerable curricular continuity from the "old PUMC"?

What is especially valuable about this essay are the results of a survey sent to PUMC alumni enrolled in PUMC from 1956 - 2008. Although only 26.4% responded this survey provides invaluable information on PUMC's alumni cohort. The surveys chart an increase in the number of women graduates from approximately 30% in the 1950s to over 50% in the most recent cohort, 2000 - 2008, as well as an expected increase in their professional levels. Most significant are the ways in which the careers of the graduates of 1979 - 1989 differ from both those who came before and after them. Those graduating in this first post-Cultural Revolution cohort tended to study and live abroad, or elsewhere in China: very few returned to PUMC. These figures correspond with other professional groups who studied abroad during this period. The shift to more China-based careers, including at PUMC, was partially a result of better providing with residency, internship and research opportunities in China after 1990.

Liu Depei, president from 2001 – 2012, brought a medical research focus to his PUMC leadership which is reflected in his chapter on the major scientific and technological advances under the Chinese Academy of Medical Sciences and PUMC. By highlighting the most notable research contributions Liu reminds us that researchers at CAMS/PUMC were critical to China's independent medical breakthroughs made during the period 1956 to 1980. In epidemics and infectious diseases these included developing a vaccine for polio, advances in leprosy treatment, and, later, innovative treatments for AIDS. The treatment of cardiovascular disease and esophageal cancer was greatly improved by research at CAMS' Cancer and Fuwai Hospitals. Other advances have been made by CAMS/ PUMC faculty in cytogenetics, the study of the human genome and multiple areas of gene therapy. Often overlooked, Liu includes a section on pharmacology, demonstrating multiple instances in which research led to the successful development of new drugs, including those from traditional Chinese herbs.

Ba Denian, who presided over PUMC from 1992 – 2001, was the president who introduced some of the changes that encouraged more PUMC graduates to remain in China. He also was responsible for PUMC's first major new building program since the 1920s which built a large new teaching and research facility. His chapter focuses in some detail on the institutional contributions of PUMC faculty and graduates both to PUMC and CAMS but also significantly to many other medical institutions and government ministries and research facilities. His extensive list of names demonstrates in very specific ways how

PUMC's influence was felt across China since 1950. He also provides an overview of some of the major research contributions.

The final chapter in this volume, "Rising Up to Our Shared Challenges," is written by Ke Yang, immediate past president of Peking University Health Science Center and a noted oncologist. While noting PUMC's many contributions, she uses its centennial to draw attention to the continued challenges of Chinese medical education. She cites the need for medical education to become more comprehensive, encompassing the many different health professionals. The changes in people's lives - including technology and globalization - are cited as background for the need to reestablish trust between patient and physician, and to attend to the multi-dimensional requirements for training today's doctors:

> ...medical students are experiencing greater anxiety amid conflicts of values, collapse of trust, diversified career paths and temptation of materialism. This is an urgent call for holistic education and professionalism cultivation which will help students grow into mature, confident and committed human beings. The days are gone when stepping into medical school meant a life devoted to the career, and so are the days when medical education meant nothing more than training of skills. We cannot sit back and wait for society and its institutions to perfect themselves; we must push for change from the educational front. [11]

With such calls for continued educational transformation Ke Yang reminds all celebrating PUMC's first hundred years not to be complacent, but to forge ahead with renewed vigor and leadership in its second century.

Bibliography

1. Quoted in Mary Ferguson, *China Medical Board and Peking Union Medical College* (China Medical Board: New York, 1970), 40.

2. Berghout, 132.

3. Yang Chongrui graduated in 1917 from PUMC's predecessor institution.

4. Tina Johnson, 54.

5. Hu Cheng, 253.

6. Mary Brazleton, 342.

7. Jiang Yuhong, 302.

8. Ibid.

9. Brazelton, 342

10. Ibid.

11. Ke Yang, 501.

致　谢

　　本书得以在协和百年校庆庆典前出版，要感谢很多人默默的支持和鼓励。特别感谢北京协和医学院的各位领导 —— 曹雪涛院长慨然作序，两位老院校长巴德年和刘德培两位院士百忙之中很早就完成了文稿。也感谢李国勤、姚龙山、王云峰、张勤、张抒杨、张学对两位主编一直以来的关心和支持。

　　感谢中外作者在长期研究的基础上，为本书提供了学术价值很高的稿件。

　　同时还要感谢院校办公室主任朱成斌及办公室的同事、科技管理处处长王建伟及同事、档案室张霞、陈建辉、人文学院前任院长翟晓梅、现任院长何仲等给予的指导和协助。还要感谢协和八年制 2003 级同学王诗蕊同学及另一位译者孙爱平出色的翻译工作、外教 Sam Seery 的校对工作及中国协和大学出版社同事加班加点的工作。还有感谢美国中华医学基金会（China Medical Board，CMB）等其他国际友好人士的关心和支持。

　　以及热爱协和并为协和默默奉献的同仁们！

　　由于本书从策划到出版时间非常有限，没有能做索引，在英文翻译方面不免存在某些瑕疵。敬请读者批评指正！

蒋育红　玛丽·布朗·布洛克（Mary Brown Bullock）

Acknowledgment

The timely publishing of this book before the centennial celebration of Peking Union Medical College owed a great deal to the contribution by many people. We would like to express our deep appreciation for the leaders of Chinese Academy of Medical Sciences(CAMS)& Peking Union Medical College(PUMC), especially President Cao Xuetao for writing the preface for this book, as well as former President Ba Denian and Liu Depei who finished their own chapters ahead of schedule in spite of their tight schedule. We also express our gratitude to the long standing support from other leaders of CAMS and PUMC: Li Guoqin, Yao Longshan, Wang Yunfeng, Zhang Qin, Zhang Shuyang, and Zhang Xue.

We are grateful to the contributors of this book-Chinese or foreign for their timely submission of manuscripts of high academic quality.

Meanwhile, we would love to thank the director of the President's office CAMS/PUMC Zhu Chengbin and his colleagues, Dr. Wang Jianwei, director of the Office for Science and Technology Administration and his colleagues, Prof. Zhang Xia and Chen Jianhui from PUMC archive, Dean Zhai Xiaomei and Dean He Zhong of the School of Humanities and Social Sciences PUMC and the colleagues from the School. Wang Xirui-a student of class 2021 of PUMC 8 - year curriculum and translator Sun Aiping helped a lot in providing the quality translation. PUMC's foreign teacher-Sam Seery offered proof reading for the English version. PUMC press worked hard during the summer vocation to make the publishing of this book possible. We also appreciate the great support from China Medical Board.

We would love to acknowledge the gratitude to all the faculties and staffs of PUMC who dedicate their hardworking to the PUMC and CAMS.

Due to the time constraint, we did not have time to do the index. There might be flaws or errors in translating the manuscripts from Chinese to English. We appreciate your understanding and your comment!

Jiang Yuhong and Mary Brown Bullock

目　录

第一部分　传统 LEGACY ⋯⋯⋯⋯⋯⋯⋯⋯⋯⋯⋯⋯ 1

"对医学教育的国际贡献"：北京协和医学院的全球化背景 ⋯⋯⋯ 3

"An International Contribution to Medical Education"：The Global Context of the Peking Union Medical College ⋯⋯⋯⋯⋯⋯ 19

杨崇瑞、林巧稚与 20 世纪中国妇女健康 ⋯⋯⋯⋯⋯ 37

Yang Chongrui, Lin Qiaozhi, and Women's Health in 20th-Century China ⋯⋯⋯⋯⋯⋯⋯⋯⋯⋯⋯⋯⋯⋯⋯⋯ 54

北京协和医学院早期的中药研究：从 1910 年到 1941 年 ⋯⋯⋯ 76

Traditional Chinese Medical（TCM）Research at Peking Union Medical College：1910 – 1941 ⋯⋯⋯⋯⋯⋯ 89

斯乃博：二战时期在北京协和医学院的荷兰医生 ⋯⋯⋯⋯ 107

Isidore Snapper and PUMC During the Second World War ⋯⋯⋯ 132

第二部分　传承 Transition ⋯⋯⋯⋯⋯⋯⋯⋯⋯ 163

"老协和"的回忆 ⋯⋯⋯⋯⋯⋯⋯⋯⋯⋯⋯⋯⋯⋯⋯ 165

Memories of Old PUMC ⋯⋯⋯⋯⋯⋯⋯⋯⋯⋯⋯⋯⋯ 177

北京协和医学院的两代内分泌宗师——刘士豪和史轶蘩 ⋯⋯⋯ 192

Liu Shihao and Shi Yifan – The Two Generations of Masters in Endocrinology at Peking Union Medical College ⋯⋯⋯⋯ 207

"新协和"的医学专业化（1951 – 1966） ⋯⋯⋯⋯⋯ 231

The New PUMC and Its Professionalism（1951 – 1966） ⋯⋯⋯⋯ 253

中国医学科学院的成立及其早期运作（1956 – 1966） ⋯⋯⋯ 287

Establishing and Strengthening the Chinese Academy of Medical Sciences
　（1956 – 1966） ·· 302

收归国有之后的北京协和医学院（1949 – 1985） ······················· 326

Peking Union Medical College after nationalization，1949 – 1985 ········· 342

第三部分　新生 REVITALIZATION ····································· 363

协和学子：百年回顾 ··· 365

PUMC Alumni：A Centennial Review ·· 393

建院以来的主要科技成就及其影响 ·· 431

CAMS's Major Scientific and Technological Achievements since its
　Establishment ··· 445

协和的创造力和影响力——纪念协和建校 100 周年 ··················· 468

Creativity and Influence of Peking Union Medical College ·············· 479

让我们共同迎接挑战——写在协和百年之际 ····························· 496

Rising Up to Our Shared Challenges ·· 501

第一部分　传统 LEGACY

"对医学教育的国际贡献"[1]：北京协和医学院的全球化背景

达尔文·斯塔普顿（Darwin H. Stapleton, Ph. D., C. A.）

达尔文·斯塔普顿（Darwin H. Stapleton）在宾夕法尼亚长大，在斯沃斯莫尔学院（Swarthmore College）学习历史和经济发展，并获得了历史学硕士；在特拉华大学（University of Delaware）获得技术史博士学位。他在凯斯西储大学（Case Western Reserve University）教过科技史和美国研究，并在波士顿马萨诸塞大学教授档案科学。在担任洛克菲勒档案中心执行馆长时开始研究和撰写二十世纪中国和东亚科学技术与医学史。

北京协和医学院（PUMC，以下简称"协和"）是洛克菲勒最重要的慈善事业之一。在约翰·D·洛克菲勒（John D. Rockefeller）的全球视野的启发下，以及一群相信西方科学的普世功效的"医学人"[2]的驱动下，创立了协和。洛克菲勒搭建的各项事业组成了一个庞大的网络，在其运行的最初三十年，协和一直是这个网络的主要结点之一。它被规划并被视为"中国的约翰·霍普金斯大学"——即一所致力于高端医学教育和高端研究的西式大学，激励并促进全中国的卫生事业的发展。本文将回顾协和所实现的洛克菲勒的愿景规划，然后转而讨论协和之后的作用，并在国际化背景下考量两个方面的效果。

几名颇有建树的历史学家都谈及过协和成立的历史背景，最著名的是玛丽·布朗·布洛克（Mary Brown Bullock）的《洛克菲勒基金会与协和模式》（An American Transplant）。[3]需要指出的是，成立协和的想法来自洛克菲勒慈善事业中两股强大力量的交汇——其一是约翰·D·洛克菲勒传教精神的驱动，要在中国创造一个伟大的事业；其二则是新的洛克菲勒慈善机构——洛克菲勒基金会的国际卫生委员会愿望，在更加科学的基础上改革和引导西方医学，使其朝更科学的基础的方向上发展。世界已知的最伟大的慈善力量越来越多地笃信这样的想法，即在欧洲和美国发展起来的实验科学是战胜重大疾病痛苦的基础。[4]

在 20 世纪最初的二十年，洛克菲勒在卫生领域所制定的战略聚焦在塑造或者推动卓越的医学教育中心的发展：为已有建树的机构提供大量的新资源——众所周知，用洛克菲勒的说法，这一点被称为"让顶峰更高"；但在少数情况下则成立全新的机构。特别是在美国、东欧、南欧、巴西和日本成立公共卫生机构。[5] 洛克菲勒期望这些机构既作为国家疾病问题研究的场所，又作为医疗和公共卫生人员的培训之地。

约翰·霍普金斯大学是被选定的得到进一步加强的"顶峰"机构之一，但它也被选择成为一所公共卫生研究机构。霍普金斯大学成立于1876 年，并迅速成为少数在世纪更替之前重点放在师资和研究生研究项目而不是本科教育的凤毛麟角的美国大学之一。受到 19 世纪德国大学的发展的启发，特别是在科学方面以及在基于科学的医学方面的启发，渴望在科学方面接受高端培养的美国人纷纷去往诸如保罗·埃尔利希（Paul Ehrlich）、罗伯特·科赫（Robert Koch）和卡尔·路德维希（Carl Ludwig）等杰出人物的实验室工作。[6]

这些美国人的其中一个就是韦尔奇（William H. Welch）。他毕业于耶鲁大学，随后到德国与卡尔·路德维希这位杰出的生理学家一起做研究，返回美国后在约翰·霍普金斯大学促进基于实验室细菌学的医学研究核心方法。当洛克菲勒的慈善机构开始为高等教育和医学提供大量的资助时，随着 1901 年洛克菲勒医学研究所的成立、1902 年普通教育委员会的成立及 1909 年成立的洛克菲勒根除钩虫病委员会（该委员会在 1913 年演变成国际卫生委员会），在监管洛克菲勒慈善事业的人士圈中他经常提供顾问咨询。[7]

在 1914 年，普通教育委员会意识到，在公共卫生最基层方面的工作因为缺乏受过培训的工作者而遇到阻碍，因此开始探索找到适当的地方来培养公共卫生人才。最终，韦尔奇与罗时（Wickliffe Rose）共同撰写了一份关于公共卫生教育的报告，该报告最终促成了洛克菲勒对美国马里兰州（Maryland）巴尔的摩市（Baltimore）的霍普金斯大学的公共卫生学院的资助。该学院于 1918 年开课，并立即为全美公共卫生教育树立了标准，且成为洛克菲勒资助的世界上其他公共卫生学院的榜样。[8]

需要指出的是，创办协和的计划是与霍普金斯大学成立新的公共卫生学院的计划同时进行的。其教学理念、现代医学和科学的远见卓识以及学院目标都是一样的。洛克菲勒基金会（它自身创立于 1913 年）在 1914 年设立了一个附属机构，即罗氏驻华医社（简称 CMB），并于 1915 年派出两个考察团到中国考察中国医学教育状况。韦尔奇是第二个考察团的领导成员，其陪同人员包括洛克菲勒医学研究所所长西蒙·福勒克斯纳（Simon Flexner）和普通教育委员会主任鲍垂克（Wallace Buttrick）。在中国时，他们同一位在华的美国教授的私人会议中透露了他们对中国局势的看法。在叙述这次会面时，西蒙·福勒克斯纳强有力地为考察团说明来意：

> 他们认为，他们可以提供的最伟大的工作是能够在中国教授现代医学。在他们考察的所有机构中，他们没有看到一所机构在他们看来是在教授现代医学的。在有些地方，只有寥寥一两个人试图这样做，但也只有一个或两个而已。一个现代的教师队伍必须完全由专家组成，每门课程都能用现代方法、并全部都用现代化的手段来教授。[9]

最终，考察团建议罗氏驻华医社收购协和医学堂（Union Medical College）的建筑物和地皮，并创建一个新的学院，即北京协和医学院（Peking Union Medical College，即 PUMC），目的是复制在霍普金斯大学已经开展了将近四十年的基于实验室的高水平的科学医学教育项目。

在决定创立北京协和医学院（PUMC，以下仍简称为"协和"）之后，创立协和的计划的愿景是：将协和建成一所与洛克菲勒的其他机构水平相当的学院。建筑师之前为位于纽约的洛克菲勒医学研究所、位于美国俄亥俄州克利夫兰市的西储大学（Western Reserve University）医学院以及哈佛大学医学院设计了首批建筑物。在协和建设完工后被描述为"其他医学院校的样板……比之前的任何一所都要完善的示范学院，具有现代医学院的所有必备要素的典范"。[10]一名协和教授在访问了几所欧洲的大学和研究所之后评论说："在参观完这些实验室及其条件后，我愈发感到我们在东方的巨大责任与机会。"[11]协和的设施情况在《医学教育的方法和问题》的一系列文章中有详细的描述，此书系洛克菲勒的出版物，在世界各地发行。这些文章里包括建筑规划图、照片、课程讨论和实验室设备描述。文章还勾勒出协和的先进教育工作及基础设施。其中一篇文章指出，协和的研究往往是"其员工们在国外业已开展了的研究工作"的延续。[12]

1921 年 9 月在北京协和医学院的校园的开业仪式强调了对国际接轨的期望。来自欧洲、亚洲和美国的演讲嘉宾作报告，介绍了不同主题的最新医学研究，洛克菲勒二世（John D. Rockefeller Jr.）和其他杰出人士讨论了他们对未来的展望。洛克菲勒二世将协和的目的描述为"在中国建立（或正在建立）一所与西方文明世界中众所周知的领先机构的标准相媲美的医学院与医院……给中国人民提供（或正在提供）西方科学医学方面全面的知识和教育的机构"。[13]韦尔奇对洛克菲勒二世的言论做了进一步补充，他告诉参加仪式的协和教师和政要们：

> 各位的最高抱负应当是在现代化的、科学的医学方面培养中国学生……这些学生日后将在中国传播知识、践行最好的疾病预防和治疗的医学知识；这些学生日后将创建新的教育、研究、伤病的医疗中心。意识到你们正在推动这一崇高目标，由此促使这个伟大的国家的健康与繁荣、实际上也是全世界文明的健康和繁荣，一定将是对各位的最高报答……

在某些方面，那些在开业式上表达的对协和的国际接轨的期待和展望已在实现的过程中。洛克菲勒基金会所提供的第一批研究资助就给予了 1914 年想到国外深造的中国人，另外 1915~1916 年还为协和未来的工作人员提供了进修的资助金。这些资助计划为 1917 年洛克菲勒学者资助项目的正式启动打下了基础。[15] 1918 年，在其总共 68 名资助者当中，给中国学者的就有 65 个。[16] 随着该资助项目在 20 世纪 20 年代和 30 年代不断扩张，给中国学生、中国教师和中国官员的资助总是十分充足，通常比任何其他国家得到的都要多。[17] 在洛克菲勒基金会看来，这些资助不仅能形成一批"训练有素和经验丰富的专家队伍"，而且还能"给每个国家的进步都做出重大贡献，并能成为促进国际间理解和善意的手段。"[18]

在那些给协和学生和教师提供的资助中，大多数人受到资助去了霍普金斯大学、哈佛大学或洛克菲勒医学研究所进修。[19] 这些举措提高了协和在国际间的联系和声誉。接受资助者的一个杰出例子是袁贻谨，他于 1928～1931 年在霍普金斯大学进修。除了在那里的学习之外，他还在芝加哥大学参加了一个夏季课程；并访问了美国纽约州首府奥尔巴尼（Albany）、罗德岛州首府普罗维登斯（Providence）和密歇根州底特律市（Detroit）的城市卫生部门；还考察了哈佛大学公共卫生学院和多伦多大学的卫生学院；并出席了在波士顿举办的第 13 届国际生理学大会。[20] 最初是得到一个为期两年的资助，后来在里德（Lowell Reed）教授的推荐下，他又延期了一年。在他到达霍普金斯大学后仅仅几个月内，有一位教授就说："袁博士是一位超凡的人，是从协和来到霍普金斯的所有人员中素质最好、最优秀的人之一。"[21] 他回国时，可以看出"袁博士在霍普金斯大学的履历令人非常满意。生物统计学系主任里德教授和生物系的佩尔（Raymond Pearl）教授也对他做了最高评价。"[22] 引用佩尔教授曾经说过的话，"在我长期任教的职业生涯中，很少有学生在我看来拥有与袁（博士）旗鼓相当或者超过他的能力"。[23]

一些协和教师得到资助在欧洲进修。协和生理学系的张锡钧就获得了资助，并于 1931～1932 年的秋冬季节与海斯（W. R. Hess）一起在瑞士的苏黎世大学生理学院开展了为期六个月的研究工作，随后访问了位于德国、法国和英国的生理学部门以及实验室。他参加完 1932 年 8 月在意大利罗马举行的国际生理学大会之后完成了进修计划。[24] 许雨阶是协和的寄生虫学系教授，1933 年得到资助，其中包括资助他去欧洲旅行的费用。他马不停蹄地报告说："我花了两周时间来疯狂访问了不同的寄生虫研究机构。我见到了这一领域同我研究的大多数课题相关的著名人士及活生生的权威，并同他们进行了讨论。与这些人交流比较各自的研究记录是非常有启发的，我发现法国所教授的（钩虫病）以及发现疟疾学在英国有激烈的争议……另外，我发现在罗马被认为是正统的思想，到了伦敦却令人憎恶。"[25]

有趣的是，洛克菲勒资助项目也资助了一些日本学生或日本官员到协和学习。在洛克菲勒的管理者看来，20 世纪 20 年代和 30 年代，日本的公共卫生管理部门也需要改革，而协和的公共卫生项目可以给日本提供效仿的榜样。[26]这些最早期的日本研究员中，有两位——Ikuko Kawamura 和 Yoshi Kitade 被送到协和的护理学校学习一年。1927 ~ 1928 年，Takeo Inouye 去协和的 X 光部门实习。后来，两名日本研究人员在到国外旅行期间安排时间对协和进行了短期访问。[27]

协和的教师是协和与国际接轨的又一个例子。虽然在协和的教学都要求用英语，但教师都是全球招聘的，因此大多数教师都来自美国与其他母语为英语的国家。虽然教师来自其他高等教育机构，但是协和与洛克菲勒医学研究所有着特别的关系。作为美国的第一家生物医学研究机构，该研究所于 1901 年由洛克菲勒一世成立，借鉴了欧洲 19 世纪的典范性机构，即巴斯德研究所、李斯特研究所和科赫研究所。但是，虽然这些研究所的成立是为了支持某一位杰出科学顶尖人才的工作，但洛克菲勒医学研究所旨在进行疾病的基础研究。它按照实验室来组织建构，每个实验室都有自己的某个研究方向。

在 20 世纪 20 年代和 30 年代，协和和洛克菲勒医学研究所保持着稳定的相互交流。几名洛克菲勒医学研究所的教师来到协和一年或者甚至更长时间，几名协和毕业生则去洛克菲勒医学研究所获取研究生阶段的实验室经验。最早的学生之一是刘瑞恒，他在 1921 年在詹姆斯·墨非（James B. Murphy）的癌症研究实验室工作。[28]当刘瑞恒完成他的进修之后，墨非报告说：

> 他非常遗憾自己的实验室失去了刘博士，因为他已经成为一名非常有用的工作人员——是独一无二的，他原本希望能够永久留住刘成为自己的员工……通常是那些甚至来自更好学校的毕业生都需要几个月时间才能真正在研究工作中发挥作用。刘博士到达仅一个月之后，就开始崭露头角。刘博士的个性也显然让他在研究所的同事印象十分深刻，对其褒奖有加。[29]

洛克菲勒医学研究所教师交换的著名例子是凡思莱克（Donald Van Slyke）和路易·皮尔斯（Louise Pearce）。凡思莱克自 1907 年以来就一直在洛克菲勒医学研究所工作，主要从事血液化学研究。洛克菲勒医学研究所的所长西蒙·福勒克斯纳也是洛克菲勒基金会的董事。1922 年，应他的邀请，凡思莱克在协和度过了一个学期。在那里，他与教师吴宪合作，证明"在红细胞和血浆二者之间，电解质在血液中的分布符合道南平衡（Donnan equilibrium），并且在这种分布下，氧和二氧化碳二者的变化的效果对分布的影响可以通过生理化学法来解释和预测"。[30]凡思莱克向西蒙·福勒克斯纳报告说："从科学研究的角度看，我在这里的访问是激动人心的。"[31]路易斯·皮尔斯（Louise Pearce）从霍普金斯大学博士毕业来到洛克菲勒医学研究所，加入了西蒙·福勒克斯纳自己的实验室，后来也建立了她自己的实验室。她有广泛的兴趣，但皮肤病是她的专长。她于 1931~1932 年在协和担任客座教授，并在后来与协和教授合作出版了一系列出版物。[32]

最后，重要的是回到协和的洛克菲勒框架。虽然它在某些方面是一个相对孤立的机构，但是对于洛克菲勒更广泛的全球疾病控制战略来说，协和总是承载着一些基本要素。尤其是，协和发展成为一个健康中心，这是洛克菲勒项目在世界各地的典型元素。1925 年，北京第一卫生事务所在北京一个区域开业，其服务范围包括各种健康问题，其中也涵盖工业环境。虽然该站为其指定区域的大约十万名居民提供了大量的预防服务和治疗服务，但它也是协和学生、其中特别是那些公共卫生领域的学生的重要培训场所。此外，该事务所的示范功能不仅仅是体现在名称上：

洛克菲勒基金会打算把它建成一个潜在的、本地的疾病控制和健康教育的卫生部门。北京第一卫生事务所日后可以启发中国政府和中国卫生官员开展国家项目。协和医学院的校长胡恒德（Henry Houghton）评论过："如果要全面有效的话，那么有必要在大的卫生管理体系下使卫生中心的工作在微观环境下开展起来。"[33]

显然，北京第一卫生事务所确实对中国的国家卫生体系产生了重大影响。1935 年，袁贻谨在一篇重要文章中评论说："许多现在［政府］负责卫生事务的官员曾经是［协和公共卫生系］以及其培训中心［北京第一卫生事务所］的学生。"[34]协和毕业生陈志潜在北京第一卫生事务所接受过培训。他在回忆录中写道："通过兰安生（John B. Grant）的工作和其他现任和前任的学生与教职员工的工作，洛克菲勒基金会和协和能够对［中国的］卫生政策和管理的发展施加重大影响。"[35]除此之外，北京第一卫生事务所还有一些国际影响。与大多数洛克菲勒示范站一样，它位于首都，不仅国家的政要易于视察，国际人士也能很方便地进行考察——其中也包括那些想要考察基层公共卫生项目的洛克菲勒官员。

考虑了协和作为一所学院的国际化之后，让我们转而谈谈协和的全球效应。协和对全球科学医学贡献的最重要证据是保留下来的协和教师和学生大量的重要出版物。根据罗氏驻华医社（CMB）的档案所收集的抽印本，对这些出版物的所做的选择性回顾（selective review）表明，它们大多发表在英文版的中国期刊和美国期刊上，但也在世界各地传播，其中也包括一些德国、法国、英国和荷兰的期刊。到 20 世纪 20 年代中期，协和的教师每年发表一百多篇论文，见于二、三十种专业期刊上。虽然这些论文较为分散，但协和的文章最常出现的出版物有洛克菲勒医学研究所出版的《实验医学杂志》（Journal of Experimental Medicine）以及《实验医学与生物学学会论文集》（Proceedings of the Society for Experimental Medicine and Biology），该出版物与洛克菲勒医学研究所的教员密切相关。[36]1922 年，实验生物学与医学学会的一个分支在协和由麦可林（Franklin McLean）创建。麦可林在来协和之前曾经一直都是洛克菲勒医学研究所的工作人员。[37]毫无疑问，协和与洛克菲勒医学研究所的密切联系使这些期刊乐于接受来自协和的论文。

有关协和研究的一份有价值的摘要于 1941 年由斯乃博（Isidore Snapper）发表，他在 1938 年至 1942 年担任协和的内科学教授。斯乃博认为协和医院是世界上"最好的现代化教学医院之一"，后来他描述在协和的时间是"我生命中最美好的几年"。[38] 他的书回顾了协和所研究的、经治疗减轻的以及经常得到治愈的各种疾病。[39] 在回顾大量协和的出版物之后，他研究了在协和的门诊和医院观察到的传染病和系统性疾病，并始终关注患者的营养情况和社会条件。他思辩性的、基于研究的研究结果使他的书在全球畅销。三十年后，约翰·鲍尔斯（John Bowers）指出，斯乃博的书"将［他的］名字与协和紧密联系在一起；当今医学界一提及协和，大家脑海里立刻想起的名字就是斯乃博。"[40]

虽然协和出版物针对的是全球的学术型读者，但是协和的另一项开拓性工作吸引了国内外更多人士的注意。此项工作是协和参与了在定县的"平民教育运动"——晏阳初（Y. C. Yen）的心血结晶。定县是北京以南约 200 公里的一个县，大约 400 个村庄，人口 40 万左右。经中国政府许可，"平民教育运动"试图通过教育、农业改革和基本卫生项目来改革中国的农村社会。这个草根项目使一些协和毕业生，特别是那些在北京第一卫生事务所积累了经验的人，转而前往定县开展农村公共卫生工作。最后，洛克菲勒基金会提供资金支持协和在定县的学生培训，而且在那里工作成为协和公共卫生课程的常规组成部分。[41]

定县的工作蜚声中外。据报道，早在 1931 年，"访问者络绎不绝"。[42]当协和毕业陈志潜于 1932 年接管定县卫生项目的监督工作时，他可能招待了那一年的两个重要访问者：美国驻华使馆商务随员安诺德（Julean Arnold）和洛克菲勒基金会国际卫生部的主任葛莱格（Allan Gregg）。[43] 陈志潜后来回忆说："好多国际卫生领导人来到定县视察我们的工作。"[44] 最终，由于晏阳初擅于在美国筹集资金，定县的工作也变得更加广为人知。美国杂志《读者文摘》（Reader's Digest）的一篇文章以及赛珍珠（Pearl

Buck）的传记进一步扩大了它的知名度。[45]

最后，协和也在某种程度上参与到国际联盟卫生组织（League of Nations' Health Organization）的工作。国际联盟是在第一次世界大战结束后不久成立的，为国际间的合作和协助提供了一个平台。1921年，该联盟成立了国际联盟卫生组织（Health Organization，以下称为"国联卫生组织"）。国联卫生组织逐步开发了疾病控制国际项目，并且特别关注中国，因为中国很有可能成为疫情的源头，特别是因为（国联卫生组织的调查者认为）中国在其非常活跃的港口城市很少有或者根本没有疾病检疫制度。1928年，国联卫生组织高兴地注意到，中国政府开始采取措施，即成立了卫生部，协和毕业生刘瑞恒担任次长。国联卫生组织表示，"我们希望新成立卫生部与我们的［东方的］办事处之间将建立密切的合作关系。"[46]1929年初，国联卫生组织的医疗主任路德维希·瑞驰曼（Ludwig Rajchman）访问中国，他一心想为中国制定国家医疗规划。1930年3月，在日内瓦召开的国联卫生组织会议上，代表中国政府参会的有两位——协和的兰安生和陈志潜，此外还有米尔班克纪念基金（Milbank Memorial Fund）的艾德格（Edgar Sydenstricker）。在这次会议上，路德维希·瑞驰曼展示了他为期两个月的中国之旅的结果。[47]

路德维希·瑞驰曼提请国联卫生组织考虑能向中国提供什么样的援助。当意识到"中国的卫生重组必须与国家的经济复苏同时实现"时，国联卫生组织认识到中国是一个经济不发达地区，将受益于西方医学和公共卫生的影响，并设想信息和知识的流动主要是单向的。会议记录表明参与中国的问题影响了全球卫生政策，因为此政策是由国联卫生组织制定的。在他关于访问中国的报告的官方讨论中，路德维希·瑞驰曼评论说，他希望国联卫生组织能够在"对中国和其他国家有价值的改革"方面合作发展，而且他建议中国可以给其他地方的卫生项目当样板。[48]整个20世纪30年代期间国联卫生组织继续为中国的卫生管理的发展提供支持，包括在美国和欧洲为中国的卫生官员组织的"考察"，但改变很缓慢，抗战开始之后就停止了。[49]

有趣的是，协和的许雨阶也为国联卫生组织提供了一些支持。当罗马尼亚的米海·丘卡（Mihai Ciuca）教授在 1931 年被卫生组织派到中国，研究长江流域在灾难性的洪水之后疟疾暴发情况时，许雨阶与米海教授一起合作，米海教授表示"对许雨阶博士最近关于疟疾问题的研究工作深感钦佩"。[50]许雨阶随后得到资助，去欧洲和美国旅行，途中结识了知名疟疾学家，并从 1937 年开始加入国联卫生组织的疟疾委员会。[51]

结论

有位研究北京协和医学院历史的学者曾经声称协和已经"成为整个亚洲最著名的医学教育和研究中心"。在二十世纪上半叶，更进一步说，协和已经"享誉全球"。[52]由于本文回顾了协和在出版、洛克菲勒基金会进修资助及师资交流的国际网络中所扮演的角色，以及协和的各类工作所引起的广泛兴趣，这当然看上去是一个准确的评估。当然协和的公开的角色，是在科学的、基于实验室的医学下引导中国的医学教育，但是不管是从概念上还是从功能上来说，协和都是洛克菲勒机构国际网络中的一个重要节点。

参考书目

1. I-chin Yuan to John B. Grant, 1 July 1930, folder 542, box 77, China Medical Board Inc. Archives, Rockefeller Archive Center, Sleepy Hollow, New York, USA.

2. "医学人"这个词是通过 Richard Brown 的著作应用到洛克菲勒慈善的语境中的，我并不赞同其批判性的作者，但认同其对这个主题的学术贡献。E. Richard Brown, *Rockefeller Medicine Men: Medicine and Capitalism in America* (Berkeley, CA: University of California Press, 1979)

3. Mary Brown Bullock, *An American Transplant: The Rockefeller Foundation and the Peking Union Medical College* (Berkeley, CA: University of California Press, 1980). See also: Mary Brown Bullock, *The Oil Prince's Legacy: Rockefeller Philanthropy in China* (Washington: Woodrow Wilson Center Press, 2011); John Z. Bowers, *Western Medicine in a Chinese Palace: Peking Union Medical College, 1917 – 1951* (Philadelphia: Josiah Macy, Jr. Foundation, 1972); Raymond B. Fosdick, *The Story of the Rockefeller*

Foundation (New York: Harper & Brothers, 1952), ch. 7; and Qiusha Ma, "The Peking Union Medical College and the Rockefeller Foundation's Medical Programs in China," in William H. Schneider, ed., *Rockefeller Philanthropy and Modern Biomedicine: International Initiatives from World War I to the Cold War* (Bloomington, IN: Indiana University Press, 2002), pp. 159 – 183.

4. John Farley, *To Cast Out Disease: A History of the International Health Division of the Rockefeller Foundation (1913 – 1951)* (New York: Oxford University Press, 2004), esp. ch. 10; Howard S. Berliner, *A System of Scientific Medicine: Philanthropic Foundations in the Flexner Era* (New York: Tavistock Publications, 1985).

5. Farley, To Cast Out Disease, pp. 203 – 263. For one example, see: Darwin H. Stapleton, "Internationalism and nationalism: the Rockefeller Foundation, public health, and malaria in Italy, 1923 – 1951," *Parassitologia* 42 (2000): 127 – 134.

6. Elizabeth Fee, *Disease and Discovery: A History of the Johns Hopkins School of Public Health, 1916 – 1939* (Baltimore: Johns Hopkins University Press, 1987).

7. Fee, *Disease and Discovery*, ch. 3.

8. Fee, *Disease and Discovery*, ch. 2.

9. Harold Balme to (?) Cormack, 12 September 1915, folder 663, box 93, China Medical Board Inc. Archives, Rockefeller Archive Center, Sleepy Hollow, New York, USA.

10. Roger S. Greene, "China Medical Board: Report of the Director," *Rockefeller Foundation: Annual Report for 1921* (New York: Rockefeller Foundation, 1922), p. 247.

11. Davidson Black to George Vincent, 21 August 1924, folder 71, box 11, China Medical Board Inc. Archives, RFA.

12. Davidson Black, "Peking Union Medical College: Department of Anatomy," *Methods and Problems of Medical Education*, first series (New York: Rockefeller Foundation, 1924), pp. 25 – 39, quote on p. 38; Hsien Wu, "Peking Union Medical College: Department of Biochemistry," *Methods and Problems of Medical Education*, third series (New York: Rockefeller Foundation, 1925), pp. 205 – 208; Ernest W. H. Cruickshank, "Peking Union Medical College: Department of Physiology," *Methods and Problems of Medical Education*, fifth series (New York: Rockefeller Foundation, 1926), pp. 65 – 75; O. H. Robertson, "Peking Union Medical College: Department of Medicine," *Methods and Problems of Medical Education*, eighth series (New York: Rockefeller Foundation, 1927), pp. 101 – 108; John B. Grant, "Department of Public Health and Preventive Medicine: Peking Union Medical College," *Methods and Problems of Medical*

Education, fourteenth series (New York: Rockefeller Foundation, 1929), pp. 109 – 145; Gertrude E. Hodgman, "School of Nursing: Peking Union Medical College," *Methods and Problems of Medical Education*, twenty-first series (New York: Rockefeller Foundation, 1932), pp. 135 – 142.

13. John D. Rockefeller Jr. , "Response for the Rockefeller Foundation," in *Addresses and Papers: Dedication Ceremonies and Medical Conference*, *Peking Union Medical College*, *September 15 – 22, 1921* (Concord, NH: Rumford Press, 1922), p. 59.

14. William Henry Welch, "Pathological Problems in the Orient," in *Addresses and Papers*, p. 381.

15. Thomas B. Appleget, "Report on Fellowship Programs of the Rockefeller Foundation," 1932, folder 318, box 43, series 100E, Record Group (hereafter RG) 1. 2, Rockefeller Foundation Archives (hereafter RFA), Rockefeller Archive Center, Sleepy Hollow, New York, USA.

16. Rockefeller Foundation, *Annual Report for 1918* (New York: Rockefeller Foundation, 1919), p. 48.

17. 比如，1928 年洛克菲勒基金会医学教育分部管理了 383 名进修人员，其中 125 名是从中国来的学生或研究者，占 33% "Rockefeller Foundation Fellowships Active during 1928," folder 279, box 37, series 100E, RG 1. 2, RFA.

18. Rockefeller Foundation, *Annual Report for 1918*, p. 49. See also: Darwin H. Stapleton, "Fellowships and Field Stations: The Globalization of Public Health Knowledge, 1920 – 1950," read for "Explorations in Public Health History" conference, Bellagio Conference Center, Bellagio, Italy, October 27-November 1, 2003.

19. Bullock, *An American Transplant*, p. 126.

20. I. C. Yuan to Margery Eggleston, 17 November 1929, folder 541, box 77, China Medical Board Inc. Archives, RAC; I. C. Yuan to John B. Grant, 1 July 1930, folder 542, box 77, China Medical Board Inc. Archives, RAC.

21. Extract from WSC diary, 26 February 1929, folder 541, box 77, China Medical Board Inc. Archives, RAC.

22. China Medical Board, Executive Committee, action on I-chin Yuan, 1932, personnel record for Yuan, I-chin, volume #3620, Peking Union Medical College Archives (hereafter PUMCA), Beijing, Peoples Republic of China.

23. Quoted in memorandum from Department of Hygiene, PUMC, 17 March 1932, personnel record for Yuan, I-chin, volume #3620, PUMCA.

24. Personnel record for Chang, His-chun, volume #494, Peking Union Medical

College Archives (hereafter PUMCA), Beijing, Peoples Republic of China.

25. O. K. Khaw to Roger Greene, 6 August 1933, personnel record for Oo-Keh Khaw, volume #1312, PUMCA.

26. Darwin H. Stapleton, " 'Removing the obstacles to public health work', Context for the Rockefeller philanthropies and public health in China and Japan, 1920 – 1950," in Liping Bu, Darwin H. Stapleton, and Ka-che Yip, eds. , *Science*, *Public Health and the State in Modern Asia* (London: Routledge, 2012), pp. 103 – 104.

27. Fellowship recorder cards for Takeo Inouye, Ikuko Kawamura, Yoshi Kitade, Yoshio Kusama, and Chieta Mitsuhori, RFA.

28. George W. Corner, *A History of the Rockefeller Institute*, *1901 – 1953*: *Origins and Growth* (New York: Rockefeller Institute Press, 1964), pp. 217 – 218.

29. R. S. Greene to H. S. Houghton, 26 January 1922, folder 496, box 70, China Medical Board Inc. Archives, RAC.

30. Corner, *A History of the Rockefeller Institute*, p. 276.

31. Donald Van Slyke to Simon Flexner, 5 December 1922, reel 119, Simon Flexner papers, American Philosophical Society, Philadelphia, PA, USA.

32. " Dr. Louise Pearce," at cfmedicine. nlm. nih. gov/physicians/biography _ 248. html, accessed 2 November 2016. Co-authored publications appeared as late as 1936 in *Archives of Dermatology and Syphilis*, *Journal of Experimental Medicine*, *Journal of Immunology*, and *Journal of Pathology and Bacteriology*: reprints are in the China Medical Board Inc. Archives.

33. "Excerpt from Memorandum, HSHoughton to RSGreene-December 17, 1924, Subject: Department of Hygiene and Public Health (PUMC)," folder 465, box 66, China Medical Board Inc. Archives, RAC.

34. I-chin Yuan, "Progress of State Medicine in China," reprint from the *Chinese Recorder*, January 1935, copy in vol. 3632, PUMCA.

35. C. C. Chen, *Medicine in Rural China*: *A Personal Account* (Berkeley, CA: University of California Press, 1989), p. 61.

36. 这些评论是作者在其收集的 CMB 档案中保存的 1924 – 25 及 1936 – 37 协和教师及学生选刊的回顾基础上做出的。马秋莎统计了 1926 年协和师生发表了 168 篇文章。Qiusha Ma, "The Peking Union Medical College and the Rockefeller Foundation's Medical Programs in China," p. 181 n. 40.

37. "Program: First Meeting, Society for Experimental Biology and Medicine, Peking Branch, Peking, China," attached to Donald Van Slyke to Simon Flexner, 5 December

1922, reel 119, Simon Flexner Papers, American Philosophical Society, Philadelphia, PA, USA; George C. Corner, *A History of the Rockefeller Institute, 1901 - 1953: Origins and Growth* (New York: Rockefeller Institute Press, 1964), pp. 275 - 276.

38. Bowers, *Western Medicine in a Chinese Palace*, pp. 183 - 85, quote on p. 184.

39. I. Snapper, *Chinese Lessons to Modern Medicine: A Contribution to Geographical Medicine from the Clinics of Peiping* [sic] *Union Medical College* (New York: Interscience Publishers, 1941), p. 8.

40. Bowers, *Western Medicine in a Chinese Palace*, p. 183.

41. Bullock, *An American Transplant*, pp. 149 - 150; Chen, *Medicine in Rural China*, pp. 96 - 98.

42. Extract of letter, G. E. Hodgman to M. Beard, 23 June 1931, folder 70, box 7, series 601, RG 1.1, RFA.

43. John B. Grant to Victor G. Heiser, 6 August 1932, and Allan Gregg diary entries, 30 September-2 October 1932, both in folder 70, box 7, series 601, RG 1.1, RFA.

44. Chen, *Medicine in Rural China*, p. 58. Yen later commented that Edgar Sydenstricker of the Millbank Memorial Fund visited Ding Xian: Pearl S. Buck, *Tell the People: Talks with James Yen about the Mass Education Movement* (New York: International Mass Education Movement, 1959, originally published in 1945), pp. 48 - 49.

45. J. P. McEvoy, "Jimmy Yen: China's Teacher Extraordinary," *Reader's Digest* (November 1943): 38 - 44; Buck, *Tell the People.*

46. Société des Nations. Organisation d'Hygiène. Bureau d'Orient. Report Annuel de l'Année 1928 et Procès-Verbaux de la Quatrième Session du Comité Consultatif, Tenue a Singapour du 14 au 16 février 1929 (Geneva: League of Nations, 1929), doc. No. C-48-M-28-1929-III. Translation by the author. For a discussion of the Health Ministry see: Xi Gao, "Between the State and the Private Sphere: Chinese State Medicine Movement, 1930 - 1949," in Bu, Stapleton, and Yip, eds., *Science, Public Health and the State*, pp. 144 - 160.

47. League of National Health Committee, *Minutes of the Fifteenth Session Held at Geneva from March 5th to 8th, 1930* (Geneva: League of Nations, 1930), pp. 6 - 22.

48. League of National Health Committee, *Minutes of the Fifteenth Session Held at Geneva from March 5th to 8th, 1930*, p. 8.

49. Iris Borowy, "Thinking Big-League of Nations Efforts towards a Reformed National Health System in China," in Iris Borowy, ed., *Uneasy Encounters: The Politics of Medicine and Health in China, 1900 - 1937* (Frankfurt am Main: Peter Lang, 2009), pp. 211,

213; Bullock, *An American Transplant*, pp. 154 – 155.

50. Borowy, "Thinking Big," 213 – 215; J. Heng Liu to Roger Greene, 4 January 1932, volume #1312, PUMCA.

51. Personnel file for Oo-Keh Khaw, volume #494, PUMCA; O. K. Khaw to Roger Greene, 1 April 1932, 12 September 1932, 20 November 1932, 6 June 1933, volume # 1312, PUMCA.

52. Ma, "The Peking Union Medical College and the Rockefeller Foundation's Medical Programs in China," p. 179.

"An International Contribution to Medical Education"[1]:
The Global Context of the Peking Union Medical College

Darwin H. Stapleton, Ph. D. , C. A.

Darwin H. Stapleton grew up in Pennsylvania, studied history and economic development at Swarthmore College, and got an M. A. in history and Ph. D in the history of technology at the University of Delaware. He taught the history of technology and science, and American studies, at Case Western Reserve University, and taught archival science at University of Massachusetts Boston. While Executive Director of the Rockefeller Archive Center he began research and writing about the history of science, technology and medicine in China and east Asia in the 20th century.

Peking Union Medical College was one of the most significant undertakings of Rockefeller philanthropy. Inspired by the global vision of John D. Rockefeller, and driven by a corps of "medicine men" who believed in the universal efficacy of Western science, PUMC was created and sustained as one of the major nodes of the Rockefeller network for its first three decades of existence. [2] It was planned and viewed as a "Johns Hopkins for China" -a Western-style university dedicated to advanced training and advanced research in medicine that would stimulate and promote improved health throughout China. This chapter will review the planning of PUMC actuated by the Rockefeller vision, and will then turn to the consequential effects of PUMC – considering both in an international context.

The historical framework for the founding of PUMC has been admirably related by several historians, most notably by Mary Brown Bullock in An American Transplant. [3] It is important to understand that the idea for PUMC came from the confluence of two powerful forces in Rockefeller philanthropy – John D. Rockefeller's missionary impulse to create a great work in China, and the desire of the new Rockefeller philanthropic institutions, the International Health Board and the Rockefeller Foundation, to reform and redirect Western medicine toward a more scientific basis. The greatest philanthropic force that the world had ever known increasingly committed itself to the idea that laboratory science, as developed in Europe and the United States, was fundamental to overcoming historic scourges of disease. [4]

The Rockefeller strategy in the health field that developed in the first two decades of the 20th century focused on creating or furthering centers of excellence in medical education: already excellent institutions were given substantial new resources – known in Rockefeller parlance as "making the peaks higher"; but in a few cases entire new institutions were established. In particular, institutes of public health were founded in the United States, eastern and southern Europe, Brazil and Japan. [5]These institutes were expected to function both as sites of research on national problems of disease, and to serve as training sites for medical and public health personnel.

Johns Hopkins University was one of the peak institutions that was chosen to be strengthened, but it was also selected as a site for a public health institute Johns Hopkins University was founded in 1876 and quickly became one of the few American universities that, before the turn of the century, focused on faculty and post-graduate research programs rather than undergraduate education. Inspired by 19th-century developments in German universities, particularly in science and science-based medicine, Americans who desired the advanced training in the sciences went to work in the laboratories of such luminaries as Paul Ehrlich, Robert Koch, and Carl Ludwig. [6]

One such American was William H. Welch, a Yale graduate who

subsquently studied in Germany with Carl Ludwig, an outstanding physiologist, and returned to promote laboratory-based bacteriology as the core methodology for medical research at Johns Hopkins. When John D. Rockefeller's philanthropies began providing substantial funds for both higher education and medicine, with the founding of the Rockefeller Institute for Medical Research in 1901, the General Education Board in 1902, and the Rockefeller Commission for the Eradication of Hookworm Disease in 1909 (which evolved into the International Health Board in 1913), Welch became a frequent advisor to the circle of men who were overseeing Rockefeller's largess. [7]

In 1914 the General Education Board, recognizing that grass-roots work in public health was impeded by the lack of trained workers, began exploring the creation of a suitable place to educate them. Ultimately, Welch, in collaboration with Wickliffe Rose, wrote a report on public health education that led to the Rockefeller funding of the School for Hygiene and Public Health at Johns Hopkins University in Baltimore, Maryland (USA). The School opened in 1918 and immediately set a standard for public health education throughout the United States, and became a model for other Rockefeller-funded schools of public health throughout the world. [8]

It is important to understand that plans that led to the creation of the Peking Union Medical College were being carried out in parallel with plans for the new school at Johns Hopkins. The pedagogical ideas, the visions of modern medicine and science, and the institutional goals were the same. The Rockefeller Foundation (itself created in 1913) established a subsidiary organization, the China Medical Board in 1914, and sent two commissions to China in 1915 to investigate the state of medical education there. Welch was a leading member of the second commission, and was accompanied by Simon Flexner, Director of the Rockefeller Institute for Medical Research, and Wallace Buttrick, Director of the General Education Board. Their view of the situation in China was revealed in a private meeting with an American professor then in China. As he recounted the meeting, Simon Flexner spoke forcefully for the group.

> *They consider that the greatest service they can render is to make it possible for Modern Medicine to be taught in China. Of all the institutions they have visited, they have not seen one which, in their opinion, is teaching Modern Medicine. In a few places only one or two men are attempting to do so, but only one or two. A modern faculty must be composed wholly of experts, so that every subject is taught by modern methods and with all modern facilities.* [9]

Ultimately the commission recommended that the China Medical Board acquire the buildings and grounds of the Union Medical College, and create a new institution, the Peking Union Medical College, with the goal of duplicating the high-level program of laboratory-based scientific medicine that had been practiced at Johns Hopkins University for nearly four decades.

After the decision was made to create the Peking Union Medical College, the plans for the college were always made with a vision to establish it at a level comparable to other Rockefeller-related institutions. The architect had previously designed the initial buildings for the Rockefeller Institute for Medical Research in New York, the medical campus for Western Reserve University (Cleveland, Ohio, USA), and the Harvard University medical school. The completed facilities at PUMC were described as "a model for other medical schools... a demonstration more nearly adequate than any that has preceded it, of the essential elements of a modern medical school."[10] One PUMC professor, after visiting several universities and institutes in Europe commented that "The more I see of other laboratories and conditions the more impressed I am with the greatness of our responsibilities and opportunities in the East."[11] PUMC's facilities were lavishly described in a series of articles in *Methods and Problems of Medical Education*, a Rockefeller publication that was distributed throughout the world. Including building plans, photographs, discussions of coursework, and descriptions of laboratory equipment, the articles laid out the advanced programs and facilities at PUMC. One article noted that research at PUMC was often a continuation of "work [which] had already been begun abroad by staff members. "[12]

The dedication of the PUMC campus in September 1921 underlined expectations of its international connectivity. Speakers from Europe, Asia, and the United States gave presentations on various topics of recent medical research, and John D. Rockefeller Jr. and other luminaries discussed their hopes for the future. JDR Jr. described the purpose of PUMC as "develop[ing] in China a medical school and hospital of a standard comparable with that of the leading institutions known to Western civilization... offer[ing] to the Chinese people facilities for acquiring a thorough knowledge of and training in Western scientific medicine. "[13] William H. Welch expanded on JDR Jr'. sremarks by telling the assembled PUMC faculty and dignitaries that

> *Your highest ambition should be to train Chinese students in modern, scientific medicine... who will spread in their country the knowledge and the practice of the best that medicine can offer for the prevention and treatment of disease, and who will create new centers for education, investigation, and the care of the sick and injured. The consciousness that you are furthering this high purpose and thereby the health and prosperity of this great country, indeed of the civilization of the world, must be your supreme reward...*[14]

In some ways the expectations and hopes for PUMC's international connectivity that were expressed at the dedication were already in the process of being fulfilled. The very first cohort of fellowships offered by the Rockefeller Foundation were for was for Chinese who were seeking advanced training abroad in 1914, with additional fellowships given to future PUMC staff members in 1915 and 1916. These set the stage for the initiation of a formal Rockefeller fellowship program in 1917. [15] In 1918 sixty-five fellowships were awarded to

China of the total of sixty-eight fellowships. [16] As the fellowship program expanded in the 1920s and 1930s awards to Chinese students, faculty and officials were always substantial, and usually more than any other country received. [17] In the view of the Rockefeller Foundation, fellowships not only developed a corps of "well-trained and experienced experts," but also made "a fundamental contribution to progress in each nation, and may be made a means of promoting international understanding and good will." [18]

Of the fellowships going to PUMC students and faculty, most were directed to studies at Johns Hopkins University, Harvard University or the Rockefeller Institute for Medical Research. [19] These fellowships heightened the international connections and reputation of PUMC. An outstanding example of the fellowship experience was that of I-chin Yuan, who studied at Johns Hopkins in 1928 – 1931. In addition to his studies there, he had a summer course at the University of Chicago; visited city health departments at Albany (New York), Providence (Rhode Island), and Detroit (Michigan); observed the programs at Harvard University's School of Public Health and the University of Toronto's School of Hygiene; and attended the 13th International Congress of Physiology at Boston. [20] Originally granted a two-year program, he was given a one-year extension on the recommendation of Professor Lowell Reed. Within a few months after his arrival at Johns Hopkins one of his professors "state [d] that Dr. Y [uan] is a superior man, one of the very first quality and one of the best who has come to Hopkins from P. U. M. C. " [21] On his return it was noted that "Dr. Yuan's record while at Johns Hopkins was very satisfactory. Professor L. J. Reed, head of the department of biostatistics and Professor Raymond Pearl, of the department of biology, have spoken of him in the highest terms. " [22] Professor Pearl was also quoted as stating that "in my long career as a teacher I have had few students who seemed to me to equal or to surpass Yuan in ability. " [23]

Some PUMC faculty had fellowships for study Europe. Hsi-chun Chang, of the Physiology Department at PUMC took a fellowship to study with W. R. Hess at the Physiology Institute of the University of Zurich (Switzerland) for six months in the fall and winter of 1931 – 32 , and subsequently visited physiology departments and laboratories in Germany, France and Britain. He completed his fellowship by attending the International Congress of Physiology in Rome, Italy, in August 1932. [24] Oo-Keh Khaw, a professor of parasitology at PUMC, had a fellowship in 1933 that included travel in Europe. He reported breathlessly that he had "spent a hectic fortnight visiting the various institutes of research on parasitology. I saw and discussed most of the problems of my subject with the most famous names and living authorities. It was very instructive to compare notes with these people and to find out that what was being taught in France on [hookworm disease] and malariology was warmly contradicted...in England and what was orthodoxy in Rome was anathema in London. "[25]

Interestingly, in a few instances Rockefeller fellowships were granted to Japanese students or officials to study at PUMC. In the view of Rockefeller officials the public health administration in Japan in the 1920s and 1930s needed reform, and the PUMC public health program provided a model that the Japanese could emulate. [26] Two of the earliest Japanese fellows were Ikuko Kawamura and Yoshi Kitade, who were sent to the nursing school at PUMC for a year. In 1927 – 1928 Takeo Inouye went to PUMC for an internship in the Roentgenology (X-ray) Department. Later two Japanese fellows made brief visits to PUMC during their allotted travels abroad. [27]

The faculty of PUMC is a further example of PUMC's international connectivity. It was recruited globally, although with the requirement that education was taking place in English, most came from the United States and other English-speaking countries. Although faculty came from other institutions of higher education, the connection with the Rockefeller Institute for Medical Research was particularly strong. The Institute was founded in 1901 by John D. Rockefeller as the first biomedical research organization in the United States, drawing on the European examples of the latter 1800s – the Pasteur Institute,

Lister Institute, and Koch Institute. But, while those institutes had been founded to support the work of one outstanding leader, the RIMR was intended to conduct fundamental research on diseases. It was organized into laboratories, each pursing promising lines of investigation.

The interchange between PUMC and RIMR was constant throughout the 1920s and 1930s, when several RIMR faculty came to PUMC for a year or more, and several PUMC graduates went to the Institute for post-graduate laboratory experience. One of the earliest students was Jui-heng Liu, who worked in James B. Murphy's cancer-research laboratory in 1921.[28] When Liu completed his program Murphy reported that

> *He was extremely sorry to lose Dr. Liu from his laboratory as she had become an extremely useful worker – one of the kind that he would like to retain permanently on his staff... it usually took graduates even of the better schools several months to become really effective in research work but that a month after Dr. Liu's arrival he was beginning to get results. Dr. Liu's personality also evidently impressed his fellow workers in the Institute very favorably.*[29]

Notable examples of the RIMR faculty exchange were Donald Van Slyke and Louise Pearce. Van Slyke had been at the Institute since 1907, working largely on blood chemistry. In 1922, at the invitation of the Director of the Institute, Simon Flexner, who was also a trustee of the Rockefeller Foundation, Van Slyke spent a semester at PUMC. There he collaborated with faculty member Hsien Wu to demonstrate that "the distribution of electrolytes in the blood, between red cells and plasma, conforms to the Donnan equilibrium and that the effects of oxygen and carbon dioxide changes on this distribution could be explained and predicted by physiochemical laws. "[30] Van Slyke reported to Flexner that "scientifically I have found my visit her stimulating. "[31] Louise Pearce came to the Institute with a doctorate from Johns Hopkins, joined Simon Flexner's own laboratory, and later established her own laboratory. She had a wide range of interests, but skin diseases were her specialty. She was a visiting professor at PUMC in 1931 – 1932, and co-authored a series of publications with PUMC faculty that appeared afterward. [32]

Finally, it is important to return to the Rockefeller framework of PUMC. Although it was in some ways a stand-alone institution, it always carried some elements of the broader Rockefeller strategy for global disease control. Notably, PUMC spawned a health center that was a typical element of the Rockefeller program throughout the world. In 1925 the Peking Health Demonstration Station was opened in a district of Beijing that included a variety of health problems, including industrial environments. Although the Station provided substantial preventative and curative services to the approximately 100, 000 residents of its designated area, it was also an important training facility for PUMC students, particularly those in the public health field. Moreover, the demonstration function of the station was not in name only: the Rockefeller Foundation intended it to be a demonstration of the potential of local health units for disease control and health education. Primarily the Peking Health Demonstration Station was to be an inspiration to the Chinese government and Chinese health officials to undertake a national project: Henry Houghton, Director of PUMC, remarked that "it is necessary that the health center work be undertaking in a miniature setting of a whole scheme of health administration if it is to be fully effective. "[33]

Clearly the Health Demonstration Center did have a substantial influence on the national health infrastructure in China. In 1935 I-chin Yuan commented in a major article that "many of the [government] health officers who are now in responsible positions were at one time or another students [in the PUMC Department of Hygiene] and its training center, the [Peking] First Health Station. "[34] C. C. Chen, a PUMC graduate who had experience at the Health Station, noted in his memoirs that "through Grant's activities and those of other current and former students and faculty members, the Rockefeller Foundation and the PUMC were able to exercise a substantial influence on evolving health policy and administration [in China] . "[35] Beyond that, the Health Station had some international influence. Like most Rockefeller demonstration stations, it was located near a capital city so that it not only could be visited easily by national leaders, but also by international figures – which included Rockefeller officers – who wanted to observe a grass-roots public health program.

Having considered the international connectivity of PUMC as an institution, let us turn to PUMC's global effects. The most consequential evidence of PUMC contributions to scientific medicine globally is the very substantial record of publication by PUMC faculty and students. A selective review of its publications, based on the collected offprints in the archives of the China Medical Board, shows that they appeared largely in English-language Chinese and American journals, but also reached around the world, including several in German, French, British and Dutch journals. By the mid-1920s the faculty of PUMC was publishing well over a hundred articles a year, appearing in several dozen professional publications. Although the publications were widely scattered, the most frequent locations for PUMC publications were the *Journal of Experimental Medicine*, published at the Rockefeller Institute for Medical Research, and the *Proceedings of the Society for Experimental Medicine and Biology*, which was closely associated with the Institute's faculty. [36] (In 1922 a branch of the Society for Experimental Biology and Medicine was founded at PUMC by Franklin McLean, who had been on the staff of the Institute before coming to PUMC. [37]) Undoubtedly, the close connection of PUMC with the Institute made those journals receptive.

A valuable compendium of PUMC research was published in 1941 by Isidore Snapper, who was a professor of medicine at PUMC, 1938 to 1942. Snapper regarded PUMC's hospital "as one of the best modern teaching hospitals" in the world, and in later years described his time at PUMC as "the best years of my life. "[38] His book reviewed the wide variety of diseases that were investigated, ameliorated, and often cured, at PUMC. [39] Drawing heavily on PUMC's record of publications, he looked at infectious diseases and systemic diseases observed in the clinics and hospitals of PUMC, always keeping an eye on the nutritional and social circumstances of the patients. His critical, research-based study gave his book a global readership, such that thirty years later John Bowers could comment that it "linked [Snapper's] name inseparably with PUMC; for the general medical community, any reference to the college today immediately brings to mind the name of Isidore Snapper." [40]

While PUMC publications reached a global scholarly audience, another outreach of PUMC attracted the attention of a broader community, ranging from officials of national and international health organizations to the general public. That outreach was PUMC's involvement in the Mass Education Movement's operations at Ding Xian, the brainchild of Y. C. Yen. Ding Xian was a county about 200 kilometers south of Beijing, containing about 400,000 people in some 400 villages. With the permission of the Chinese government, the Mass Education Movement was attempting to reform rural Chinese society through education, agricultural reform and basic health initiatives. This grassroots program led some PUMC graduates, especially those with experience at the Peking Health Demonstration Station, to move on to village public health work at Ding Xian. Eventually the Rockefeller Foundation provided funds to support PUMC student training at Ding Xian, and work there became a regular element of PUMC's public health curriculum. [41]

The work at Ding Xian became known internationally. As early as 1931 it was reported to have been "swamped with visitors." [42] When PUMC graduate C. C. Chen took over supervision of the health program at Ding Xian in 1932 he likely hosted two important visitors of that year, Julean Arnold, the commercial attaché to the United States Embassy to China, and Allan Gregg, the head of the Rockefeller Foundation's International Health Division. [43] Chen later recalled that "more than a few international health leaders had come to Dingxian to observe our work. " [44] Ultimately the work at Ding Xian became more widely known as Y. C. Yen became adept at fund-raising in the United States. An article in *Reader's Digest*, and a biography by Pearl Buck cemented his fame. [45]

Finally, PUMC was peripherally, but significantly, involved with the League of Nations' Health Organization. The League, founded just after World War I to create a forum for international cooperation and collaboration, established the Health Organization in 1921. The Health Organization gradually developed programs for international disease control, and took a special interest in China as a likely source of epidemic disease, particularly because (in the view of the Health Organization's investigators) China had little or no disease quarantine provision at its very active port cities. In 1928 the Health Organization had been pleased to note that the Chinese government had taken steps to create a ministry of hygiene, with PUMC graduate Liu Ruiheng (Jui-heng Liu) as vice-minister. The Health Organization expressed "our hope that a close collaboration will be established between this new Ministry and our 〔Eastern〕 Bureau. " [46] When the Health Organization's medical director, Ludwig Rajchman, visited China for early in 1929, he became absorbed with the idea of promoting a national medical strategy there. In a meeting of the Health Organization in Geneva in March 1930, attended by two representatives of the Chinese government, John B. Grant and C. C. Chen of PUMC, and Edgar Sydenstricker of the Millbank Memorial Fund, Rajchman laid out the results of his two-month tour of China. [47]

Rajchman asked the Health Organization to consider what aid it might provide to China, while recognizing that "the health reorganization of China must be achieved concomitantly with the economic revival of the country. " While it is clear that the Health Organization saw China as an underdeveloped area that would benefit from the influence of Western medicine and public health, and envisioned the flow of information and knowledge as primarily unidirectional, there are suggestions in the record that engagement with the problems in China influenced global health policy as it was being developed by the Health Organization. In the official discussion of his report on his visit to China Rajchman commented that it was his hope that the Health Organization could collaborate in "reforms which would be valuable both to China and to other countries," suggesting that work in China could provide a model for health programs elsewhere. [48] The Health Organization continued to provide support for the development of health administration in China through the 1930s, including providing "study tours" in the United States and Europe for Chinese health officials but changes were slow and matters came to a halt with the beginning of the Japanese War. [49]

Interestingly, Oo-keh Khaw of PUMC provided some support for the League of Nations Health Organization. When Professor Mihai Ciuca of Romania was sent by the Health Organization to study a malaria outbreak in the Yangtze valley following devastating floods there in 1931, Khaw collaborated with Ciuca, who expressed "admiration of the services provided by Dr. O. K. Khaw during his recent survey of the malaria problem." [50] Khaw subsequently made the acquaintance of leading malariologists while traveling through Europe and the United States on a fellowship, and beginning in 1937 was appointed to the Malaria Commission of the Health Organization. [51]

Conclusion

One scholar of the history of the Peking Union Medical College has stated that it "became the most famous medical education and research center in all of Asia" in the first half of the twentieth century, and further that it had a "worldwide reputation." [52] Considering this chapter's review of PUMC's role in the international network of publications, fellowships and faculty exchanges fostered by the Rockefeller Foundation, and the widespread interest in the activities of PUMC, that certainly appears to be an accurate assessment. While formally the role of PUMC was to direct medical education in China in the direction of scientific, laboratory-based medicine, in conception and in its functions the Peking Union Medical College was an important node in the international network of Rockefeller institutions.

Bibliography

1. I-chin Yuan to John B. Grant, 1 July 1930, folder 542, box 77, China Medical Board Inc. Archives, Rockefeller Archive Center, Sleepy Hollow, New York, USA.

2. The term "medicine men" entered the discourse on Rockefeller philanthropy through the work of E. Richard Brown, whose very critical work I do not agree with substantially, but recognize as a contribution to scholarship on the subject: E. Richard Brown, *Rockefeller Medicine Men: Medicine and Capitalism in America* (Berkeley, CA: University of California Press, 1979).

3. Mary Brown Bullock, *An American Transplant: The Rockefeller Foundation and the Peking Union Medical College* (Berkeley, CA: University of California Press, 1980). See also: Mary Brown Bullock, *The Oil Prince's Legacy: Rockefeller Philanthropy in China* (Washington: Woodrow Wilson Center Press, 2011); John Z. Bowers, *Western Medicine in a Chinese Palace: Peking Union Medical College, 1917 - 1951* (Philadelphia: Josiah Macy, Jr. Foundation, 1972); Raymond B. Fosdick, The Story of the Rockefeller Foundation (New York: Harper & Brothers, 1952), ch. 7; and Qiusha Ma, "The Peking Union Medical College and the Rockefeller Foundation's Medical Programs in China," in William H. Schneider, ed., *Rockefeller Philanthropy and Modern Biomedicine: International Initiatives from World War I to the Cold War* (Bloomington, IN: Indiana University Press, 2002), pp. 159 - 183,

4. John Farley, *To Cast Out Disease: A History of the International Health Division of the Rockefeller Foundation (1913 - 1951)* (New York: Oxford University Press, 2004), esp. ch. 10; Howard S. Berliner, *A System of Scientific Medicine: Philanthropic Foundations in the Flexner Era* (New York: Tavistock Publications, 1985).

5. Farley, To Cast Out Disease, pp. 203 - 263. For one example, see: Darwin H. Stapleton, "Internationalism and nationalism: the Rockefeller Foundation, public health, and malaria in Italy, 1923 - 1951," *Parassitologia* 42 (2000): 127 - 134.

6. Elizabeth Fee, *Disease and Discovery: A History of the Johns Hopkins School of Public Health, 1916 - 1939* (Baltimore: Johns Hopkins University Press, 1987),

7. Fee, *Disease and Discovery*, ch. 3.

8. Fee, *Disease and Discovery*, ch. 2.

9. Harold Balme to (?) Cormack, 12 September 1915, folder 663, box 93, China Medical Board Inc. Archives, Rockefeller Archive Center, Sleepy Hollow, New York, USA.

10. Roger S. Greene, "China Medical Board: Report of the Director," *Rockefeller Foundation: Annual Report for 1921* (New York: Rockefeller Foundation, 1922), p. 247.

11. Davidson Black to George Vincent, 21 August 1924, folder 71, box 11, China Medical Board Inc. Archives, RFA.

12. Davidson Black, "Peking Union Medical College: Department of Anatomy," *Methods and Problems of Medical Educatiion*, first series (New York: Rockefeller Foundation, 1924), pp. 25 – 39, quote on p. 38; Hsien Wu, "Peking Union Medical College: Department of Biochemistry," *Methods and Problems of Medical Education*, third series (New York: Rockefeller Foundation, 1925), pp. 205 – 208; Ernest W. H. Cruickshank, "Peking Union Medical College: Department of Physiology," *Methods and Problems of Medical Education*, fifth series (New York: Rockefeller Foundation, 1926), pp. 65 – 75; O. H. Robertson, "Peking Union Medical College: Department of Medicine," *Methods and Problems of Medical Education*, eighth series (New York: Rockefeller Foundation, 1927), pp. 101 – 108; John B. Grant, "Department of Public Health and Preventive Medicine: Peking Union Medical College," *Methods and Problems of Medical Education*, fourteenth series (New York: Rockefeller Foundation, 1929), pp. 109 – 145; Gertrude E. Hodgman, "School of Nursing: Peking Union Medical College," *Methods and Problems of Medical Education*, twenty-first series (New York: Rockefeller Foundation, 1932), pp. 135 – 142.

13. John D. Rockefeller Jr., "Response for the Rockefeller Foundation," in *Addresses and Papers: Dedication Ceremonies and Medical Conference, Peking Union Medical College, September 15 – 22, 1921* (Concord, NH: Rumford Press, 1922), p. 59.

14. William Henry Welch, "Pathological Problems in the Orient," in *Addresses and Papers*, p. 381.

15. Thomas B. Appleget, "Report on Fellowship Programs of the Rockefeller Foundation," 1932, folder 318, box 43, series 100E, Record Group (hereafter RG) 1.2, Rockefeller Foundation Archives (hereafter RFA), Rockefeller Archive Center, Sleepy Hollow, New York, USA.

16. Rockefeller Foundation, *Annual Report for 1918* (New York: Rockefeller Foundation, 1919), p. 48.

17. For example, in 1928 the Rockefeller Foundation's Division of Medical Education

was administering 383 fellowships, of which 125, or 33% were for students or researchers from China: "Rockefeller Foundation Fellowships Active during 1928," folder 279, box 37, series 100E, RG 1.2, RFA.

18. Rockefeller Foundation, *Annual Report for 1918*, p. 49. See also: Darwin H. Stapleton, "Fellowships and Field Stations: The Globalization of Public Health Knowledge, 1920 – 1950," read for "Explorations in Public Health History" conference, Bellagio Conference Center, Bellagio, Italy, October 27-November 1, 2003.

19. Bullock, *An American Transplant*, p. 126.

20. I. C. Yuan to Margery Eggleston, 17 November 1929, folder 541, box 77, China Medical Board Inc. Archives, RAC; I. C. Yuan to John B. Grant, 1 July 1930, folder 542, box 77, China Medical Board Inc. Archives, RAC.

21. Extract from WSC diary, 26 February 1929, folder 541, box 77, China Medical Board Inc. Archives, RAC.

22. China Medical Board, Executive Committee, action on I-chin Yuan, 1932, personnel record for Yuan, I-chin, volume #3620, Peking Union Medical College Archives (hereafter PUMCA), Beijing, Peoples Republic of China.

23. Quoted in memorandum from Department of Hygiene, PUMC, 17 March 1932, personnel record for Yuan, I-chin, volume #3620, PUMCA.

24. Personnel record for Chang, His-chun, volume #494, Peking Union Medical College Archives (hereafter PUMCA), Beijing, Peoples Republic of China.

25. O. K. Khaw to Roger Greene, 6 August 1933, personnel record for Oo-Keh Khaw, volume #1312, PUMCA.

26. Darwin H. Stapleton, " 'Removing the obstacles to public health work,' Context for the Rockefeller philanthropies and public health in China and Japan, 1920 – 1950," in Liping Bu, Darwin H. Stapleton, and Ka-che Yip, eds. , *Science*, *Public Health and the State in Modern Asia* (London: Routledge, 2012), pp. 103 – 104.

27. Fellowship recorder cards for Takeo Inouye, Ikuko Kawamura, Yoshi Kitade, Yoshio Kusama, and Chieta Mitsuhori, RFA.

28. George W. Corner, *A History of the Rockefeller Institute*, *1901 – 1953*: *Origins and Growth* (New York: Rockefeller Institute Press, 1964), pp. 217 – 218.

29. R. S. Greene to H. S. Houghton, 26 January 1922, folder 496, box 70, China Medical Board Inc. Archives, RAC.

30. Corner, *A History of the Rockefeller Institute*, p. 276.

31. Donald Van Slyke to Simon Flexner, 5 December 1922, reel 119, Simon Flexner

papers, American Philosophical Society, Philadelphia, PA, USA.

32. "Dr. Louise Pearce," at cfmedicine. nlm. nih. gov/physicians/biography_ 248. html, accessed 2 November 2016. Co-authored publications appeared as late as 1936 in *Archives of Dermatology and Syphilis*, *Journal of Experimental Medicine*, *Journal of Immunology*, and *Journal of Pathology and Bacteriology*; reprints are in the China Medical Board Inc. Archives.

33. "Excerpt from Memorandum, HSHoughton to RSGreene-December 17, 1924, Subject; Department of Hygiene and Public Health (PUMC)," folder 465, box 66, China Medical Board Inc. Archives, RAC.

34. I-chin Yuan, "Progress of State Medicine in China," reprint from the *Chinese Recorder*, January 1935, copy in vol. 3632, PUMCA.

35. C. C. Chen, *Medicine in Rural China: A Personal Account* (Berkeley, CA: University of California Press, 1989), p. 61.

36. These comments are based on the author's review of the collected offprints of PUMC faculty and students for the years 1924 – 25 and 1936 – 37, as found in the China Medical Board, Inc. Archives. Qiusha Ma counted 168 articles published by PUMC faculty and students in 1926; Qiusha Ma, "The Peking Union Medical College and the Rockefeller Foundation's Medical Programs in China," p. 181 n. 40.

37. "Program: First Meeting, Society for Experimental Biology and Medicine, Peking Branch, Peking, China," attached to Donald Van Slyke to Simon Flexner, 5 December 1922, reel 119, Simon Flexner Papers, American Philosophical Society, Philadelphia, PA, USA; George C. Corner, *A History of the Rockefeller Institute*, *1901 – 1953: Origins and Growth* (New York: Rockefeller Institute Press, 1964), pp. 275 – 276

38. Bowers, *Western Medicine in a Chinese Palace*, pp. 183 – 85, quote on p. 184.

39. I. Snapper, *Chinese Lessons to Modern Medicine: A Contribution to Geographical Medicine from the Clinics of Peiping* [sic] *Union Medical College* (New York: Interscience Publishers, 1941), p. 8.

40. Bowers, *Western Medicine in a Chinese Palace*, p. 183.

41. Bullock, *An American Transplant*, pp. 149 – 150; Chen, *Medicine in Rural China*, pp. 96 – 98.

42. Extract of letter, G. E. Hodgman to M. Beard, 23 June 1931, folder 70, box 7, series 601, RG 1. 1, RFA.

43. John B. Grant to Victor G. Heiser, 6 August 1932, and Allan Gregg diary entries, 30 September-2 October 1932, both in folder 70, box 7, series 601, RG 1. 1, RFA.

44. Chen, *Medicine in Rural China*, p. 58. Yen later commented that Edgar Sydenstricker of the Millbank Memorial Fund visited Ding Xian: Pearl S. Buck, *Tell the People: Talks with James Yen about the Mass Education Movement* (New York: International Mass Education Movement, 1959, originally published in 1945), pp. 48 – 49.

45. J. P. McEvoy, "Jimmy Yen: China's Teacher Extraordinary," *Reader's Digest* (November 1943): 38 – 44; Buck, *Tell the People.*

46. Société des Nations. Organisation d'Hygiène. Bureau d'Orient. Report Annuel de l'Année 1928 et Procès-Verbaux de la Quatrième Session du Comité Consultatif, Tenue a Singapour du 14 au 16 février 1929 (Geneva: League of Nations, 1929), doc. No. C – 48 – M – 28 – 1929 – III. Translation by the author. For a discussion of the Health Ministry see: Xi Gao, "Between the State and the Private Sphere: Chinese State Medicine Movement, 1930 – 1949," in Bu, Stapleton, and Yip, eds., *Science, Public Health and the State*, pp. 144 – 160.

47. League of National Health Committee, *Minutes of the Fifteenth Session Held at Geneva from March 5ᵗʰ to 8ᵗʰ, 1930* (Geneva: League of Nations, 1930), pp. 6 – 22.

48. League of National Health Committee, *Minutes of the Fifteenth Session Held at Geneva from March 5ᵗʰ to 8ᵗʰ, 1930*, p. 8.

49. Iris Borowy, "Thinking Big-League of Nations Efforts towards a Reformed National Health System in China," in Iris Borowy, ed., *Uneasy Encounters: The Politics of Medicine and Health in China, 1900 – 1937* (Frankfurt am Main: Peter Lang, 2009), pp. 211, 213; Bullock, *An American Transplant*, pp. 154 – 155.

50. Borowy, "Thinking Big," 213 – 215; J. Heng Liu to Roger Greene, 4 January 1932, volume #1312, PUMCA.

51. Personnel file for Oo-Keh Khaw, volume #494, PUMCA; O. K. Khaw to Roger Greene, 1 April 1932, 12 September 1932, 20 November 1932, 6 June 1933, volume # 1312, PUMCA.

52. Ma, "The Peking Union Medical College and the Rockefeller Foundation's Medical Programs in China," p. 179.

杨崇瑞、林巧稚与 20 世纪中国妇女健康[1]

蒋菲婷（Tina Phillips Johnson）

蒋菲婷（Tina Phillips Johnson），宾夕法尼亚拉贝托·圣文森特学院（Latrobe Saint Vincent College）历史学教授及中国研究中心主任，也是匹兹堡大学（University of Pittsburgh）亚洲研究中心副研究员。她的研究重要在二十世纪中国妇女健康及医疗历史。她目前正在研究中国农村公共卫生项目。

引言

杨崇瑞（1891－1983）与林巧稚（1901－1983）出生相差十年，并且一个来自北方，一个来自南方。上世纪 20 年代，她们成为北京协和医学院（简称"协和"）的医学生，随后成为协和医院的医生，在她们之前，没有几个中国女性取得如此成就。通过培养医务工作者，诊治各行各业的病人，开展各种关于妇婴疾病的研究，影响政府的卫生政策，北京协和医学院在中国妇女健康促进事业上发挥了重要作用。而杨崇瑞与林巧稚，这两位终身未婚的基督徒，为医学事业奉献终生。作为榜样，她们扩大了协和在妇女健康领域的影响力。她们的事业与一生，揭示出 20 世纪大部分时期中国妇女健康事业的挑战与变化。

民国时期的妇产专业的塑形

杨崇瑞在位于北京东南部的通县的一个知书达礼的基督教家庭长大。她家有两个孩子，杨崇瑞排行老大。其父在 18 岁时中了举人，后来在通州（华北）协和大学教书。从很小的时候开始，杨崇瑞就在父亲的教导下学习英语，并被送入传教士兴办的北京贝满女中就读。[2]1917 年，杨崇瑞从北京协和医学院的前身协和女子医学堂毕业，来到山东德州、之后又到天津妇婴医院从事临床和教学工作。[3]1921 年，北京协和医学院开业之后，杨崇瑞回到北京，最终选定了公共卫生和妇产科专业。在协和，她和同事兰安生（John B. Grant）一起开展了一些母婴健康项目，并深受其影响。[4]

1927 年，在北京协和医学院的资助下，杨崇瑞在位于马里兰州巴尔的摩的约翰·霍普金斯大学的公共卫生学院进修之后，她游历了北美和欧洲的数个城市，其间还在英国伍尔里齐助产士机构（Midwives Institute in Woolrich）进行了访学。[5]回到北京后，她担任了北京协和医学院公共卫生系的助理教授，同时担任第一卫生事务所的负责人。第一卫生事务所是以母婴保健为主的城市公共卫生试验中心。正是在第一卫生事务所，她希望提升中国人卫生水平的想法开始成型。她不断遇到新生儿感染破伤风或产后败血症的病例，这两种本可以避免的疾病却是导致中国母婴死亡率高的罪魁祸首。尽管难以核实，但民国时期婴儿死亡率大约为每千名新生儿有 115～300 例死亡，而每千个产妇中有 4～15 例死亡。[6]杨崇瑞断定，生产过程中过高的母婴死亡率主要归咎于未经训练的助产妇，即"旧式接生婆"。据她估算，全国范围内有大约四十万个这样的接生婆。[7]她意识到，保证母婴健康对于提升中国人的整体健康水平具有重要意义。

杨崇瑞的观点可能受到国际上优生学理论的大背景的影响。上世纪20 年代，中国在数次同外国列强的战争中失败，中国人被很多外国列强视为"东亚病夫"。清朝灭亡后，中国陷入军阀割据，被蒋介石这样的军人统治。然而他们并没能实现对整个国家的控制。从清朝晚期开始，梁启超、康有为等早期改革者就开始用无数笔墨描绘一个愿景，希望有朝一日能建成一个健康强大、不受外国奴役的新中国。他们的关注点常落在中国妇女身上。几个世纪以来，中国妇女在封建父系家族的禁锢下，缺少教育、缠足而懦弱。甚至在 20 世纪早期，人们对妇女的期待仍然是拥有三寸金莲的贤妻良母，早早结婚生子，最好能生男孩子以传宗接代。如果家庭经济条件允许，妇女们通常隐匿在幽深宅院，很少出门。此外，当时的妇女也很少接受教育。

　　然而，上世纪 20 年代，由于西方传教士、教育精英、政治家、作家以及想要改革或破除大多数中国传统习俗的知识分子等现代化思潮的影响下，中国妇女的社会地位也在变化中。当时，关于妇女健康、科学持家、胎教的杂志、期刊、手册等出版物在城市中迅速涌现，而妇女受教育机会的增加则为这些读物培养了更大的读者群。在北京、上海等中心城市，胡适、陈独秀、鲁迅等新文化作家在前辈思想家的基础上著书立说，批判中国的保守主义阻碍了国家的进步并实际上禁锢了占一半人口的妇女。他们提倡将妇女从封建家族的禁锢中解放出来，倡导婚姻自由和女子教育。所有这一切都以建设一个更强大的新中国为名。发生在文化思想和社会习俗上的变化，无论是剧变还是逐步的改变，都赋予了中国妇女上学甚至上大学的可能。

　　此外，从 19 世纪起教会和慈善组织就开始建立学校和医院，这给予了更多人接受教育的机会，女孩也从中获益。这类学校用英文授课，传播细菌学说、公共卫生和西方生物医学知识。他们也选拔最优秀的中国学生前往欧洲或北美进一步深造，许多学生学成归国后在国民政府就职，在新的政府中担任领导职务。通过这种方式，接受西方教育的学生、医生成为沟通中西方文化的媒介。

　　杨崇瑞正是在这样的背景下学成回国，开始在北京第一卫生事务所和周边区域接诊病人。与之后会提到的林巧稚一样，杨崇瑞成长在一个特别的革新与进步的年代，为她们提供了机会，能够实现多数中国妇女难望其项背的成绩，独立自主并接受西方生物医学的精英教育。不过，受限于传统的性别角色，她们仍停留在主要以为妇女儿童提供医疗服务的女性职业。

　　为降低新生儿高死亡率，杨崇瑞展开了关于新生儿破伤风的研究。[8] 在南京国民政府的帮助和协和医学院同仁的帮助下，她开始规划一项生殖健康改革的国家项目。从培训助产士开始，最终于 1929 年成立了全国助产士协会这一官方机构来对助产士进行管理。政府通过了法律，要求助产士必须接受训练并注册。1929 年，杨崇瑞还在北京建立了国立第一助产学校，这是一所培训新老助产士的示范学校。[9]该学校设立在北京北部麒麟胡同的一个传统四合院里，这一区域一直以来都是接生婆聚集的地方。在中国传说中，麒麟是生育的象征，它同鹳一样能够产子。随后不久，杨崇瑞还协助建立了位于南京的国立中央助产士学校。

杨崇瑞对助产士们的训练分等级进行。较低水平的培训是对旧式助产士即接生婆的再培训，训练他们无菌的接生方法，包括洗手、使用清洁的器具并用硝酸银滴眼液控制婴儿眼部感染。这些接生婆们必须考过执照登记在册，才能合法工作。尽管如此，大部分接生婆仍然逃避法律的要求私自接生。中等程度的培训是面向护理学生、实习护士和护士的短期培训，时长从两周到两个月不等。最高等级的训练则是助产士培训班，为期两年的课程涵盖助产士需要掌握的助产方法，接受了这种训练的助产士在今天被称为助产护士。大多数接受了高水平助产士训练的女性在全国各地帮助建立类似的助产士学校。除此之外，北平[10]和新首都南京的公共卫生示范站、育儿班、公共卫生护士家访等，提供围产期检查，收集人口信息，分发教育材料，预防接种，教授产妇最新的科学育儿法。

然而，助产士项目也面临着问题。在中国，分娩被视为肮脏和不洁的事情。对于年轻女性而言，助产士不被看作是个合适的职业。人们固有的观念是，助产士都是由自己生过好几个孩子的接生婆担任。为驱除人们对生孩子的迷信和不信任，杨崇瑞致力于通过公众宣传，改变了接生服务者的形象：从没有文化的、依赖自己多次生产经验的文盲或半文盲老太太，转变成年轻、未婚、有文化的青年女性，即新的职业从业者——助产士。宣传运动面向大众展开，杨崇瑞鼓励更多的怀孕妇女和家庭在受过正规生物医学训练的助产士的帮助下分娩，而不是依赖于传统的被认为是迷信的、肮脏的老式接生婆。但这有些曲高和寡，因为大多数孕妇和他们的家庭并不愿意接受年轻妇女接生，他们认为这些女性没有结婚、缺乏自己生孩子的经验。除此之外，助产士们还使用神秘的器械，而她们的制服的白颜色，也让人联想到死亡。

尽管如此，生育改革运动依然在北京、南京等城市取得了一定成功。事实上，产妇照护与分娩常常让中国家庭第一次接触西方医学。换言之，生物医学概念下的分娩促进了西方生物医学在全国各地的传播。截止到1934 年，在中国有 1，883 名受到专业训练的注册助产士、134 所注册在案的助产士学校，每年接生超过两百万次，[11]而这仅仅是一个开始。

1929 年，杨崇瑞在协和医学院迎来了一位新学生，这位年轻女生来自南方省份福建。与杨崇瑞一样，林巧稚出生在一个富裕的基督教家庭。她成长的厦门鼓浪屿是 1842 年鸦片战争后中国开放的第一批通商口岸之一。林巧稚的父亲是一位翻译家和教师，他曾经和其祖父一起在新加坡生活，并在那习得多种外语。林巧稚的父亲从孩子很小的时候起就教他们英文，在厦门，他们使用一种由东南亚传教士发明的独特闽南语书写方式。因此，林巧稚到北京后才开始学习普通话，此前她并不会用普通话书写或交流。

林巧稚曾就读于厦门的国际学校。上学期间，她深受一位叫做玛丽·卡林（Mary Carling）的英国女教师的影响。[12]卡林被林巧稚的聪慧和决心打动，鼓励林巧稚学习医学。1921 年，林巧稚参加了北京协和医学院的入学考试，这次考试成为了林巧稚一生诸多传奇故事中极为经典的一个：在考试期间，林巧稚的一位同学晕倒了，林巧稚冒着考试不及格的风险选择帮助晕倒的姑娘而没有完成考试。最终林巧稚被协和医学院录取了，这不仅因为她的英语十分出色，完成的那部分考试分数足以达到协和的录取标准，也因为她展现出了无私奉献的精神并且在压力面前沉着冷静。1929 年，林巧稚以全班最优成绩毕业，决定从事妇产科工作，有许多故事记载，林巧稚 5 岁时她的母亲罹患宫颈癌去世是她选择妇产科的原因。林巧稚跟随杨崇瑞实习，随后，杨崇瑞邀请林巧稚在国立第一助产学校教授科学分娩课程。[13]同杨崇瑞一样，林巧稚获得了资助出国深造。她于1932 年进入伦敦医学院和曼彻斯特医学院，之后还前往维也纳和芝加哥大学学习。[14]1939 年，林巧稚被聘任为北京协和医学院妇产科学系主任，她是协和医学院历史上第一位担任学科主任的女性。[15]

　　两位女性都思考了中国高生育率所导致的身体和经济问题。她们认为太多的例子显示无计划的、不情愿的生育不仅会导致子宫脱垂等生理疾病，还会导致贫穷及对产妇和婴儿都会产生的不理想的生育结果。因此，她们都提倡家庭的计划生育、节育、生育之间拉开间隔。杨崇瑞与燕京大学社会系及北京协和医学院社会福利与慈善部门合作，以玛格丽特·桑格（Margaret Sanger）的节育委员会为蓝本，于 1930 年创建了北平母亲健康委员会。[16]不仅如此，杨崇瑞曾于 1936 年邀请桑格来华演讲。然而，由于桑格生病，再加之 1937 年日军入侵中国，这次邀约未能成行。[17] 20 世纪 30 年代，协和医学院还开办了由林巧稚负责的节育门诊。[18]然而，在 1934 年杨崇瑞关于该委员会的报告中，她悲叹道，当时的节育措施（主要是避孕膜或海绵，有时使用杀精药剂）并不可靠，且大多数来节育门诊就诊的妇女并不希望控制家庭人数，反而是希望能够多生育，想要生男孩不想生女孩。[19]

战争挑战

　　抗日战争（1937－1945）及中国内战（1945－1949）给中国妇女的健康造成了巨大挑战，但也带来了新的机遇。林巧稚与杨崇瑞在创办和开展母婴健康项目上展现出的专业才能使她们名扬中外。1937 年，杨崇瑞被委任为国际联盟卫生组织妇婴健康部门的成员，该职务使她有机会亲自考察欧亚诸多国家的公共卫生设施和政策。[20]杨崇瑞回国时，抗日战争已经开始，她加入了抗日红十字会，并于 1938 年被任命为中央卫生局（Central Health Bureau）专家协助建立贵阳医学院和位于汉口及战时首都重庆的伤兵医院，[21]此外她还参与了宋美龄的战争孤儿援助计划。[22] 1941年，在前往约翰·霍普金斯大学医学院短暂进修后，杨崇瑞出任位于重庆的中央卫生研究院（中央卫生署附属机构）妇婴健康部主任，访问全国各地致力于促进妇婴卫生保健的改善工作。[23]同时，杨崇瑞还独自或与他人合作撰写了许多关于母婴健康的文章或书籍，包括一本家庭健康手册和两本供助产士学校使用的教科书。[24]第二次世界大战结束后，国际联盟重组成立世界卫生组织（World Health Organization，WHO）。1947 年，杨崇瑞加入 WHO 国际妇婴卫生部门，最终荣升为该部副负责人。凭借这项工作她得以游历欧洲多个城市并搬至日内瓦工作。

战争期间，林巧稚则留在北京专注于临床工作。1941 年，北京协和医学院受抗日战争影响关闭，林巧稚在协和附近的东堂子胡同 10 号开办了一家私人诊所，接诊社会上各行各业的病人，并为无法负担诊费的病人减免费用。与病人的工作生活在一起使得林巧稚深切体会到了困扰女性的问题与疾病。

生育健康领域的变化：科学与人民共和国

1949 年中华人民共和国成立时，杨崇瑞仍然在日内瓦 WHO 工作，但她的同学、"基督将军"冯玉祥遗孀、时任卫生部部长的李德全代表毛泽东和周恩来向她发出了邀请，杨崇瑞回国担任卫生部妇婴健康部门的负责人，她在该岗位上工作到 1957 年，致力于降低母婴死亡率的健康网络的建设。[25]杨崇瑞继续开展培训助产士、分娩护理、围产保健等工作，该健康网络培养了大约二十七万名助产工作者、九千名产科护士。此外，在杨崇瑞的指导下，在中国各地成立了 13 家分支机构和 34 家妇婴保健门诊的二级诊所，由此，孕产妇死亡率得以从 1949 年的 0.7% 下降到 1954 年的 0.05%，同期婴儿死亡率则从 11.7% 下降到 4.6%。1966 年，杨崇瑞报告全国婴儿死亡率下降至 2%，不过该数字难以证实。[26]

战后，北京协和医学院复校。林巧稚回到协和医院重新出任妇产科学系主任，协和医院于改名为首都医院（1966～1976 年"文化大革命"期间，短暂改名为反帝医院）之后，她继续担任这一职务。相较于杨崇瑞，林巧稚更多地参与到了政治中，事实上，杨崇瑞在民国时期最为活跃，而林巧稚的事业则是在中华人民共和国时期快速腾飞。1951～1952 年"三反"运动期间，林巧稚就自己在协和的角色发表了自我批评文章，还在

1956～1957 年反"右"运动中批判了时任协和校长的李宗恩。[27]与自己接受的帝国主义教育决裂后，林巧稚公开宣誓要为新中国奉献终生。1953年，林巧稚加入北京妇女联合会，并被选为中华全国妇女联合会委员，随后担任北京妇联副主席。1978 年，当选为全国妇联主席。[28] 1955 年，林巧稚被选为全国人大代表，1978 年，林巧稚再次当选人大代表，并围绕妇女健康、儿童健康、职业健康、传染病防治等重要性发表讲话。随后林巧稚还入选了全国人大常委会。1955 年，林巧稚当选为中国科学院学部委员；她还担任了中华医学会副会长（1956）、《中华妇产科杂志》总编辑及国务院科学规划委员会医学组成员（1957）。[29]

无痛分娩

民国时期，生物医学科学具有政治敏感性，而考察这个问题最好的领域就是生育健康。战时在国民党的统治下，杨崇瑞曾撰写文章，指出妇幼健康在国家工作中的重要性，而女性被认为是个人、家庭和公共卫生的主要维护者。[30]杨崇瑞的这种观点来源于她所接受的西方教育以及当时关于优生学和人种卫生学的广泛讨论。20 世纪 50 年代初，中国领导人远离西方理念而转向按照苏联模式设置政府机构及制定政策。科学是为国家服务的，但是掺杂了较大的政治内容。例如，作为"向巴甫洛夫学习"的科学运动中的一部分，中国卫生部于 1952 年开始提倡苏联的"精神无痛分娩法"，该方法在不使用麻醉剂或止痛剂的情况下解除妇女分娩的疼痛，主要方法是基于细致的言语暗示、所有人——医护工作者及家属对产妇的悉心照看及特别的呼吸技巧。从本质上看，妇女被灌输分娩是一个无痛的自然过程，应该顺其自然地接受该过程；若是在分娩中感受到了疼痛，则说明产妇缺乏正确的政治观念和/或行动。[31]这种精神方法是当时主流政治意识形态在医学领域的表达：中国共产党解放了中国人民，不仅仅将人民从压迫中解放了出来也将妇女从分娩的痛苦中解放。林巧稚在《中华妇产科杂志》和英文宣传杂志《中国建设》上发表文章提倡这种无痛分娩方法。[32]然而，无痛分娩——这个短命的运动随着 1960年中苏关系破裂而告终。

计划生育

计划生育是政治影响科学的另一个典型代表。恰如前文提到的，在协和医学院，杨崇瑞和林巧稚都是计划生育的早期支持者，她们的一生都致力于这个事业。从 1949 年起，她与杨崇瑞就紧密配合卫生部及全国妇联的工作推动家庭自愿的生育控制政策。20 世纪 50 年代，林巧稚还曾在北京及河南、河北部分地区开展控制生育调查和宣教。然而，20 世纪 50 年代早期，卫生部决定鼓励生育，因为社会主义制度从理论上并不受马尔萨斯人口压力和食物短缺的影响，更不必考虑分娩的疼痛。卫生部对于避孕的反对在 50 年代末逐渐松动，然而，当几位女性共产党员在 1953 年向全国妇联写信呼吁，要求实施避孕以更好地参与"共产主义建设"。[33]刘少奇在 1954～1955 年期间在国家和党的层面召开一系列会议讨论生育控制。参加会议的包括卫生部部长李德全、林巧稚和杨崇瑞，1956 年林巧稚私下同毛泽东讲需要控制人口。[34]早在 1957 年，林巧稚就开始在当时备受欢迎的妇女杂志《中国妇女》上发表文章间接地提倡晚婚。[35]这些讨论的结果是，尽管一些妇女选择使用节育措施，但全国妇联并未发起任何针对性的控制生育运动。共产党和卫生部在控制生育的问题上未做任何决定，也未做任何承诺。

次年 6 月，林巧稚在第一届全国人大第四次会议上做了关于加强计划生育作为控制人口的手段的论证。她的讲话排在北京大学校长、经济学家马寅初之后。马寅初在同次会议提出"新人口理论"，提出倘若中国人口不受控制地持续增长，势必有害于国家的经济发展。他提倡政府采取节育和计划生育的措施来控制生育率。[36]林巧稚和杨崇瑞联名在《人民日报》上发表了两篇文章支持马寅初的观点。[37]最终，马寅初对计划生育的提倡被视为批评社会主义，反对者认为他支持马尔萨斯主义，并轻视人民。1957 年，马寅初被打为右派。杨崇瑞遭受了同样的命运，她被送入社会主义学院接受再教育，远离了医学岗位，降职到中华医学会为外文书籍分类。之后，她虽得以在妇产科杂志担任编辑、为妇婴健康组当顾问，但直到 1979 年她的右派帽子才被摘去。[38]实际上，她的职业生涯就此结束了。

"文化大革命"（1966 – 1976）

林巧稚在反"右"运动中并未受到严重迫害。然而，在"文化大革命"中，林巧稚被打为"反动学术权威"并被指控为美国间谍。[39]她被迫暂时离开了行政管理岗位而干起实习生的活。林巧稚的几位家庭成员支持国民党政府并为其工作，还在 1949 年后逃至台湾。这种家庭背景加上林巧稚在协和医学院的西式教育和职业经历，她本应受到更为严酷的对待。据记载，林巧稚是周恩来总理及总理夫人邓颖超的密友，他们在那个动荡的年代保护了林巧稚。此外，林巧稚还有一些身居要职的医生兼朋友，如李德全、康克清（军队领袖朱德的夫人），因此林巧稚的政治危机历时较为短暂。[40]

林巧稚很快恢复了之前的工作，并在政府卫生政策的制定和宣传中扮演了重要角色。1965 年，在一次经常被提起的讲话中，毛泽东公开批评中国卫生部只为 15% 的人口服务，意指有大量没有门路或财力的人无法享有高质量的医疗。[41]这次讲话促使城市卫生系统开展运动，促进医务人员下乡服务。卫生部在全国建立了农村卫生合作医疗体系和卫生中心，派遣城市的医疗卫生专业人员到农村培训并为农村人口服务。[42]在这次运动中，林巧稚和医疗队 30 多名医护工作者一起于 1965 年去湖南省湘阴县农村开展了四个多月的医疗工作。该医疗队接诊了超过三万名患者，并在"干校"培训了当地的卫生工作者和助产士。这是赤脚医生运动的早期形式。赤脚医生在 1970 年代被世界卫生组织树立为全民初级医疗保健的典范。他们在湖南农村的工作以中英文分别发表在《中国妇女》和《中华医学杂志》上，突出了全民医疗卫生及解放后的职业女性的作用：她们是半边天——她们是新的、现代化的中国的一份子。[43]

对很多人说，林巧稚是一个可信任的属于公众的专家。他们可以向她咨询并得到诚恳的健康意见（也许除了短暂的"无痛分娩"运动外）。林巧稚在大众的杂志和《人民日报》上发表了一系列关于育儿、营养、怀孕、产后护理、体育运动、青少年、婴儿和妇女健康的文章。[44]20 世纪 60 年代末，林巧稚定期出现在大众杂志和书籍中。在大众心目中，林巧稚代表新中国的现代的、职业的、解放的无私与奉献的女性。[45]在"文化大革命"的大部分时间和之后的岁月中，林巧稚非但没有受到迫害，反而成为了一个偶像，一个代表着职业女性、科学和现代化的模范工作者。[46]她无私照顾贫穷和需要帮助的人们，为广大人民群众提供医疗服务。

当林巧稚的朋友兼同事杨崇瑞在 1957 年从其之前的国际交往中悄然隐退后，林巧稚越来越多地出现在国际交往中。参加医学及各类友好代表团访问世界各地，与来华的外国领导人会面。林巧稚体现了中国公共卫生制度的美誉，并且体现了新政权下男女平等与中国女性所受的良好教育。1953 年，林巧稚出访了前苏联，次年，作为中国代表团成员之一出席了在维也纳召开的世界健康大会。[47]虽然林巧稚的国际出访活动在"文化大革命"初期短暂中断，但 1972 年，林巧稚成为中华医学会访美代表团的唯一女性成员，该访美团是 1971 年"乒乓外交"后中国第二个官方访美代表团。[48]1974 年，她担任友好代表团团长，出访伊朗以庆祝德黑兰－北京直航的开通；1978 年，她也是友好代表团的成员出访欧洲。[49]林巧稚还是记者埃德加·斯诺（Edgar Snow）的朋友，斯诺在其关于中国共产党革命的书中提到了她。[50]当外国代表团在 1970 年代来到中国访问时，例如 1954 赫鲁晓夫和尼赫鲁访华时，总会有林巧稚的身影。[51]1974 年，美国儿童早期发展代表团访华，随后印发的出版物中，有大量篇幅是写林巧稚在母婴健康和围产保健方面的工作。[52]1973 年至 1977 年，林巧稚担任世界卫生组织医学研究顾问委员会顾问。[53]在国际舞台上，她在政治一端代表了中国最好的一面，是中华人民共和国所取得的卓越成绩的模范代表——被解放的女性、全民医疗保健以及令人瞩目的医学和科学研究。正是像她这样的杰出女性稳固了中国在现代世界的地位。

尽管林巧稚以妇产科大夫的身份闻名，但事实上她对中国妇女健康的最大贡献很多是在研究和学术上。20 世纪 60 年代，林巧稚开展了大样本调查及普及大众对宫颈癌的认识，宫颈癌的发病率得以大幅降低。[54]她还针对新生儿溶血、先天畸形、妇科肿瘤、不孕不育展开了一系列科学研究并发表论文。20 世纪 60 年代末，她设计发明了塑料和金属材质的宫内器具（"宫内节育环"）。[55]林巧稚还编写了一本广泛使用的妇科肿瘤教科书，该书的第 4 版在 2006 年发行。[56]林巧稚的研究为中华人民共和国所取得的科学成就作出了杰出贡献，同时也强调了社会主义制度人民大众的健康保健。

遗产

1983 年，杨崇瑞和林巧稚相隔数月在北京相继离世。在第一助产学校的所在地——麒麟胡同旁边的东四妇产医院里的人们纪念着杨崇瑞。协和医学院妇产科学系的同事——严仁英于 1990 年编纂了纪念杨崇瑞贡献的文集，收录了杨的学生与同事所写的文章。[57]杨崇瑞在东四妇产医院的继任者们都对她的一生及事业非常敬重。然而，杨崇瑞在默默无闻中离开人世。与之相反，人们对林巧稚的纪念却多种多样：电影、两部电视系列片、纪念邮票、至少十多本传记和上百篇文章。[58]北京协和医学院、北京妇女儿童博物馆、中华世纪坛、北京妇产医院和厦门林巧稚妇幼保健院都在纪念着林巧稚。此外，在林巧稚的故乡厦门鼓浪屿，建起了一座林巧稚纪念馆，馆中的花园里竖立了孩子的雕像、镌刻着林巧稚的名言。她的骨灰埋葬在鼓浪屿的林巧稚的石膏雕像下，让人想起大慈大悲的观世音菩萨。

21 世纪的中国医疗体系问题颇多，而林巧稚作为关爱病人的医生榜样，再次被人们纪念。医师的超负荷工作、腐败贿赂、即使身患小病也排长队苦等专家诊治、不时发生的伤医甚至杀医事件，常常充斥在 21 世纪报刊的头条。[59]至少从 2010 年起，林巧稚以其无私奉献、淡泊名利、一心关注患者健康，再次出现在大众媒体中。北京妇产医院的学生和员工每年清明节依然会悼念林巧稚，厦门市妇幼保健院的继任者们都会在就职时宣誓成为林巧稚那样的医生。2012 年，广西医学院设立"林巧稚奖"，奖励杰出的妇产科医师。[60]林巧稚书写的病历也被当作准确、详细、全面的典范供医生们学习。[61]

从在协和学习开始，杨崇瑞与林巧稚倾尽一生致力于中国妇女健康保健、教育、政策制定及科学研究。她们的医学专业给其职业发展和个人成长打开了通道，是从事其他行业如商业、法律等难以达到的。她们两位都为事业牺牲了家庭——这是她们必须做出的选择。在那个时代，已婚女性不可能出门工作（事实上，杨崇瑞开设的助产学校的入学要求即是年轻、未婚）。尽管如此，她们依然在更广的概念上符合女性抚育、自我牺牲的标准。林巧稚有"万婴之母"的美誉，虽然没有自己生过孩子，但她是全国孩子的母亲。林巧稚在动荡的政治风波中波澜不惊，而杨崇瑞则始终未能成功转变成为新中国公共卫生事业的一分子。这也许是因为杨崇瑞更具反叛精神，更有现代意识，因此她难以融入一个未改家长制的社会。从杨崇瑞和林巧稚的一生可以看出，她们有着相似的背景却走向了不同的结局，她们的经历折射出二十世纪医学和公共卫生的大景观的风云变幻，反映二十世纪的政治、妇女生活及社会期许。

参考书目

1. 本章部分内容受蒋经国基金会和 China and Inner Asia Council of the Association for Asian Studies 资助。

2. Wang Bing, "Yang Chongrui," in *Biographical Dictionary of Chinese Women*: *The Twentieth Century* 1912 – 2000, ed. Lily Xiao Hong Lee, A. D. Stefanowska, and Sue Wiles, trans. Jennifer Zhang (Routledge, 2002), 611 – 13.

3. Zhao Liangfeng, "Yang Chongrui: Pioneer in China's Modern Obstetrics," *www. womenofchina. cn*, (March 12, 2013), http: //history. cultural-china. com/en/ 48History14254. html.

4. Liping Bu and Elizabeth Fee, "John B. Grant: International Statesman of Public Health," *Am J Public Health* 98, no. 4 (April 2008): 628 – 29.

5. Nicole Elizabeth Barnes, "Protecting the National Body: Gender and Public Health in Southwest China during the War with Japan, 1937 – 1945" (PhD dissertation, University of California at Irvine, 2012), 295.

6. Marion Yang, "Midwifery Training in China," *China Medical Journal* 42 (1928): 768 – 75.

7. Ibid. , 769.

8. Marion Yang and I-Chin Yuan, "Report of an Investigation on Infant Mortality and Its

Causes in Peiping," *Chinese Medical Journal*, no. 47 (1933): 597 –604.

9. Tina Phillips Johnson, *Childbirth in Republican China: Delivering Modernity* (Lanham, MD: Lexington Books, 2011), Chapter Three.

10. 字面上北京是北方的首都的意思。1927 年首都迁到南京后，北京改称北平（北方和平）。1949 年，中华人民共和国在北京建都后，北平又改回称北京。

11. First National Midwifery School, "Fifth Annual Report, First National Midwifery School, Peiping, July 1, 1933-June 30, 1934," Annual Report, (September 15, 1934).

12. 张清平，*林巧稚传*，天津：百花文艺出版社，2005，13 –17。

13. Wright, Guowei, "Lin Qiaozhi: The Steady Pulse of a Quiet Faith," in *Salt and Light: Lives of Faith That Shaped Modern China*, ed. Hamrin, Carol Lee and Stacy Bieler (Eugene, OR: Wipf and Stock Publishers, Pickwick Publications, 2008), 114 –32.

14. 厦门市林巧稚大夫纪念活动筹备委员会)，*林巧稚大夫：卓越的人民医学家* 厦门市林巧稚大夫纪念活动筹备委员会，1984）；Zhuhong, "Lin Qiaozhi: Guardian Angel of Mothers, Babies," *All-China Women's Federation*, December 6, 2007.

15. Lily Xiao Hong Lee, "Lin Qiaozhi," in *Biographical Dictionary of Chinese Women: The Twentieth Century 1912 –2000*, ed. Lily Xiao Hong Lee, A. D. Stefanowska, and Sue Wiles (Routledge, 2002), 343 –46.

16. Wang Bing, "Yang Chongrui."

17. Mirela Violeta David, "Free Love, Marriage, and Eugenics: Global and Local Debates on Sex, Birth Control, Venereal Disease and Population in 1920s-1930s China" (PhD dissertation, New York University, 2014).

18. Mary Brown Bullock, *An American Transplant: The Rockefeller Foundation and Peking Union Medical College* (Berkeley: University of California Press, 1980), 179; Lin Qiaozhi, "Around the World for Birth Control," *China Medical Journal* 59 (1936): 38 –41.

19. Marion Yang, "Birth Control in Peiping: First Report of the Peiping Committee on Maternal Health," *The Chinese Medical Journal* 48 (1934): 786 –91.

20. David, "Free Love, Marriage, and Eugenics"; Wang Bing, "Yang Chongrui."

21. 杨崇瑞，"我的自传，一九四九年十月，"见 *杨崇瑞博士：诞辰百年纪念*，严仁英主编，北京：北京医科大学中国协和医科大学联合出版社，1990，143 –53；Zhao, "Yang Chongrui: Pioneer in China's Modern Obstetrics."

22. Barnes, "Protecting the National Body," 291 –92.

23. Wang Bing, "Yang Chongrui"; Barnes, "Protecting the National Body", Chapter Six.

24. 杨崇瑞，王诗锦，*婦婴衛生學*，重庆：中央卫生实验院妇婴卫生组，1944；杨崇瑞，*第一助產學校十週年紀念刊*，1939；杨崇瑞，*中國婦婴衛生過去與現在*，

1940；杨崇瑞，主婦須知：家庭衛生及家政概要，南京：衛生署中央健康實驗院 1947）；杨崇瑞，婦嬰衛生概要，1943；婦嬰衛生講座，新运妇女指导委员会文化事业组编，1945）；杨崇瑞，第一助產學校十週年紀念刊.

25. Wang Bing，"Yang Chongrui"；Zhao，"Yang Chongrui：Pioneer in China's Modern Obstetrics. "

26. Zhao，"Yang Chongrui：Pioneer in China's Modern Obstetrics. "

27. 林巧稚，"打开'协和'窗户看祖国，"人民日报，9 月 27 号，1952；林巧稚，"我的思想装变"，中华医学杂志38. 9（9 月 1952）：749 – 54；林巧稚，"李宗恩应及早悔悟，"健康报3（8 月 6 号，1957）.

28. Zhuhong，"Lin Qiaozhi：Guardian Angel of Mothers，Babies"；Lee，"Lin Qiaozhi. "

29. Lee，"Lin Qiaozhi. "

30. 杨崇瑞，主婦須知：家庭衛生及家政概要；杨崇瑞婦嬰衛生講座；See Barnes，"Protecting the National Body"，Chapter Six.

31. Paula Michaels，"Childbirth Pain Relief and the Soviet Origins of the Lamaze Method，" National Council for Eurasian and East European Research Working Paper（Seattle，WA：NCEEER，October 16，2007）；Gao Xi，"Learning from the Soviet Union：Pavlovian Influence on Chinese Medicine，1950s，" in *Public Health and National Reconstruction in Post-War Asia：International Influences，Local Transformations*（Routledge，2014），72 – 89.

32. Lim，Kha-Ti，"Painless Childbirth，" *China Reconstructs*，1952；林巧稚，"参观苏联的医学科学几个主要特点的简单介绍，"中华妇产科杂志4（1953）：289 – 303.

33. Susan Greenhalgh and Edwin A. Winckler，*Governing China's Population：From Leninist to Neoliberal Biopolitics*（Stanford：Stanford University Press，2005），65.

34. Lee，"Lin Qiaozhi"；Wright，Guowei，"Lin Qiaozhi：The Steady Pulse of a Quiet Faith. "

35. 林巧稚，"从生理上谈结婚年龄，"中国妇女 4（1957）：25 – 26.

36. 马寅初，"新人口论，"人民日报，7 月 5 号，1957.

37. 王历耕等，"广泛宣传迟婚和计划生育"，人民日报，3 月 15 号 1957；王淑贞，"妇产科大夫王淑贞、林巧稚、何碧辉、俞霭峰 对于实行计划生育的意见，"人民日报，7 月 20 号，1957.

38. Wang Bing，"Yang Chongrui. "

39. Lee，"Lin Qiaozhi. "

40. 姚远，周恩来与"东方圣母"林巧稚，中国共产党新闻网，12 月 15 号，2010，http：//dangshi. people. com. cn/GB/85040/13515215. html.

41. David M. Lampton, "Public Health and Politics in China's Past Two Decades," *Health Services Report* 87, no. 10 (December 1972): 895 – 904.

42. Early rural cooperative medical systems were established in various locations as early as 1955, with brigade health auxiliaries called Barefoot Doctors. These programs went nationwide in 1965. Naisu Zhu et al., "Factors Associated with the Decline of the Cooperative Medical System and Barefoot Doctors in Rural China," *Bulletin of the World Health Organization* 67, no. 4 (1989): 431 – 32.

43. Huang Chia-ssu, "Our Medical Team in the Countryside," *Chinese Medical Journal* 84, no. 12 (December 1965): 799 – 803; "坚持卫生工作的革命方向, 促进卫生队伍的革命化: 巡回医疗队在农村," *中国妇女* 7 月1965.

44. 林巧稚, *农村妇幼卫生常识问答*, 北京: 人民卫生出版社, 1975; 林巧稚, 秦牧, *家庭教育顾问*, 北京: 中国青年出版社: 新华书店北京发行所发行, 1981; 林巧稚, 王元萼, *妇科肿瘤*, 北京: 人民卫生出版社, 1982.

45. Tina Mai Chen, "Female Icons, Feminist Iconography? Socialist Rhetoric and Women's Agency in 1950s China," *Gender and History* 15, no. 2 (2003): 268 – 95.

46. Huang Chia-ssu, "Our Medical Team in the Countryside."

47. Zhuhong, "Lin Qiaozhi: Guardian Angel of Mothers, Babies."

48. 姚远, "周恩来与'东方圣母'林巧稚"; UPI, "Chinese View U. S. Medicine," *Desert Sun*, November 3, 1972, California Digital Newspaper Collection.

49. Wolfgang Bartke, "Lin Qiaozhi," in *Who Was Who in the People's Republic of China* (Walter de Gruyter, 1997), 270.

50. Edgar Snow, *The Long Revolution* (Vintage Books, 1973), especially Chapter Three, "Medical Care and Population Control."

51. 新华社, "周总理招待尼赫鲁总理," 人民日报), 10 月 20 号 1954; 新华社, n" 苏联驻我国大使尤金举行招待会," *人民日报*, 10 月 13 号, 1954.

52. William Kessen, ed., *Childhood in China*, American Delegation on Early Childhood Development (New Haven and London: Yale University, 1975), especially Chapter 8, "Health and Nutritional Factors."

53. 厦门市林巧稚大夫纪念活动筹备委员会, *林巧稚大夫*

54. Lee, "Lin Qiaozhi"; Lim, Kha-Ti, Kao, JC, and Chang, CF, "Mass Survey for the Cancer of Cervix Uteri in China," *Acta Unio Int Contra Cancrum* 19 (1963): 902 – 5.

55. Lim, Kha Ti and Snyder, Franklin F., "The Effect of Respiration Stimulants in the Newborn Infant," *Am. J. Obst. & Gynec.* 50 (1945): 1460153; Lim, Khati (Lin Qiaozhi), "Obstetrics and Gynecology in the Past Ten Years," *Chinese Medical Journal* 79,

no. 5（November 1959）：375 – 83；Lee，"Lin Qiaozhi"；Gao Xi，"Learning from the Soviet Union."

56. 林巧稚，连利娟，*林巧稚妇科肿瘤学*，第四版（北京：人民卫生出版社，2006.

57. 严仁英，主编，*杨崇瑞博士：诞辰百年纪念*

58. 高力强，*大爱如天*，2007，http：//movie. douban. com/subject/2279571/，http：//jq. tvsou. com/introhtml/699/1_ 69943. htm；冯雪松，*二十世纪中国女性史：生育革命*)（中国中央电视台，1999），http：//v. youku. com/v_ show/id_ XNDUwMTM4ODQw. html？old&from = y1. 2 – 2. 4. 15；王韧，*大师*中国中央电视台，2008）.

59. Chris Buckley，"A Danger for Doctors in China：Patients' Angry Relatives，" *New York Times*，May 18，2016，sec. Asia Pacific；Adam Jourdan，"China Investigates Former Top Healthcare Official for Bribery，" *Reuters*，May 27，2015，sec. World News；See，for example，Kazunori Takada，"Bribery Serves As Life-Support for Chinese Hospitals，" *Reuters*，July 23，2013，sec. Lifestyle.

60. "新员工入职宣誓 缅怀林巧稚大夫，"*厦门日报*，7 月 28 号，2015；"林巧稚：'万婴之母'，大医之魂，"*新华每日电讯*，12 月 11 号，2015；北京妇产医院，"教育处组织全体研究生瞻仰首任院长林巧稚铜像，" *Health. Sohu. Com*，April 1，2016，http：//health. sohu. com/20160401/n443189093. shtml.

61. "年前林巧稚手书病历亮相，"*海西晨报*，7 月 29，2015.

Yang Chongrui, Lin Qiaozhi, and Women's Health in 20th-Century China[1]

Tina Phillips Johnson

Tina Phillips Johnson is Associate Professor of History and Director of Chinese Studies at Saint Vincent College in Latrobe, Pennsylvania; and a Research Associate with the University of Pittsburgh Asian Studies Center. Her research focuses on women's health and the history of medicine in twentieth-century China, and she also works on contemporary public health projects in rural China.

Introduction

Yang Chongrui (1891 – 1983) and Lin Qiaozhi (1901 – 1983) were born a decade apart, one a northerner and the other from the South. In the 1920s they achieved what few women before them had: they became medical students and later physicians at Peking Union Medical College. This institution has influenced women's health in China in significant ways - by training medical personnel, serving patients of all walks of life, sponsoring research on women's and infant's diseases, and shaping government health policy. These two women, both unmarried, Christian, and dedicated to the medical profession, exemplify PUMC's impacts on the health of women. Their lives and careers illustrate the challenges and changes to women's health in China for much of the twentieth century.

Shaping the Profession in Republican China

The eldest of the two, Yang Chongrui, was raised in Tong County, southeast of Beijing, in an educated Christian family. Her father had attained the provincial scholar (*juren*) degree at age 18 and taught at the Union Academy in Tong County. He began teaching her English at a young age and then sent her to the missionary-run Bridgeman Girls' High School in Beijing. [2] In 1917, Yang graduated from the Women's Union Medical College, a precursor to the Peking Union Medical College, and took clinical and teaching positions in Dezhou, Shandong province, and at Tianjin Women's and Children's Hospital. [3] After PUMC was established in 1921, Yang returned to Beijing and eventually specialized in public health and obstetrics and gynecology. There she was influenced by the work of fellow physician John B. Grant, with whom she worked on several maternal and child health projects. [4]

In 1927, Yang completed a PUMC-sponsored fellowship at the Johns Hopkins University School of Hygiene and Public Health in Baltimore, Maryland, followed by a tour of several North American and European cities including study at the Midwives Institute in Woolrich, England. [5] After returning to Beijing, she assumed a joint post as assistant professor of public health and head of the First Health Demonstration Station, an urban experimental public health center that focused on maternal and infant work. It was here that she began to formulate her ideas about improving the health of China's population. She repeatedly encountered cases of tetanus neonatorum and puerperal sepsis, two preventable diseases that greatly contributed to the country's high maternal and infant mortality rates. While difficult to verify, estimates of infant mortality during the Republican period range from 115 to 300 per 1000 births; maternal mortality from 4 to 15 per 1000 births. [6] Yang asserted that " the main responsibility for the excessive deaths among the mothers and babies may be laid on the untrained group" of old-style midwives, which she estimated to number 400,000 nationwide. [7] She knew that maternal and infant health were crucial factors in improving the overall health of China's population.

Her thinking was likely shaped by the global discourse of eugenics. By the 1920s, China had lost several wars with foreign powers, many of whom considered the Chinese population as "sick men of Asia" (*dongya bingfu*). The Qing empire had fallen, replaced by bellicose warlords and military men like Chiang Kai-shek who were unable to consolidate control over the entire country. Since the late Qing, early reformers like Liang Qichao and Kang Youwei had devoted countless words to creating a viable vision of a new, healthy China independent from foreign control. Much of their attention was turned towards women, who for centuries had suffered from the weakening effects of patriarchal seclusion, lack of education, and foot binding. Women in the early 20th century were still expected to bind their feet and be "good wives, wise mothers" (賢妻良母 *xian qi liang mu*), to marry young and have children, preferably male; and to remain relatively secluded if the family finances allowed. Education for girls was not common.

However, by the 1920s women's place in society was in flux due to modernizing influences of western missionaries, educated elites, politicians, writers, and intellectuals who wanted to reform or remove some of China's most traditional customs. Magazines, journals, and handbooks dedicated to women's health, scientific housekeeping, and prenatal education (*taijiao*) proliferated in the cities, as increased educational opportunities of women proffered a wider readership. In urban centers like Shanghai and Beijing, New Culture writers like Hu Shi, Chen Duxiu, and Lu Xun built on works by earlier thinkers who lamented the conservatism that kept the country from moving forward and virtually imprisoned half of its population. They advocated for emancipation from authoritarian patriarchal structures, for free marriage, and for women's education, all in the name of building a new and stronger China. These changes in cultural ideas and norms, some cataclysmic and others gradual, gave women of certain elite status the opportunities go to school and even college.

Furthermore, missionary outfits and philanthropic organizations had established schools and hospitals since the late 1800s, giving more people, including girls, the chance for education. These schools propagated English-language education and new concepts of germ theory, public health, and western biomedicine. They also sent their best Chinese students back to Europe or North America for additional schooling. Many who returned filled positions in the Nationalist government and became leaders in the new nation. In this way, western-trained students and physicians became intermediaries between two cultures.

This was the environment in which Yang Chongrui found herself after returning from abroad as she saw patients at Beijing's health demonstration station and surrounding areas. Yang - and Lin, as we will see shortly - came of age in a particularly innovative and progressive time that provided opportunities to achieve what was considered most unusual for women: independence, and an elite education in western biomedical sciences. They also remained constrained by traditional gender roles in a feminine caring profession that focused on women and children.

Yang undertook a tetanus neonatorum study to better understand how to alleviate the problem of high infant mortality. [8] With the help of the Nationalist government in Nanjing and others at PUMC, she began to formulate a national program of reproductive health reforms for China, beginning with midwifery education and culminating in the creation of a government agency to regulate midwifery, the National Midwifery Board, established in 1929. The government passed new laws requiring that midwives be trained and licensed. She also established the First National Midwifery School in Beijing in 1929 as the model school for educating midwives old and young. [9] The school was set in a traditional courtyard home in Qilin Alley in northern Beijing, an area historically known as a place where midwives gathered. The mythical *qilin*, according to Chinese folklore, is a symbol of fertility and, like the stork, also delivered babies. Shortly afterwards, Yang helped to found the Central National Midwifery School in Nanjing.

Yang implemented a tiered system of midwifery training. The lower level retrained old-style midwives (*jieshengpo*, *laopo*) in aseptic birth methods, namely hand washing, using clean implements, and administering silver nitrate eye drops to curb infant eye infections. These women had to be licensed and registered to work legally, though the majority of old-style midwives continued to work while evading legal requirements. The middle levels of midwifery training were short courses in midwifery of two weeks to two months to nursing students, nursing apprentices, and nurses. At the top of this pyramid was a class of midwives who received two years of instruction in midwifery methods. Today we may call them nurse-midwives. Many of these highly trained women helped to establish similar midwifery programs throughout the country. Additional public health demonstration stations, mothercraft classes, and home visits by public health nurses in both Beiping,[10] and in the new Nationalist capital of Nanjing provided pre-and post-natal checkups, collected population information, distributed educational materials, administered inoculations, and taught new mothers about the latest scientific child care.

But there was a problem. Childbirth was considered polluting and unclean. And midwifery was certainly not an appropriate vocation for proper young ladies. For as long as anyone could remember, midwifery had been a job of old *jieshengpo* who themselves had had many children. To dispel the mistrust and superstition surrounding childbirth, Yang engaged in a sort of publicity campaign, transforming the image of birth attendants from apprenticed multiparous, often semi-literate or illiterate older grannies, to a new profession, *zhuchanshi*, populated by young, unmarried, and educated young women. This campaign extended to the public, as she encouraged parturient women and their families to utilize these biomedically-trained midwives rather than relying on what she considered superstitious and dirty old-style birth attendants. This was a tall order, because most pregnant women and their families were unwilling to submit to the services of young ladies who were not married and who had had no personal experience with childbirth. Furthermore, the *zhuchanshi* utilized mysterious implements and dressed in white uniforms, a color associated with death.

Nonetheless, the birth reform campaign was moderately successful in cities like Beijing and Nanjing. And, in fact, parturient care and childbirth were oftentimes the first introduction of Chinese families to western biomedical health care. To put it plainly, biomedical childbirth helped to spread western biomedicine throughout the country. By 1934 there were 1883 trained, registered midwives in China and 134 licensed midwifery schools to attend the more than two million births per year. It was a beginning.

In 1922, Yang Chongrui had welcomed a new student at PUMC, a young woman from the southern province of Fujian. Like Yang, Lin Qiaozhi was from an affluent Christian family, growing up on the island of Gulangyu in Xiamen (Amoy), one of the first treaty ports opened in China after the Opium War's end in 1842. Lin's father was a translator and teacher who had lived in Singapore with his grandfather, where he picked up many languages. He taught his children English from a young age, and being from Xiamen they used the unique Minnan POJ written vernacular developed by missionaries in Southeast Asia. In fact, Lin was unable to speak or write Mandarin, learning the language only after moving to Beijing.

Lin attended international schools in Xiamen, where she was greatly influenced by one of her teachers, an Englishwoman named Mary Carling. Ms. Carling was impressed by Lin's intelligence and determination, and she encouraged Lin to pursue medicine. In 1921 Lin sat the examination to enter PUMC, which is the basis of one of the many legendary stories of Lin's life:

during the entrance examination, one of Lin's classmates fainted. Lin risked failure by helping the ill girl rather than finishing her own exam. She was admitted to PUMC anyway, not only because her partially completed exam was sufficient and her English was excellent, but also because of her dedication, selflessness, and calm demeanor under stress. Lin graduated at the top of her class in 1929 and decided to focus on obstetrics and gynecology. Many stories recount Lin's mother's death from cervical cancer when Lin was five years old as the stimulus for this decision. Lin worked under Yang Chongrui for her practicum; later, Yang invited Lin to teach scientific childbirth classes at the First National Midwifery School. Like Yang, Lin received fellowships for further study abroad. She attended London Medical College and Manchester Medical College in 1932, and later studied in Vienna and at the University of Chicago. In 1939, Lin was appointed head of PUMC's obstetrics and gynecology department, the first woman ever to hold a departmental head position at the college.

Both women were troubled by the physical and economic problems resulting from high fertility rates in China. Together they advocated for family planning, promoting birth control and birth spacing with the belief that numerous unplanned and unwanted births created not only physical ailments like prolapsed uterus, but also poverty and substandard birth outcomes for both mothers and infants. In collaboration with Yenching University's Sociology Department and PUMC's Charity and Welfare Department, Yang had helped to found the Peiping [Beiping] Committee on Maternal Health in 1930, an organization modeled on Margaret Sanger's birth control committees. In fact, Yang invited Sanger on a lecture tour to China in 1936, though it never materialized due to Sanger's illness and later the Japanese invasion in 1937. PUMC also operated a birth control clinic in the 1930s run by Lin Qiaozhi. However, in Yang's 1934 report on the Committee's activities, she lamented existing birth control methods (primarily diaphragms or sponges, sometimes with a spermicidal agent) were unreliable, and that most women came to the clinic in the hopes of increased fertility, and to give birth to sons instead of daughters, rather than to limit their family size.

Wartime Challenges

The Sino-Japanese War (1937 – 45) and China's civil war (1945 – 49) created challenges for women's health, yet also offered new opportunities. Both Lin's and Yang's expertise extended broadly and internationally in their abilities to create and administer new maternal and child health projects. In 1937, Yang was appointed a member of the League of Nations-Health Organization Women's and Infants' Health Section, which offered the opportunity to observe first-hand the public health infrastructure and policies in many countries in Asia and Europe. When she returned to China the war with Japan had already begun, and she joined China's Anti-Japanese Red Cross Unit. She was appointed to the Central Health Bureau as a specialist in 1938 and was sent to help establish a medical college in Guiyang, the Wounded Soldiers' Hospital in Hankow, and a hospital in the wartime capital of Chongqing. She also worked with Song Meiling's war orphan relief efforts. Following additional brief training at Johns Hopkins Medical College in 1941, Yang assumed the directorship of the Maternal and Child Health Section of the National Institute of Health (a subsidiary branch of the National Health Administration) in Chongqing, and she traveled throughout China advocating for improved health care for women and children. She also wrote or coauthored numerous articles and books on maternal and child health during this time, including a family health manual and two textbooks for use in midwifery schools. After the end of WWII, the League of Nations was reorganized as the World Health Organization, and in 1947 Yang joined their International Women's and Infants' Health Section, where she was eventually made deputy director. This provided opportunity for more travel to several European cities, and she moved to Geneva to work.

Lin remained in Beijing focused on clinical work during the war. When PUMC closed in 1941 because of the Sino-Japanese War, Lin opened a private clinic nearby at 10 Dongtangzi Alley, seeing patients from all walks of life and decreasing or omitting fees for patients who could not afford her services. Living and working among her patients gave Lin a greater understanding of the troubles and illnesses of women.

Reproductive Health in Transition: Science and the People's Republic

At the founding of the People's Republic in 1949, Yang was still working in Geneva with the WHO, but she returned to China that year at the request of former classmate and now Health Minister Li Dequan, the widow of "Christian general" warlord Feng Yuxiang, on behalf of Mao Zedong and Zhou Enlai. Yang became director of the Women's and Infants' Section of the Ministry of Health, a post she held until 1957, working to establish a network to decrease infant and maternal mortality. Yang continued her work training mid-wives, attending births, and advocating pre-and post-natal care. This network trained nearly 270, 000 childbirth assistants and 9000 obstetric nurses. In addition, under her guidance 13 branches and 34 sub-clinics of the maternal and child health clinics were established throughout China, helping to decrease the maternal mortality rate from 0. 7 percent in 1949 to 0. 05 percent in 1954, and infant mortality from 11. 7 percent to 4. 6 percent in the same time period. By 1966 Yang reported that the infant mortality rate nationwide had dropped to 2 percent, though these numbers are difficult to verify.

When PUMC reopened after the war, Lin Qiaozhi resumed her post as head of the obstetrics and gynecology department and continued in that position after the hospital was renamed Capital Hospital in 1951 (and, briefly, the Anti-Imperialist Hospital during the Cultural Revolution, 1966 – 76). But Lin was more actively involved in politics than Yang. In fact, while Yang Chongrui was most active in the Republican period, Lin Qiaozhi's career rapidly accelerated under the People's Republic of China. During the Three-Antis

Campaign in 1951 – 52, she published self-criticisms about her role within PUMC, as well as critiques of PUMC president Li Zong'en during the Anti-Rightist Movement in 1956 – 57. Revoking her imperialist education, she publicly vowed to dedicate her life to the new People's Republic. In 1953, Lin attended the Beijing Women's Conference and was elected a member of the All-China Women's Federation, later serving as deputy chair of the Beijing association and, in 1978, chair of the national organization. In 1955, she was elected to the National People's Congress and reelected until 1978, giving speeches about the importance of women's health, child health, occupational health, infectious disease prevention, and other topics. She was later appointed to its Standing Committee. Lin also held posts as member of the Chinese Academy of Sciences (1955), deputy president of the Chinese Medical Association (1956), chair and chief editor of the *Journal of Chinese Gynecology and Obstetrics*, and member of the Medical Section of the State Council's Scientific Planning Committee (1957).

Painless Childbirth

As in the Republican era, biomedical science was politically charged, and there is no better place to examine this than in the realm of reproductive health. Under the Guomindang and during wartime, Yang had written about the importance of proper maternal and child health in the service of the state, with women targeted as the primary caretakers of individual, family, and public health. These ideas drew from Yang's western education and widespread discussions of eugenics and racial hygiene. In the early 1950s, Chinese leadership distanced itself from Western concepts and modeled their government and policies on the Soviet Union. Science remained in the service of the state but was imbued with greater political import. For example, as part of the "Learn from Pavlov" scientific movement, China's Ministry of Health in 1952 began promoting the Soviet "psychoprophylactic painless childbirth method" (*wu tong fenmian* 无痛分娩) that was to free women from the pain of childbirth without the use of chemical anesthesia or analgesia. The methods are based on careful word suggestion, meticulous care of the patient by all medical staff and family, and specialized breathing techniques. In essence, women were taught that childbirth is a natural pain-free process and to allow that process to occur unimpeded; women who experienced pain during this natural process were lacking the correct political mindset and/or actions. This psychoprophylactic method was a medical expression of the dominant political ideology: the CCP had liberated the Chinese people, and this freedom from oppression extended to the birth experience. Lin published articles advocating painless childbirth in the *Chinese Journal of Obstetrics and Gynecology* aimed at the profession, and also in the English-language propaganda magazine *China Reconstructs*. The movement was short-lived, however, ending with the Sino-Soviet split by 1960.

Birth Control

Birth control is another important example of the ways politics impact science. As we have seen, at PUMC both Yang and Lin were early active supporters of family planning methods. This dedication continued throughout their careers. In the 1950s, Lin conducted surveys and educational campaigns for birth control in Beijing and in parts of Hebei and Henan, and both she and Yang worked closely with Ministry of Health and the All-China Women's Federation to liberalize birth control policies after 1949. However, the Ministry of Health of the early 1950s was decidedly pro-natalist, as a socialist system was theoretically immune from Malthusian population pressures and food shortages, not to mention painful childbirth. Initial ministry opposition to contraception gradually softened over the 1950s, however, as several female CCP members wrote in 1953 to the All-China Women's Federation demanding contraception in order to participate in "socialist construction. " Liu Shaoqi arranged a series of meetings in 1954 – 55 to discuss birth control at the national Party level. Present at these meetings were Minister of Health Li Dequan, Lin Qiaozhi, and Yang Chongrui; and in 1956 Lin personally spoke to Mao Zedong about the need for population control. Lin also began publishing articles as early as 1957 in the popular women's magazine *Women of China* (*Zhongguo funu*) that indirectly advocated late marriage. The outcome of the discussions was that although women may choose to utilize birth control, the All-China Women's Federation would not undertake any targeted birth control campaigns. The CCP and the Ministry of Health remained undecided and uncommitted on the issue of birth control.

The following year in June, Lin argued atthe fourth session of the First National People's Congress to strengthen family planning as a means to control the population. She was following economist and president of Beijing University Ma Yinchu, who at the same meeting had presented his "New Population Theory" in which China's growing population, if left unchecked, would be detrimental to the country's economic development. He advocated government control of fertility using birth control and family planning measures. Lin and Yang further supported Ma's work by co-authoring two articles in *People's Daily*. In the end, Ma's support of family planning was seen as criticism of socialism, support of Malthusian doctrine, and contempt for the people. In 1957 he was denounced as a rightist. Yang suffered the same fate. She was sent to the Academy of Socialism (社会主义学院) for reeducation, removed from her medical posts, and demoted to cataloguing foreign language books for the Chinese Medical Association. Later she was able to work as editor of the journal *Gynecology* (妇产科杂志) and advise the Women's and Infants' Health Department, though her rightist label was rescinded only in 1979. Her career was over.

The Cultural Revolution (1966 – 76)

Lin escaped the Anti-Rightist Campaign without serious harm. However, during the Cultural Revolution Lin was criticized as a "reactionary academic authority" and accused of being an American spy. She was forced to temporarily step down from her executive administrative positions and to perform the duties of an intern. Several of Lin's family members supported or worked for the Nationalist government and had fled to Taiwan after 1949. This, coupled with Lin's western educational and professional background at PUMC, could have resulted in even harsher treatment. However, according to several accounts, Lin was a close friend of Premier Zhou Enlai and his wife Deng Yingchao, both of whom protected her throughout these turbulent years. She was also physician and friends with many others in powerful positions like Li Dequan and Kang Keqing (wife of military leader Zhu De), and Lin's political problems were short lived.

Lin soon reassumed her previous posts and became an important actor in formulating and propagating government health policies. In 1965, in an often-recounted speech, Mao Zedong publicly criticized the Chinese Ministry of Health for ministering to only 15% of China's population, meaning that those without means or money could not access quality health care. This speech prompted the movement of urban health systems and professionals to the countryside. The Ministry of Health established the Rural Cooperative Medical System and health centers nationwide, and sent health care professionals from the cities to train and provide services to the rural populations. As part of this campaign, Lin traveled with a team of 30 nurses and doctors to do medical work in Xiangyin County in the Hunan countryside for more than four months in 1965. This medical team treated over 30,000 patients and trained local health workers and midwives in "farm-study schools." This was an early form of the barefoot doctor movement that the World Health Organization heralded in the 1970s as a model for universal primary health care. Their activities in rural Hunan were published in Chinese in *Zhongguo Funu* and in English in the *Chinese Medical Journal*, highlighting healthcare for all and the usefulness of emancipated professional women who would soon hold up half the sky - the actors in a new and modern China.

For many, Lin was a trusted public professional, someone to turn to for honest information about healthcare (save for, perhaps, the short-lived "painless childbirth" campaign). Lin published dozens of articles in popular magazines and *People's Daily* on childrearing, nutrition, pregnancy and postpartum; physical culture; and adolescent, children's and women's health. By the late 1960s, Lin had become a regular feature in the popular press. To the public, Lin represented a modern, professional, emancipated yet selfless and devoted woman of the People's Republic. Instead of being persecuted, during most of the Cultural Revolution and afterward Lin became an icon, a model worker representing professional women, science, and modernity. She was a selfless caregiver who ministered to the poor and needy, and she provided health care to the masses.

While her friend and colleague Yang Chongrui lived quietly after 1957 and relinquished her previous international connections, Lin's public face extended internationally. Traveling around the world on medical and goodwill delegations, and meeting foreign leaders in China, Lin represented the acclaimed Chinese public health care system and further showed that China's women were educated and equal under the new order. In 1953 Lin toured the Soviet Union and later that year attended a world health conference in Vienna as a member of the China delegation. After a hiatus in international travel during the early years of the Cultural Revolution, in 1972 Lin was the only woman on the Chinese Medical Association delegation to the United States, the second official delegation to the US after the "ping-pong diplomacy" exchange the previous year. In 1974, she was the head of a goodwill delegation to Iran commemorating a direct air link between Tehran and Beijing; and in 1978 was part of a friendship delegation to Europe. She was a friend of journalist Edgar Snow, who wrote about her in his book on China's communist revolution. When foreign delegations came to China in the 1970s, Lin was invariably present, for example at Kruschev's and Nehru's visits in 1954. The American Delegation on Early Childhood Development visited in 1974, and the resulting publication dedicates many pages to Lin's work on maternal health and pre-and postnatal care. From 1973 to

1977, Lin was a consultant to the WHO's Medical Research Advisory Committee. She was a global intermediary representing the best of China for political ends, a model for all that was remarkable about the People's Republic-emancipated women, health care for all, stellar medical and scientific research. Women like her helped to solidify China's place in the modern world.

Although Lin is best known as a clinical obstetrician/gynecologist, some of her greatest contributions to women's health in China come from her research and scholarship. She is credited with a considerable drop in cervical cancer rates in China based on a massive survey and widespread awareness of the disease in the 1960s. She also conducted scientific research and published articles on hemolytic disease of newborns, congenital deformities, gynecological tumors, and female infertility; and she designed a plastic and metal intrauterine device in the late 1960s called the intrauterine contraceptive ring (*gongnei jieyu huan* 宫内节育环). She authored a widely used medical textbook on gynecologic oncology, whose fourth edition was published in 2006. Her work underscores the importance of scientific achievements in the People's Republic, as well as the emphasis on health care for the masses under the new socialist system.

Legacy

Yang Chongrui and Lin Qiaozhi died a few months apart in Beijing in 1983. Yang has since been memorialized at Dongsi Hospital adjacent to Qilin Alley, the site of the First National Midwifery School. Fellow PUMC obstetrician/gynecologist, Yan Renying, edited a commemorative volume in 1990 on Yang's contributions, gathered from among Yang's former students and colleagues. Her successors at Dongsi Hospital continue to honor her life and career. But otherwise, Yang died in obscurity. In contrast, Lin has been commemorated in numerous ways: a movie, appearances in two television series, a commemorative stamp, at least one dozen biographies, and hundreds of articles. She is memorialized at Peking Union Medical College, the Women's and Children's Museum in Beijing, the China Millennium Monument, the Beijing Obstetrics and Gynecology Hospital, and the Xiamen Lin Qiaozhi Maternity and Child Health Care Hospital. In addition, a memorial in her birthplace of Gulangyu, Xiamen, hosts a museum and garden with statuary of children and engravings of some of Lin's famous quotes. The alabaster statue of Lin that houses her ashes on Gulangyu is reminiscent of Guanyin, the Goddess of Mercy.

In the twenty-first century, Lin is being resurrected in China as a model for the caring doctor amidst a troubled medical system. Overworked physicians, corruption and bribes, long lines to see specialists even for minor ailments, and patients attacking and even killing doctors are some of the stories that populate the headlines in newspapers in the 21st century. At least since 2010, Lin has once again appeared in the popular press as the selfless, dedicated doctor interested not in fame or money, but only in the wellbeing of her patients. Students and staff at Beijing Obstetrics and Gynecology Hospital continue to commemorate Lin Qiaozhi during Qingming festival; new hires at the obstetrics and gynecological hospital in Xiamen take an oath to be like Lin; Guangxi Medical School established a Lin Qiaozhi award in 2012 for an outstanding obstetrician/gynecologist. Even her patient case notes are held up as an example of how physicians should write accurate, detailed, and thorough patient records.

From their early days as students at PUMC, Yang Chongrui and Lin Qiaozhi dedicated their lives to women's health care, teaching, policymaking, and research. The medical profession gave them an outlet for professional development and personal growth in ways that business or law or other professions could not. Both women chose career over family - they had to make that choice, for it was unseemly for married women to work outside the home. (In fact, requirements for entrance into Yang's midwifery school were that her students be young and unmarried.) However, both women still fit within the broader norms of feminine nurturing and self-sacrifice. Lin became known as "the mother of 10,000 babies" (万婴之母), mother of the nation's children rather than of her own biological offspring. She also seemed to move more easily among the vagaries of political change, while Yang never successfully made the transition as part of the PRC's public health infrastructure. Perhaps Yang attempted to be more iconoclastic, a more modern woman, and that may be why she had trouble fitting in to an ostensibly egalitarian society that was still rigidly patriarchal. The biographies of Yang and Lin, these women of similar backgrounds yet with very different outcomes, remind us about the fluctuating landscape of medicine and public health, of politics, and of women's lives and society's expectations of them across the twentieth century.

Bibliography

1. Research for this chapter was partially funded by the Chiang Ching-Kuo Foundation and the China and Inner Asia Council of the Association for Asian Studies.

2. Wang Bing, "Yang Chongrui," in *Biographical Dictionary of Chinese Women: The Twentieth Century* 1912 – 2000, ed. Lily Xiao Hong Lee, A. D. Stefanowska, and Sue Wiles, trans. Jennifer Zhang (Routledge, 2002), 611 – 13.

3. Zhao Liangfeng, "Yang Chongrui: Pioneer in China's Modern Obstetrics," *www. womenofchina. cn*, (March 12, 2013), http: //history. cultural-china. com/en/48History14254. html.

4. Liping Bu and Elizabeth Fee, "John B. Grant: International Statesman of Public Health," *Am J Public Health* 98, no. 4 (April 2008): 628 – 29.

5. Nicole Elizabeth Barnes, "Protecting the National Body: Gender and Public Health in Southwest China during the War with Japan, 1937 – 1945" (PhD dissertation, University of California at Irvine, 2012), 295.

6. Marion Yang, "Midwifery Training in China," *China Medical Journal* 42 (1928): 768 – 75.

7. Ibid. , 769.

8. Marion Yang and I-Chin Yuan, "Report of an Investigation on Infant Mortality and Its Causes in Peiping," *Chinese Medical Journal*, no. 47 (1933): 597 – 604.

9. Tina Phillips Johnson, *Childbirth in Republican China: Delivering Modernity* (Lanham, MD: Lexington Books, 2011), Chapter Three.

10. Beijing, literally "northern capital," was changed to Beiping ("northern peace") when the capital moved to Nanjing ("southern capital") in 1927. It reverted to Beijing after the People's Republic of China was established in 1949 with Beijing as the capital city.

11. First National Midwifery School, "Fifth Annual Report, First National Midwifery School, Peiping, July 1, 1933-June 30, 1934," Annual Report, (September 15, 1934).

12. Zhang Qingping (张清平), *Lin Qiaozhi* (*Lin Qiaozhi Zhuan*, 林巧稚传) (Tianjin: Baihua Literature and Art Publishing House (百花文艺出版社), 2005), 13 – 17.

13. Wright, Guowei, "Lin Qiaozhi: The Steady Pulse of a Quiet Faith," in *Salt and Light: Lives of Faith That Shaped Modern China*, ed. Hamrin, Carol Lee and Stacy Bieler (Eugene, OR: Wipf and Stock Publishers, Pickwick Publications, 2008), 114 – 32.

14. Xiamen Lin Qiaozhi Memorial Preparation Committee (厦门市林巧稚大夫纪念活动筹备委员会), *Lin Qiaozhi Daifu: Zhuoyue de Renmin Yixuejia* (*Dr. Lin Qiaozhi: Outstanding Physician to the People* 林巧稚大夫: 卓越的人民医学家) (Xiamen: Xiamen shi Lin Qiaozhi daifu jinian huodong choubei weiyuanhui (厦门市林巧稚大夫纪念活动筹备委员会), 1984); Zhuhong, "Lin Qiaozhi: Guardian Angel of Mothers, Babies," *All-China Women's Federation*, December 6, 2007.

15. Lily Xiao Hong Lee, "Lin Qiaozhi," in *Biographical Dictionary of Chinese Women: The Twentieth Century 1912 – 2000*, ed. Lily Xiao Hong Lee, A. D. Stefanowska, and Sue Wiles (Routledge, 2002), 343 – 46.

16. Wang Bing, "Yang Chongrui."

17. Mirela Violeta David, "Free Love, Marriage, and Eugenics: Global and Local Debates on Sex, Birth Control, Venereal Disease and Population in 1920s-1930s China" (PhD dissertation, New York University, 2014).

18. Mary Brown Bullock, *An American Transplant: The Rockefeller Foundation and Peking Union Medical College* (Berkeley: University of California Press, 1980), 179; Lin Qiaozhi, "Around the World for Birth Control," *China Medical Journal* 59 (1936): 38 – 41.

19. Marion Yang, "Birth Control in Peiping: First Report of the Peiping Committee on Maternal Health," *The Chinese Medical Journal* 48 (1934): 786 – 91.

20. David, "Free Love, Marriage, and Eugenics"; Wang Bing, "Yang Chongrui."

21. Yang Chongrui (Marion Yang), "My Autobiography (Wo de Zizhuan 我的自传) (October 1949)," in *Dr. Yang Chongrui: 100 Year Commemoration* (*Yang Chongrui Boshi: Danchen Bai Nian Ji Nian* 杨崇瑞博士: 诞辰百年纪念), ed. Yan Renying 严仁英 (Beijing: Beijing yike daxue, zhongguo xiehe yike daxue lianhe chubanshe 北京医科大学, 中国协和医科大学联合出版社, 1990), 143 – 53; Zhao, "Yang Chongrui: Pioneer in

China's Modern Obstetrics. "

22. Barnes, "Protecting the National Body, " 291 – 92.

23. Wang Bing, "Yang Chongrui"; Barnes, "Protecting the National Body", Chapter Six.

24. Yang Chongrui and Wang Shijin, *The Study of Maternal and Children's Health* (*Fuying Weisheng Xue 婦嬰衛生學*) (Chongqing: National Institute of Health, 1944); Yang Chongrui, *The First National Midwifery School Tenth Anniversary Memorial Publication* (*Diyi Zhuchan Xuexiao Shi Zhounian Jinian Kan 第一助產學校十週年紀念刊*), 1939; Yang Chongrui, *The Past and Present of Maternal and Children's Health in China* (*Zhongguo Fuying Weisheng Guoqu Yu Xianzai 中國婦嬰衛生過去與現在*), 1940; Yang Chongrui, *What a Housewife Must Know*: *An Outline of Family Hygiene and Home Economics* (*Zhufu Xuzhi*: *Jiating Weisheng Ji Jiazheng Gaiyao 主婦須知：家庭衛生及家政概要*) (Nanjing: National Health Administration, 1934); Yang Chongrui, *An Outline of Maternal and Children's Health* (*Fuying Weisheng Gaiyao 婦嬰衛生概要*), 1943; Yang Chongrui, *Lectures on Maternal and Children's Health* (*Fuying Weisheng Jiangzuo 婦嬰衛生講座*) (New Life Movement Women's Advisory Council Press, 1945); Yang Chongrui, *The First National Midwifery School Tenth Anniversary Memorial Publication* (*Diyi Zhuchan Xuexiao Shi Zhounian Jinian Kan 第一助產學校十週年紀念刊*).

25. Wang Bing, "Yang Chongrui"; Zhao, "Yang Chongrui: Pioneer in China's Modern Obstetrics. "

26. Zhao, "Yang Chongrui: Pioneer in China's Modern Obstetrics. "

27. Lin Qiaozhi, "Open the 'PUMC' Window and Take a Look at the Motherland (Dakai 'Xiehe' Chuanghu Kan Zuguo 打开 '协和' 窗户看祖国)," *Renmin Ribao*, September 27, 1952; Lin Qiaozhi, "My Thinking Transformed (Wo de Sixiang Zhuangbian 我的思想装变)," *Zhonghua Yixue Zazhi* 38, no. 9 (September 1952): 749 – 54; Lin Qiaozhi, "Li Zong' en Should Repent Immediately (Li Zongen Ying Jizao Huiwu 李宗恩应及早悔悟)," *Health News* (*Jiankang Bao*) 3 (August 6, 1957).

28. Zhuhong, "Lin Qiaozhi: Guardian Angel of Mothers, Babies"; Lee, "Lin Qiaozhi. "

29. Lee, "Lin Qiaozhi. "

30. Yang Chongrui, *What a Housewife Must Know*: *An Outline of Family Hygiene and Home Economics* (*Zhufu Xuzhi*: *Jiating Weisheng Ji Jiazheng Gaiyao 主婦須知：家庭衛生及家政概要*); Yang Chongrui, *Lectures on Maternal and Children's Health* (*Fuying Weisheng Jiangzuo 婦嬰衛生講座*); See Barnes, "Protecting the National Body",

Chapter Six.

31. Paula Michaels，"Childbirth Pain Relief and the Soviet Origins of the Lamaze Method，" National Council for Eurasian and East European Research Working Paper (Seattle，WA：NCEEER，October 16，2007)；Gao Xi，"Learning from the Soviet Union：Pavlovian Influence on Chinese Medicine，1950s，" in *Public Health and National Reconstruction in Post-War Asia：International Influences，Local Transformations* (Routledge，2014)，72 – 89.

32. Lim，Kha-Ti，"Painless Childbirth，" *China Reconstructs*，1952；Lin Qiaozhi，"Introducing Several Key Features in Medicine and Science Observed on a Tour of the Soviet Union (Canguan Sulian de Yixuekexue Ji Ge Zhuyao Tedian de Jiandan Jieshao 参观苏联的医学科学几个主要特点的简单介绍)，" *Chinese Journal of Obstetrics and Gynecology* (*Zhonghua Fuchanke Zazhi* 4 (1953)：289 – 303.

33. Susan Greenhalgh and Edwin A. Winckler，*Governing China's Population：From Leninist to Neoliberal Biopolitics* (Stanford：Stanford University Press，2005)，65.

34. Lee，"Lin Qiaozhi"；Wright，Guowei，"Lin Qiaozhi：The Steady Pulse of a Quiet Faith."

35. Lin Qiaozhi，"Discussion of Marriage Age on Physiology (Cong Shenglishang Tan Jiehun Nianling 从生理上谈结婚年龄)，" *Zhongguo Funu* 4 (1957)：25 – 26.

36. Ma Yinchu，"New Population Theory (新人口论)，" *People's Daily* (*Renmin Ribao* 人民日报)，July 5，1957.

37. Wang Ligeng et al.，"Advocate for Late Marriage and Family Planning (Guangfan Xuanchuan Chihun He Jihua Shengyu 广泛宣传迟婚和计划生育)，" *People's Daily* (*Renmin Ribao* 人民日报)，March 15，1957；Wang Shuzhen et al.，"Obstetrician/Gynecologists Wang Shuzhen，Lin Qiaozhi，He Bihui，Yu Aifeng Give Their Opinions on Implementing Family Planning 妇产科大夫王淑贞、林巧稚、何碧辉、俞霭峰 对于实行计划生育的意见，" *People's Daily* (*Renmin Ribao* 人民日报)，July 20，1957.

38. Wang Bing，"Yang Chongrui."

39. Lee，"Lin Qiaozhi."

40. Yao Yuan (姚远)，"Zhou Enlai and 'Our Lady of the Orient' Lin Qiaozhi (周恩来与'东方圣母'林巧稚)，" *Chinese Communist Party News* (中国共产党新闻网)，December 15，2010，http：//dangshi. people. com. cn/GB/85040/13515215. html.

41. David M. Lampton，"Public Health and Politics in China's Past Two Decades，" *Health Services Report* 87，no. 10 (December 1972)：895 – 904.

42. Early rural cooperative medical systems were established in various locations as early

as 1955, with brigade health auxiliaries called Barefoot Doctors. These programs went nationwide in 1965. Naisu Zhu et al. , "Factors Associated with the Decline of the Cooperative Medical System and Barefoot Doctors in Rural China," *Bulletin of the World Health Organization* 67, no. 4 (1989): 431 – 32.

43. Huang Chia-ssu, "Our Medical Team in the Countryside," *Chinese Medical Journal* 84, no. 12 (December 1965): 799 – 803; Xinhua News, "Following the Revolutionary Path of Health, the Revolutionized Health Team Advances: Mobile Health Teams in Rural Areas (坚持卫生工作的革命方向, 促进卫生队伍的革命化: 巡回医疗队在农村)," *Zhongguo Funu*, 1965.

44. Lin Qiaozhi, *Questions and Answers on Rural Maternal Child Health* 农村妇幼卫生常识问答*Nongcun Fuyou Weisheng Changshi Wenda* (Beijing: Renmin weisheng chubanshe 人民卫生出版社, 1975); Lin Qiaozhi and Mu Qin, *Family Education Adviser* (*Jiating Jiaoyu Guwen* 家庭教育顾问), Qing Nian Xiu Yang Tong Xun, 8 (Beijing: 中国青年出版社: 新华书店北京发行所发行, 1981); Lin Qiaozhi and Wang Yuan'e, *Gynecologic Oncology* (妇科肿瘤*Fuke Zhongliu*) (Beijing: 人民卫生出版社, 1982).

45. Tina Mai Chen, "Female Icons, Feminist Iconography? Socialist Rhetoric and Women's Agency in 1950s China," *Gender and History* 15, no. 2 (2003): 268 – 95.

46. Huang Chia-ssu, "Our Medical Team in the Countryside. "

47. Zhuhong, "Lin Qiaozhi: Guardian Angel of Mothers, Babies. "

48. Yao Yuan (姚远), "Zhou Enlai and 'Our Lady of the Orient' Lin Qiaozhi (周恩来与 '东方圣母' 林巧稚)"; UPI, "Chinese View U. S. Medicine," *Desert Sun*, November 3, 1972, California Digital Newspaper Collection.

49. Wolfgang Bartke, "Lin Qiaozhi," in *Who Was Who in the People's Republic of China* (Walter de Gruyter, 1997), 270.

50. Edgar Snow, *The Long Revolution* (Vintage Books, 1973), especially Chapter Three, "Medical Care and Population Control. "

51. Xinhua News, "Premier Zhou Entertains Nehru 周总理招待尼赫鲁总理," *People's Daily* (*Renmin Ribao* 人民日报), October 20, 1954; Xinhua News, "Soviet Ambassador Holds Reception 苏联驻我国大使尤金举行招待会," *People's Daily* (*Renmin Ribao* 人民日报), October 13, 1954.

52. William Kessen, ed. , *Childhood in China*, American Delegation on Early Childhood Development (New Haven and London: Yale University, 1975), especially Chapter 8, "Health and Nutritional Factors. "

53. Xiamen Lin Qiaozhi Memorial Preparation Committee (厦门市林巧稚大夫纪念活

动筹备委员会）*Lin Qiaozhi Daifu*

54. Lee,"Lin Qiaozhi"; Lim, Kha-Ti, Kao, JC, and Chang, CF,"Mass Survey for the Cancer of Cervix Uteri in China,"*Acta Unio Int Contra Cancrum* 19（1963）：902 – 5.

55. Lim, Kha Ti and Snyder, Franklin F.,"The Effect of Respiration Stimulants in the Newborn Infant,"*Am. J. Obst. & Gynec.* 50（1945）：1460153; Lim, Khati（Lin Qiaozhi）, "Obstetrics and Gynecology in the Past Ten Years,"*Chinese Medical Journal* 79, no. 5（November 1959）：375 – 83; Lee,"Lin Qiaozhi"; Gao Xi,"Learning from the Soviet Union."

56. Lin Qiaozhi and Lian Lijuan, *Lin Qiaozhi's Gynecologic Oncology*, 4th ed.（*Lin Qiaozhi Fuke Zhongliu Xue, di si ban,* 林巧稚妇科肿瘤学, 第四版）（Beijing：Renmin weisheng chubanshe 人民卫生出版社, 2006）.

57. Yan Renying, ed., *Dr. Yang Chongrui*：100 *Year Commemoration.*

58. Gao Liqiang（高力强）, *Endless Love*（*Da Ai Ru Tian* 大爱如天）, 2007, http：//movie. douban. com/subject/2279571/, http：//jq. tvsou. com/introhtml/699/1 _ 69943. htm; Feng Xuesong 冯雪松, *Twentieth-Century Chinese Women's History*, *vol.* 15： *Birth Revolution*（*Ershi shiji zhongguo nuxing shi* 二十世纪中国女性史：生育革命）（China Central Television, 1999）, http：//v. youku. com/v_ show/id_ XNDUwMTM4ODQw. html? old&from = y1. 2 – 2. 4. 15; Wang Ren 王韧, *Masters*（*Da shi* 大师）（China Central Television, 2008）.

59. Chris Buckley,"A Danger for Doctors in China：Patients' Angry Relatives,"*New York Times*, May 18, 2016, sec. Asia Pacific; Adam Jourdan,"China Investigates Former Top Healthcare Official for Bribery,"*Reuters*, May 27, 2015, sec. World News; See, for example, Kazunori Takada,"Bribery Serves As Life-Support for Chinese Hospitals,"*Reuters*, July 23, 2013, sec. Lifestyle.

60. "New Employees' Oath Cherishes the Memory of Dr. Lin Qiaozhi 新员工入职宣誓缅怀林巧稚大夫,"*Xiamen Daily*, July 28, 2015; "Lin Qiaozhi：Mother of 10, 000 Babies, Soul of Medicine 林巧稚：'万婴之母', 大医之魂,"*Xinhuanet* 新华每日电讯, December 11, 2015; Beijing Obstetrics and Gynecology Hospital 北京妇产医院, "Education Department Organized All Graduate Students to Pay Tribute to First Dean Lin Qiaozhi Statue（Jiaoyuchu Zuzhi Quanti Yanjiusheng Zhanyang Shou Renyuanchang Lin Qiaozhi Tongxiang 教育处组织全体研究生瞻仰首任院长林巧稚铜像）,"*Health. Sohu. Com*, April 1, 2016, http：//health. sohu. com/20160401/n443189093. shtml.

61. "Lin Qiaozhi's Handwritten Medical Records Appear After 70 Years 年前林巧稚手书病历亮相,"*Haixi Morning News* 海西晨报, July 29, 2015.

北京协和医学院早期的中药研究：从 1910 年到 1941 年

张大庆

前北京大学医学人文研究院院长、北京大学医学史研究中心主任，教授。他也是中国科学技术史学会副理事长兼医学史专业委员会主任、国际医学史学会科学委员会委员。他的研究兴趣包括十九世纪及二十世纪中国医学文化与社会史、比较医学史及中国近代传教士医学文化。他最近的出版书籍包括《中国近代疾病社会史》（2006）《医学史》（2007）《医学史十五讲》（2007）及《医学人文导论》（2013）等。

19 世纪随着实验生理学的发展，医学家开始采用实验生理学的方法来研究药物的化学成分、性质、药理作用等。早在 18 世纪末，意大利博物学家、生理学家方塔那（F. Fontana）对千余种天然药物做过实验研究，认为天然药物中的活性成分通过作用于机体某个部位而发生作用。这一结论为德国化学家斯托勒（F. W. Serturner）首次从罂粟中分离出吗啡所证实（1806）。随后，从吐根中提取了吐根素（1817），从马钱子中提取出士的宁（1818）、从金鸡纳皮中提取出奎宁（1819），从咖啡中提取出咖啡因（1821）等，用化学方法对植物药有效成分进行提取成为 19 世纪末 20 世纪初药理研究的重要内容。此外，医学家们也开始通过实验研究药物对各器官的作用，如 F. Magendie 确定了盐酸士的宁引起肌肉僵直的作用部位在脊髓（1819），伯尔纳（C. Bernard）确定了筒箭毒碱松弛骨骼肌的作用点在神经肌接头（1856）等，对药物的作用及作用部位的研究取得了许多成果。这些研究不仅将临床药物治疗建立在实验科学的基础之上，而且也为从传统植物药中研发新药物提供了借鉴。

19 世纪末 20 世纪初来华的传教士医生大多经历了实验科学的训练，

有些医生在行医之余，对中国传统的医药知识和诊疗技术产生了兴趣，并开始研究中医药问题。20世纪初期，随着医学留学生的回国，中国学者也开始用现代科学的方法来研究传统医药的药理机制与临床价值，近代对中药物的科学研究大致可分为三个阶段，而在这三个阶段里北京协和医学院都显现出其独特的贡献。

第一阶段：对中药的认同与译介

虽然大多数来华传教士医生对中医药的价值评价不高，认为："这些药物（中医药）的制备过程非常粗糙、不纯，而且使用时很少会考虑到其已知的治疗价值。一大批其他矿物质的制备也完全不合理——比如蛤壳、鹅卵石、白垩、云母等。"[1]不过，也有一些传教士医生认为中药的治病效果还是很好的，与西药有类似之处，如道思韦德（A. W. Douthwaite）指出："（中国的）本土医生使用三硫化二砷，即'雌黄'，主要是用于外用。此外还有各种混合性的砷粉，他们通常有各种神乎其神的名字，则一般用于遏制疾病恶化，这与欧洲几年前使用的'Arsenical Pastes（砷膏）'在很大程度上大同小异。"[2]此外，他还提到白降丹（Peh-kiang-tan）、轻粉（Ch'ing-fen）、三仙丹（San-sin-tan）等中的主要成分为氯化亚汞、氯化低汞、红粉（氧化汞和硝基汞的化合物）。

中药的科学价值是传教士医生的关注点之一。汤姆逊（J. C. Thomson）较全面地研究了李时珍的《本草纲目》以及他所收集到西方学者研究中药的文献，指出："我们当时发现，中国有无穷无尽的药物，这对我们医疗传教士而言肯定有巨大价值。而且我们也已经证明了其价值。中国人在我们面前展示了很多治疗方法也已经解释了其特性，另有其他的则非常粗糙。但正如有人所说过，我们面前有一座尚未开发的宝藏，我们只需努力，就能获得知识的珍宝。"[3]不过，传教士医生对中药更大的兴趣在于其实用价值，尤为教会医院的增加并扩张到内陆地区，西药供给不足是一个严重的问题，因此需要利用本土药物作为补充。道思韦德认为："在内陆地区发展教会的一个巨大的障碍——即如何将必要的药物以及医疗器械转运到远离主要水路航道的医疗站点，有时这一困难简直难以逾越。因此有必要发现、并利用在中国国内可以获得的当地的药材以及进口药物，并考虑将现有的原料进行加工的可能性，制作出如我们所习惯的用于治疗患者的化合物。"[4]因此，在《博医会报》上常刊发传教士医生们讨论如何使用本土药材治疗疾病以及利用本土药材加工制成西药的经验。在 19 世纪末 20 世纪初传教士医生中，伊博恩（B. E. Read，1887 – 1949）对中药的研究最为全面、深入。

伊博恩 1887 年 5 月 17 日出生于英国南部城市布莱顿（Brighton），1909 年毕业于伦敦药学院（London College of Pharmacy）。毕业后受伦敦会的委派，于 1909 年来到伦敦会开办的北京协和医学堂（Union Medical College，Peking）担任化学与药剂学讲师。任教期间他开始关注在华教会医院的日常用药问题，列出了医院与诊所应必备的基本药物。1915 年洛克菲勒基金会（Rockefeller Foundation）改组北京协和医学堂，伊博恩被派往美国，曾在约翰·霍普金斯大学医学院、芝加哥大学、哈佛大学进修生物化学，以及在耶鲁大学进修了一年营养学。1918 年，伊博恩回到北京协和医学院并升任生物化学与药理学副教授。1923 – 24 年，他又去耶鲁大学深造，获得药理学博士学位，1925 年升任北京协和医学院药理学教授。回到北京后，伊博恩将精力主要集中于研究中国药物，并参与了主编《中国生理学杂志》（1927 年创刊）的工作。

伊博恩致力于中药文献的整理、译编、注释，代表作之一就是与中国植物学家刘汝强合作编撰的《本草新注》。《本草新注》又名《中国药用植物考证》（*Flora Sinensis Plantae Medicinalis Sinensis*：*Bibliography of Chinese Medicinal Plants From the Pen Ts'ao Kang Mu*，1596 A. D.）扉页上的《本草新注》为时任北平博物学学会会长的金绍基（1886 – 1949）所题。该书还请曾任北洋政府国务代总理的朱启钤作序："李氏以草莽儒臣，未窥中秘又于验药绘图不能特置多官随品设色，故于本草虽集大成而于药物形色宛隔一舍。英人伊博恩博士及京兆刘君汝强研究博物学有年，兹为沟通中西医学方术起见，就《本草纲目》所载，依盎格拉氏方式分门别类整理秩然。"对伊博恩的编译与整理工作给予了高度赞扬。

至于伊博恩本人进行这项工作的动因，从他所作的引言中可见一斑："这类书刊的发行需求是很明显的。语种的不同，以及中西方对自然历史的记录中采用的不同基本概念均造成了（中西医之间的）巨大分歧。许许多多的药用植物被声称具有不容置疑的治疗功效，尽管对它们特性的认识十分含糊，它们的化学构成被完全无视，它们对活细胞的作用也毫不明确。"为了尽可能消除这一分歧，他选择了挑战数不胜数的中药药典中最为著名的《本草纲目》，对其中的内容进行药理学与化学考察。对此，伊博恩提出并采用的研究方法就是，首先将所需要的大量各种药材的样本集中到一个中心实验室，以进行仔细的研究。

《本草新注》的有点是，该书不仅对植物性中药的植物来源成分和参考文献均有陈述，而且注重各国文献中关于中国药用植物的记录。作者收录、引用了来自德国、美国、英国、日本、中国、法国、瑞典、印度、马来西亚的学术杂志、新闻、政府官报、著述、典籍等，成为研究中药的重要参考书。该书出版后受到了学界的欢迎，不久宋大仁将该书的部分内容翻译成中文，以《中国药用植物考证：本草纲目之植物学、化学、药学的考证目录》为题，陆续登载于《中西医报》上。宋大仁指出："本草纲目为我国药物学，植物学重要书籍，惜其卷帙浩繁，旧医界多望而生畏，故只能读其节本，如本草从新，本草备要等书，即出而问世者，固无足道，而近年出版之本草书籍，亦多半是明抄暗袭，辗转失真，不脱陈腐窠臼，保存国粹之谓何？舒可叹也！译者鉴于本书关系于中西医药界甚大，尤感于国产药物西人早已研究，我人返茫昧无知，故及为逐译，以备有志中药革改者之参考。"5

除《本草新注》之外，伊博恩还对中药中的矿物类、动物类药物进行过分门别类的研究，出版了《兽类药物》（Animal Drugs，1931），《禽类药物》（Avian Drugs，1932），《鳞类药物》（Dragon and Snake Drugs，1934），《金石类、鳖蚌类药物》（Minerals and Stones；Turtle and Shellfish Drugs 1936），《中国药用植物》（Chinese Medicinal plants，1936）《鱼类药物》（Fish Drugs，1939），《虫类药物》（Insect Drugs，1941）等。他还著有《草木五谷类药物》（Vegetable and Plant Drugs，1949），但尚未刊发。

第二阶段：近代中药药理研究

北京协和医学院是中国最早开展中药药理现代研究的机构。前已述及，虽然传教士医生很早就开始关注中药的实用价值，但对中药的药理实验研究则直到陈克恢来到北京协和医学院后才正式开始。陈克恢的舅父是中医，幼年时期，他常来舅父的中药房，于是对中医药颇有兴趣。陈克恢在美国威斯康星大学药学系学习时，就曾在导师的支持下，对中药肉桂进行了实验研究，并以此研究完成了学士论文。1923 年，陈克恢获得博士学位后，受聘于北京协和医学院，任药理学助教。在协和期间，他继续从事中药研究。他和史米特（schmidt）、伊博恩首先对中药当归进行了研究。

除甘草外，在中药处方中，当归比其他任何药物都要更加常用。在治疗月经不调、产后失调，以及妇女不育症方面都很有疗效，它也用于许多其他疾病。该药物于 1899 年被默克药厂（Merck）引入西方，并被称为 Eumenol、以液体提取物的形式出售，后来则以 Eumenol 片剂的形式出售。这些制剂被推荐用于治疗月经紊乱，其效果也显著有效。陈克恢等指出：鉴于该药在中国广泛使用，及鉴于在欧洲使用该药物治疗子宫疾病方面取得的成功结果的相关报道，似乎很有可能这种药物对子宫能够产生一些明确的作用，而且也有一些明确的作用原理。经过一系列实验研究，他们的结论是：当把当归静脉注射给麻醉过的狗和兔子时，当归（Angelica polymorpha var sinensis）会抑制血液循环，有时还会经过刺激后会有利尿，以及子宫、肠、膀胱和动脉的平滑肌收缩发生。

由于当归的研究，主要是探讨其药理作用机制，虽工作颇为精详，但在化学方面未能提得有效成分，该文发表后反响不大。同年，陈克恢获知麻黄有治疗哮喘的作用后，随即开始研究麻黄素的作用机理。在几周内他就从中药麻黄中分离出左旋麻黄碱（ephedrine）并开始对麻黄碱的药理机制开展研究。他发现：适当剂量的麻黄碱会使血压升高，增加心脏活动，扩大瞳孔，缓解支气管痉挛，收缩子宫，更频繁地抑制而不是刺激胃肠道。这些效果可以通过对交感神经纤维的肌肉神经接点进行刺激来解释。[6]陈克恢与史米特于 1924 年在美国《实验生物学与医学学会通报》（Proc. Soc. Expt. Biol. Med.）上发表了其研究"麻黄素在实验性休克与出血中的作用"　（The Effect of Ephedrine on Experiment Shock and Hemorrhage），此后，陈克恢等又对麻黄素进行了一系列的实验研究，发表相关论文 10 余篇，由此，中药麻黄素的研究引起医药界的极大关注。由于麻黄素的作用与肾上腺素有相似之处，所不同的是麻黄素口服有效，且作用时间长，毒性较低，于是，麻黄素成为一个国际瞩目的拟交感神经新药。这段时间内，各国研究者纷纷对麻黄与麻黄碱开展了多方面的研究，发表相关论文数百篇，形成了一次国际中药研究的热潮。1930 年，麻黄碱被载入《中华药典》，此后，日、美、英、俄等也都将麻黄碱载入本国药典，同时也作为一种交感神经兴奋药载入教科书。陈克恢的这项从天然植物中寻找先导化合物，再进行优化，并成功开发为新药的研究，为传统的中医药研究建立了一种适宜的范式。

1923 – 24 年，伊博恩赴耶鲁大学深造，获得药理学博士学位，且在芝加哥大学进修病理学，1925 年，伊博恩返回北京协和医学院，接替史米特任药理系主任。在他的带领下，协和药理系在 1927 ~ 1933 年发表了十余篇有关麻黄素及其相关化合物的药理研究论文。伊博恩先后与林巧稚、赵承嘏、冯志东、朴柱秉等人还研究了其他中药的药理特性，使协和对中医药的研究名噪一时（见表 1）。

表 1：《中国生理学杂志》上协和医学院药物学系发表的中药相关研究论文（1927 – 1941）

Time	Authors	Title
1927	B. E. Read, Ch'iao-Chih Lin	Anesthetic mixtures of ephedrine and procaine with adrenaline and potassium sulphate
1927	Chih-Tung Feng	A method for preparing pure ephedrine hydrochloride from ephedra equisetina
1927	B. E. Read, George K. How	The iodine, arsenic, iron, calcium and sulphur content of Chinese medicinal algae
1927	Tsan-Quo Chou	Poisonous principles from Chinese Rhododendron, Nao-Yang-Hua, Rhododendron Hunnewellianum

Time	Authors	Title
1927	Kuo-Hao Lin , Chao-Chi Chen	Chemical analysis of sea slug, Stichopus japonicus Selenka (Hai Shen)
1927	Tsan-Quo Chou	Sikimitoxin, the toxic principle of Illicium Religiosum, Sieb. Mang-T'sao
1927	B. E. Read, Chih-Tung Feng	Psedoephedrine from Chinese ephedra
1927	B. E. Read	The relative toxicity of the halogen compounds of Chaulmoogra.
1927	Chih-Tung Feng	The " Biuret Reaction" as applied qualitatively and quantitatively to ephedrine mixtures
1927	Tse King, Chub-Yung Pak	A study of the effect of ephedrine on the nasal mucous membranes
1928	Chub-Yung Pak, B. E. Read	A comparative study of the bold pressor action of ephedrine, psedoephedrine and adrenaline
1928	Chih-Tung Feng, B. E. Read	A comparison of ephedra equisetina and E. sinica and their seasonal content of ephedrine
1928	Chih-Teh Loo, B. E. Read	Perfusion experiments with psedoephedrine and ephedrine
1928	Tsan-Quo Chou	The alkaloids of Chinese corydalis ambigua, cham. Et sch. (Yen-hu-so) part 1.
1928	Chih-Tung Feng, B. E. Read	Further assays of Chinese ephedras
1928	Chub-Yung Pak, B. E. Read	Comparative study of ephedrine, racemic ephedrine and psedoephedrine
1929	Tsan-Quo Chou	The alkaloids of Corydalis ambigua, cham et sch. Part II. Corydalis F, G and H.

续表

Time	Authors	Title
1929	Chub-Yung Pak, B. E. Read	Comparative studies of ephedrine, racemic ephedrine and psedoephedrine II. Comparative toxicity
1929	Tse King, Chub-Yung Pak	Comparative studies of ephedrine, racemic ephedrine and psedoephedrine III. Effects on the nasal mucous membranes
1929	Hsi-Chun Chang	The action of choline, adrenaline and ephedrine on gastric motility
1929	S. H. Li Jest Rand	The action of psedoephedrine I. On the isolated uterus and bladder.
1929	Chub-Yung Pak, B. E. Read	The action of psedoephedrine II. Its diuretic effects
1929	Tsan-Quo Chou	The alkaloids of Chinese Corydalis ambigua, cham. Et sch (Yen-hu-so). III. Corydalis I and monomethyl ethers of Corydalis F and G
1930	Chub-Yung Pak, Tse King	The action of ephedrine and psedoephedrine uponbronchial muscle
1931	Tsan-Quo Chou	The alkaloids of Chinese gelsemium, Kou Wen, Gelsemium elegans
1932	Hsiang-Ch'uan Hou	The pharmacological action of gelsemicine III. Action on circulation
1932	B. E. Read	The effect of benzyl-ephedrine on blood pressure
1932	Hsiang-Ch'uan Hou	Action of ephedrine and related substances on the blood vesselsxx
1932	T. Q. Chou	The alkaloids of Chinese drug Pei-mu, fritillaria roylei Part I. Peimine and peiminine
1932	Hsiang-Ch'uan Hou	The pharmacological action of gelsemicine IV. Action on intestine, uterus and urinary bladder

续表

Time	Authors	Title
1933	Chub-Yung Pak, B. E. Read	Action of ephedrine on the portal circulation
1933	Chub-Yung Pak, T. K. Tang	The mechanism of the mydriatic antion of ephedrine
1935	C. H. Wang, M. P. Chen	Effect of scopolamine and atropine on the muscle tonus increased by passive movements in a post-encephalitic parkinsonism patient
1938	T. P. Feng	Further observations on the propagation of veratrine contracture
1940	F. T. Dun, T. P. Feng	Studies on the neuromuscular junction XIX. Rereograde discharges from motor nerve endings in veratrinized muscle
1941	T. P. Feng, T. H. Li	Studies on the neuromuscular junction XXIV. the repetitive discharges of mammalian motor nerve endings after treatment with veratrine, barium and guanidine
1941	T. P. Feng	The production of prolonged after-discharge in nerve by veratrine

1927 – 1949 年出版的《中华生理学杂志》(Chinese Journal of Physiology) 上，发表与中药研究相关的论文 88 篇，其中 37 篇是来自北京协和医学院药物学系的研究者，发表论文较多的另外两个机构是北平研究院及中法大学药物研究所，上海雷氏德医学研究院，不过这两个机构的主要研究者也是来自原北京协和医学院药物学系的学者赵承嘏、伊博恩。

第三阶段：对中药化学的实验研究

赵承嘏是中药化学成分研究的开拓者。赵承嘏，字石民，江苏省江阴县人，生于 1885 年 12 月 11 日。1910 年获曼彻斯特大学学士学位，

1912 年获瑞士工业学院硕士学位，毕业后转入瑞士日内瓦大学，在当时著名的天然有机化学家匹克特（A. Pictet）教授指导下继续深造，1914 年获得博士学位，毕业后留校任助教。1916 年，赵承嘏受聘于法国罗克药厂研究部任职，后升为研究部主任。由于家庭经营生药铺，因此赵承嘏从小熟悉中药，这对他后来研究中药有着重要影响。1925 年，赵承嘏受聘到北京协和医学院任药物化学教授兼药理系代主任，开始了中草药研究工作，对麻黄、延胡索、莽草、贝母、钩吻等的化学成分进行了研究，发表了多篇论文，成为中国中草药化学研究的先驱者。

20 世纪初，虽然有机化学有很大的发展，植物化学的研究逐渐为化学家所重视，但在当时的中国，应用科学方法对中草药进行系统研究还是一个空白。赵承嘏运用近代化学方法，对古老的中草药进行系统的研究，为发掘和提高传统中医药学做出了卓越的贡献，并为中国医药界培养了一大批学科带头人和骨干。

赵承嘏非常重视实验室工作和实验技术，在长期的实验研究中，他对植物化学特别是生物碱的分离结晶积累了丰富的经验，创造了独特的分离方法。例如，他首次分离出了闹羊花中的毒素。[7] 当时，提取植物有效成分的经典方法是乙醇浸泡，这样得到的粗提物成分复杂，不易提纯分得结晶。鉴于植物有效成分多属生物碱，赵承嘏根据生物碱的特性，采用碱磨苯浸法，使提取物成分趋于简单，大大减少了进一步分离单体的困难。他根据不同的研究对象，设计不同的方法。他和他的学生们系统地研究了雷公藤、细辛、三七、贝母、常山、防己、延胡索、钩吻、麻黄等 30 多种中草药化学成分，得到了许多新生物碱的单体结晶，提供药理工作者进行药理研究，并选择其中有价值的推荐临床试验，从而建立了系统研究整理祖国医药学的一套科学方法。与此同时，他和学生们在国内外著名杂志中发表了许多论文，为中外学者所重视和赞赏。

赵承嘏运用自己独创的一套分离提取方法，往往能从一种植物中提得多种结晶，对植物化学做出了贡献。例如他对延胡索进行了系列研究，他首次从植物中分离得到 5 种生物碱结晶："从延胡索（Chinese Corydalis ambigua）的块茎中，迄今已有五种生物碱从非酚类部分中分离出来。它们分别被临时命名为延胡索碱 A（延胡索甲素），延胡索碱 B（延胡索乙素），延胡索碱 C，延胡索碱 D 和延胡索碱 E。其中一种与 Corydaline（延胡索甲素）是一样的，另外四种则是新的。"[8]至 1936 年，他共分离出 13 种延胡索的生物碱。

此外，他还从不同品种钩吻中分得 7 种生物碱结晶；从常山中分得 3 种在一定条件下可以相互转化的异构体。赵承嘏的提取方法在当时国际植物化学中占有重要的地位。他从三七植物中分得三七皂甙元结晶，并证明和人参二醇为同一化合物，比日本著名的化学家从人参中分得人参二醇早 20 年。[9]

赵承嘏还对已经做过研究的一些中草药重新研究，并从中分离出新的成分。例如从麻黄中分得新生物碱麻黄副素；从曼陀萝中又分得曼陀芹和曼陀芹引等新生物碱。他每得到一种生物碱，都要进行详细的药理试验。例如从常山中分得的丙种常山碱，其抗疟作用为奎宁的 148 倍；从延胡索分得的延胡索乙素现已在临床上作为镇痛、镇静剂应用，成为中国创制的新药，并载入中华人民共和国药典。

余论

1932 年之后，因多种因素的影响，北京协和医学院药物学系的几位对中药研究做出过重要贡献的学者陆续离开。赵承嘏应李石曾之邀，去创办国立北平研究院药物研究所。1927 年，国民党中央政治会议决议设立国立中央研究院，同时在筹备委员李石曾的提议下设立国立北平研究院，形成了一南一北的两个重要的国立科学研究机构。中央研究院院长为蔡元培；北平研究院院长为李石曾。在李石曾的盛情邀请下，赵承嘏出任国立北平研究院药物研究所所长，并继续开展中药研究，在中药延胡索的研究、麻黄副素的药理作用、曼陀罗的化学成分分析、细辛、防己的研究等方面都取得了重要成果。伊博恩应上海雷氏德医学研究院之邀，出任该院生理学部负责人。雷氏德医学研究院为当时国内最大的私立医学研究机构，系根据上海房产商和慈善家亨利·雷士德（Henry Lester，1840 年–1926 年）的遗嘱所创办。研究院设生理部、病理部和临床部。伊博恩在雷氏德医学研究院继续从事中药研究工作，例如他与同事研究了 80 多种《本草纲目》中提到能治疗昏盲的动植物药的化学成分，分析了中药兰草的毒性。它不同于美国的品种，E. urticaefolium 既不产生丙酮尿，也不能作为高血糖症的标志。兔子或豚鼠每天随时消耗的绿色植物的量不会引起致命的作用，但会引起慢性中毒，表现为肝脏坏死，主要是肾小管肾炎，导致虽然没有蛋白尿或高血糖发生却总是有糖尿。研究了中国治疗脚气病中药中的维生素 B_1 的含量等。（大多数植物的种子，特别是车前草的种子，含有大量的维生素。桑叶、枇杷叶和夏枯草也有很高的价值。树皮和草茎的维生素 B_1 含量则很低。）

陈克恢 1925 年就离开了协和，回到威斯康星大学医学院继续其医学教育，1926 年又转到约翰·霍普金斯大学，1927 年获医学博士学位。随后，他在药理学家约翰·阿贝尔（John J. Abel）的实验室任助教并继续开展科研。虽然陈克恢离开了中国，但他对中药研究的热情并未消退，与国内也保持着密切联系。他与赵承嘏等合作，继续开展中药研究，在 1937 年他与赵承嘏在《中华生理学杂志》（Chinese Journal of Physiology）发表了"木防己苏甲与木防己素乙之作用及毒性"（The action and toxicity of menisine and menisidine），1939 年又发表了"钩吻素己的作用方式"，（The mode of action of gelsemicine）以及"钩吻素己对兔子酸碱平衡的作用"（The action of gelsemicine on the acid-base balance in rabbits）等多篇论文。

综上，北京协和医学院药物学系对推动中国近代中药药理研究做出了重要的贡献，所开创的研究方法也为后来的中药研究提供了有益的参考。

参考书目

1. W. Jefferys & J. Maxwell，The Diseases of China，Philadelphia：P. Blakiston's Son &

Co. 1911，p 17.

2. A. W. Douthwaite，Notes on Chinese Materia Medic. CMMJ. 1889. 3（2）：53.

3. Jos. C. Thomson. Chinese Materia Medica：Its Value to Medical Missionaries. CMMJ. 1890. 4（3）：117.

4. A. W. Douthwaite，The Use of Native Drugs by Medical Missionaries. CMMJ. 1890. 4（3）：100.

5. 宋大仁，中西医报，

6. K. K. Chen and Carl F. Schmidt，Ephedrine and related substances. London：The Williams & Wilkins Company，1930. Pp. 76.

7. Tsan-Quo Chou，Poisonous Principles from Chinese Rhododendron，Nao-Yang-Hua，Rhododendron Hunnewellianum，Chinese Journal of Physiology. 1927 1（2）：157.

8. Tsan-Quo Chou The alkaloids of Chinese corydalis ambigua，cham. Et sch.（Yen-hu-so）part 1. Chinese Journal of Physiology. 1928. 2（2）：203.

9. 高怡生，忆上海药物所老所长赵承嘏教授，2009 年 09 月 23 日 11：18：35，新华网 http：//blog. sciencenet. cn/blog－43772－419630. html

Traditional Chinese Medical (TCM) Research at Peking Union Medical College: 1910 – 1941

Zhang Daqing

Zhang Daqing is Professor of History of Medicine and was the former director of the Institute of Medical Humanities at the Center for the History of Medicine, Peking University. He is also the director of the Commission for the History of Medicine, Chinese Society for the History of Science & Technology. His research interests include the cultural and social history of medicine in nineteenth-and twentieth-century china, comparative history, and medical cultures since the late nineteenth century. His recent books include A Social History of Diseases in Modern China (2006), A History of Medicine (2007), and An Introduction to the Medical Humanities (2013).

Medical professionals began using an experimental physiological approach to the study of chemical composition, nature, and pharmacological effects during the 19th Century. However, earlier during the later 18th century, F. Fontana, an Italian naturalist and physiologist, had conducted experimental research into more than a thousand kinds of natural drugs. Fontana's research led him to conclude that active ingredients found in natural drugs can be specific and have a localized pharmacological action on the body. This conclusion was confirmed in 1806 by F. W. Serturner, a German chemist who was the first to isolate morphine from the palavers somniferum L i. e. the opium poppy. Further similar research emerged and the extraction of active ingredients became common place. For example, emetine, a drug now commonly administered to induce vomiting, was first extracted from the ipecac root in 1817. Strychnine was first extracted from semen strychni in 1818, quinine was first extracted from calisaya bark in 1819, and caffeine was extracted from coffee in 1821.

During the late 19th and early 20th century, using chemical procedures to extract active ingredients from medicinal plants and herbs had become an important component in pharmacological research. In addition, medical professionals began to study the effect of drugs on various organs in the body by conducting more rigorous experiments. F. Magendie (1819) confirmed though experimentation that hydrochloric strychnine causes muscular rigidity through the spinal cord. In 1856, C. Bernard identified the location of action for tubocurarine in relaxing the musculus skeleti was the neuromuscular junction. There were many ground breaking achievements in the field during this time, not only in our understanding of drug action and the effects but also in discovering the site of function of specific drugs. These studies based clinical medication in experimental science, while at the same time providing clues for the research and development of new drugs extracted from herbs and plants.

Most of the medical missionaries who came to China in the late nineteenth century and early 20th century had obtained some training in experimental research methods. In addition to their medical practice, some of these doctors were interested in methods of diagnosis and treatment with traditional Chinese medicaments. In the early twentieth century, while some Chinese medical students who had studied abroad began to return to China, Chinese scholars also began to study the pharmacological mechanism and the clinical value of traditional medicines using a modern scientific approach. The recent history of scientific research in TCM can be divided into three stages, and in all of which Peking Union Medical College demonstrated it's own unique contribution.

Stage 1: Recognition, translation and the introduction of TCM

Most medical missionaries in China did not think highly of TCM's medical action, as they commonly believed, "the preparation of these drugs is crude and impure, and their use has little regard for their known therapeutic value. A long list of other mineral preparations is entirely irrational – clam shells, pebbles, chalk, mica, and the like. "[1] There were however some medical missionaries who thought that the therapeutic effect of TCMs was effective, and similar to that of western medication. For example, A. W. Douthwaite pointed out that, "arsenic trisulphide, or 'Orpiment' (Ts'z-hwang) is used by the native doctors, chiefly for external application, and in various compounded arsenical powders, with remarkably fancy names, are in general use for the destruction of morbid growths, in much the same way that 'arsenical pastes' were employed in Europe a few years ago. "[2] In addition, Douthwaite also mentioned that the major components of Peh-kiang-tan, Ch'ing-fen, San-Sin-tan were Hydrargyri Perchloridum, Hydrargyri Subchloridum, and Hydrargyri Oxidum Rubrum.

The scientific value of TCM became one of the interests of medical missionaries in China J. C. Thomson made a comprehensive study of Li Shizhen's master piece – "Compendium of Materia Medica" (*Pen Ts'ao Kang Mu*) and he collected literature on TCM studied by western scholars. He suggested, "We found in China an exhaustless Materia Medica which must prove of great value to us as medical missionaries. Already, we have proven its value. A goodly number of these remedies the Chinese place before us with their properties explained, others in very crude form; but as one has remarked, we have before us an undeveloped mine which only needs to be worked to yield treasures of knowledge. "[3] However, the medical missionaries placed their great interest on the practical value of TCM, especially with the increase in the number of missionary hospitals and the expansion to the inland areas, where western medication was in short supply. Therefore, practitioners needed to supplemented the shortage with locally sourced drugs. A. W. Douthwaite said, "One great hindrance to the establishment of medical missions in the interior is the difficulty — sometimes amounting to impossibility — of transit of the necessary drugs and appliances to those stations far removed from the great waterways, and hence the necessity for finding out, and making use of such native and imported drugs as can be obtained in the country, and considering the possibility of manufacturing out of the crude material at hand, such compounds as we are accustomed to use in the treatment of our patients. " [4]Therefore, in *The China Medical Journal*, many medical missionaries discussed their experiences of using local herbal remedies to treat diseases and that of processing local herbal medicines in order to make western medication. Of all those medical missionaries who came to China in the late 19th century and early 20th century, B. E. Read (1887 – 1949) 's study of TCM was the most comprehensive and in-depth.

B. E. Read was born in Brighton of south Britain on May 17, 1887. In 1909, he graduated from London College of Pharmacy. In 1909, Read was sent by the London Mission Society to Peking Union Medical College (PUMC) . At the college, Read taught materia medica and pharmacology although besides his teaching responsibilities, he began to pay more attention to the daily use of medication in the missionary hospitals in China and listed basic medicaments, essential in hospitals and clinics at the time. In 1915 the Rockefeller Foundation reorganized PUMC, and Read was sent back to the United States, where he was a fellow in biochemistry in the School of Medicine of Johns Hopkins University, University of Chicago, and Harvard University. During this time Read also studied nutrition for a year at Yale University. Then in 1918, B. E. Read returned to PUMC and was appointed associate professor of biochemistry and pharmacology. In 1923 – 24, he returned to Yale University to study and was granted a Ph. D in pharmacology. In 1925, he was promoted to the professor of pharmacology at PUMC. After, returning to Beijing, Read focused on the study of TCM and became one of the chief editors of "*Chinese Journal of Physiology*" (first issued in 1927) .

B. E. Read was committed to the sorting, translation and compiling, and giving notes on TCM literature. One of his articles was represented in the masterpiece *"New notes to materia medica"* co-authored by Liu Ju-chiang, a Chinese botanist. (*"New notes to materia medica"* was also known as *"Flora Sinensis Plantae Medicinalis Sinensis*: *Bibliography of Chinese Medicinal Plants From Pen Ts'ao Kang Mu*, 1596) The words on the flyleaf of the book were written by Jin Shaoji (1886 – 1949), the director of Peking Natural History Society. Zhu Qi Ling, who used to be the acting premier of Beiyang Government, was invited to write the preface for the book, " Li Shizhen was a scholar from grass root, so he did not know the essence of the secrets of traditional medicaments. When testing and drawing pictures of drugs, he failed to describe their shapes and colors according to specific features and qualities. Therefore, the book Pen Ts'ao Kang Mu covered a broad range of Chinese drugs; however, the content about the shape and color was not so exquisite. Professor Read and the Chinese mayor of the capital Liu Ju-chiang studied the natural history for many years. In order to maintain positive communications between Chinese and Western medicine professionals, Read and Liu Ju-chiang sorted the *Pen Ts'ao Kang Mu* into the more commonly understood Angla's method of classification and categorization" He gave high credit to B. E. Read's work.

An understanding of B. E. Read's motivation for this work can be drawn from the foreword he wrote in the book, " The demand for such books is obvious. The differences in the languages and the difference in basic concepts used in the recording of natural history between China and the West resulted in great divergence (between Chinese and Western Medicine). Many of the medicinal plants were claimed to have unquestionable therapeutic effects, although their specific features is still vaguely known. The chemical composition was completely overlooked, and the effect of them on the living cells was not clear, either. " In order to bridge the division between Western and Chinese medicine, Read challenged himself by choosing the most famous book in TCM, *Pen Ts'ao Kang Mu* and made pharmacological and chemical investigation of each of the contents. B. E. Read thereby proposed and adopted the following research method; firstly, he concentrated a large number of samples of various herbs needed to a central laboratory for rigorous and methodical study.

The advantage of "*New notes on Materia Medica*" was that this book not only reviewed medicinal herbs and plants, and the origin of active ingredients and related literature, but also focused on the records of literature around Chinese medicinal plants from other countries. The author included and quoted academic journals, news articles, official government documents, specific books, as well as quotes from the classics from Germany, the United States, UK, Japan, China, France, Sweden, India, and Malaysia. The book became an important reference for the study of TCM herbal medicine and after it was published, it became very popular in the academic community, so much so that not long after Song Daren translated a part of the content of the book into Chinese. The translation was published in the "*Chinese and Western Medicine Newspaper*" in succession under the title "*Bibliography of Research into Chinese Medicinal Plants: the Content of Research in botany, chemistry, pharmacy from the Pen Ts'ao Kang Mu*". Song Daren pointed out: "The book *Pen Ts'ao Kang Mu* is an important book on pharmacology and botany in China. Unfortunately, it is too voluminous, so that most of the people from the old medical society would be daunted by it and could only read its abridged version, such as *the Pen Ts'ao Cong Xin*, or *the Pen Ts'ao Bei Yao*. For those books that have been published at the time of the *Pen Ts'ao Kang Mu*, we have nothing to criticize; however, as for the *Pen Ts'ao* books published in recent years, most of them were just plagiarized, and had been passed through many hands and deviated extensively from the original. If we cannot get rid of the obsolete nest, how could we save the national essence? How regrettable! As the translator, considering that this book is so important for the Chinese and Western medicine society, I feel particularly lament on the fact that the westerners have been studied the Chinese medicine for a long time, while we Chinese are still not knowing it. That's why I decided to translate the book. I hope that it could of help to the people who want to reform the Chinese medicine. "[5]

In addition to the "*New notes on materia medica*", B. E. Read also studied the mineral and animal component of TCM treatments and conducted research according to the different categories. He published, "Animal Drugs" (1931), "Avian Drugs" (1932), "Dragon and snake drugs" (1934), "Minerals and Stones; Turtle and Shellfish Drugs" (1936), "Chinese Medicinal Plants" (1936), "Fish Drugs" (1939), "Insect Drugs" (1941) to name a few. He also wrote the book " Vegetable and Plant Drugs " in 1949 although this book was never published.

Stage 2: Research into the Pharmacology of TCM in modern China

PUMC was the first institution in China to conduct research into the pharmacological action of TCM treatments using modern methods. As mentioned previously, medical missionaries began to pay attention to the practical value of TCM very early, although rigorous experimental research in TCM was not seriously conducted until Chen Ko-kuei came to PUMC. Chen Ko-kuei's uncle was also a TCM practitioner. During his childhood, Chen often came to his uncle's TCM dispensary, so that he became quite interested in TCM. When Chen Ko-kuei studied in the department of pharmacology of University of Wisconsin in the United States, under the support of his supervisor, he conducted an experimental study on the TCM herbal medicine, specifically cinnamon, and he complete the Bachelor's degree thesis based on this research. In 1923, Chen Ko-kuei was granted a doctoral degree and was appointment at PUMC, working as an assistant in the pharmacology department. When he was working at PUMC, he continued his research on TCM. Chen, Schmidt, and Read initiated the study on herbal Tang-kuei.

Tang-kuei appears more frequently in Chinese prescriptions than any other drug except licorice. It is regarded as a valuable remedy in the treatment of menstrual and puerperal disorders and for female sterility, though Tang-kuei is also used for a variety of other conditions. The drug was first introduced into Western medicine in 1899 by Merck in the form of a liquid extract sold under the name of Eumenol, and later in the form of Eumenol tablets. These methods of administering Tang-kuei were recommended for the treatment of menstrual disorders, and results obtained through experimentation were apparently favorable. Chen Ko-kuei and others pointed out that, ' In view of the widespread use of the drug (Tang-kuei) in China, and the successful results reported from its use in Europe in the treatment of uterine disorders, it seemed probable that some definite action on the uterus might be expected from it, as well as some definite active principle. '[6] After a series of experiments, they concluded that, ' Tang-kuei (Angelica polymorpha var sinensis) produces circulatory depression, sometimes followed by stimulation, diuresis (increased rate of urination), and the contraction of smooth muscle of uterus, intestines, bladder, and arteries when injected intravenously in anesthetized dogs and rabbits.

The study of Tang-kuei was mainly to explore its pharmacological mechanism. Unfortunately, while this research was exquisitely done, it failed to extract any effective chemical so the publication of findings did not stimulate much interest. In the same year, Chen Ko-kuei was informed that Chinese ephedra had a positive treatment effect for asthma, and so he began to study the biological action of ephedrine. Within only a few weeks Chen had separated ephedrine from the TCM herbal medicine, Ma Huang, and then he began to study the pharmacological mechanism of ephedrine. Chen found that, ephedrine in suitable doses raises blood pressure, increases cardiac activity, dilates pupils, relieves bronchospasm, contracts the uterus, and more frequently inhibits than stimulates the gastrointestinal tract. These effects can be explained by the stimulation of the myoneural junctions of the sympathetic fibers. [7] In 1924, Chen Ko-kuei and Schmidt published their findings entitled " *The Effect of Ephedrine on Experiment Shock and*

Hemorrhage" in the *Proceedings of the Society for Experimentac Medicine and Biology*. Since then, Chen Ko-kuei and others carried out a series of experimental investigation on ephedrine, and published more than 10 papers. Thus, the study of the TCM ephedrine attracted extensive attention from the pharmaceutical sector mainly because ephedrine was found to have a similar effect as epinephrine, the only difference being that, ephedrine, if taken orally, lasts longer with a lower level of toxicity. As a result, ephedrine became a new sympathomimetic drug attracting much international interest.

During the period, researchers from different countries carried out extensive research on Chinese Ma Huang and ephedrine from different aspects, and over 100 papers were published, initiating an international craze into TCM research. In 1930, ephedrine was recorded in the "*Chinese Pharmacopoeia*", *and* later that year, it was included in the national pharmacopoeia in Japan, the United States, Britain, Russia, to name a few. At the same time, a sympathomimetic analeptic started to be included in textbooks. The research done by Chen Ko-kuei that started from looking for lead compounds from the natural plants, followed by improving and then developed into new drugs successfully established an innovative good example for the research in herbal medicine.

In 1923 – 1924, B. E. Read went to Yale University for a fellowship and obtained his Ph. D. in pharmacology and he studied pathology at the University of Chicago. In 1925, B. E. Read returned to PUMC and succeeded Schmidt to be the Dean of the pharmacology department. Under his leadership, the pharmacology department of PUMC published more than ten pharmacological research papers on ephedrine and related chemical compounds in 1927 – 1933. Working with Lim Chiao-chih, T. Q. Chou, Feng C. T. , and Phu Chu-ping, B. E. Read studied the pharmacological features of other TCM treatments, gaining further fame for PUMC's research （see Table 1）.

Table 1：Research papers related to TCM published by the pharmacology department of PUMC on "*Chinese Journal of Physiology*"（1927 - 1941）

Time	Authors	Title
1927	B. E. Read, Ch'iao-Chih Lin	Anesthetic mixtures of ephedrine and procaine with adrenaline and potassium sulphate
1927	Chih-Tung Feng	A method for preparing pure ephedrine hydrochloride from ephedraequisetina
1927	B. E. Read, GeorgeK. How	The iodine, arsenic, iron, calcium and sulphur content of Chinese medicinal algae
1927	Tsan-Quo Chou	Poisonous Principles from Chinese Rhododendron, Nao-Yang-Hua, Rhododendron Hunnewellianum
1927	Kuo-Hao Lin, Chao-Chi Chen	Chemical analysis of sea slug, Stichopus japonicus Selenka（Hai Shen）
1927	Tsan-Quo Chou	Sikimitoxin, the toxic principle of Illicium Religiosum, Sieb. Mang-T'sao
1927	B. E. Read, Chih-Tung Feng	Psedoephedrine from Chinese ephedra
1927	B. E. Read	The relative toxicity of the halogen compounds of Chaulmoogra.
1927	Chih-Tung Feng	The " Biuret Reaction " as applied qualitatively and quantitatively to ephedrine mixtures
1927	Tse King, Chub-Yung Pak	A study of the effect of ephedrine on the nasal mucous membranes
1928	Chub-Yung Pak, B. E. Read	A comparative study of the boldpressor action of ephedrine, psedoephedrine and adrenaline

Time	Authors	Title
1928	Chih-Tung Feng, B. E. Read	A comparison of ephedraequisetina and E. sinica and their seasonal content of ephedrine
1928	Chih-Teh Loo, B. E. Read	Perfusion experiments with psedoephedrine and ephedrine
1928	Tsan-Quo Chou	The alkaloids of Chinese corydalisambigua, cham. Et sch. (Yen-hu-so) part 1.
1928	Chih-Tung Feng, B. E. Read	Further assays of Chineseephedras
1928	Chub-Yung Pak, B. E. Read	Comparative study of ephedrine, racemic ephedrine andpsedoephedrine
1929	Tsan-Quo Chou	The alkaloids of Corydalisambigua, cham et sch. Part Ⅱ. Corydalis F, G and H.
1929	Chub-Yung Pak, B. E. Read	Comparative studies of ephedrine, racemic ephedrine andpsedoephedrine Ⅱ. Comparative toxicity
1929	Tse King, Chub-Yung Pak	Comparative studies of ephedrine, racemic ephedrine andpsedoephedrine Ⅲ. Effects on the nasal mucous membranes
1929	Hsi-Chun Chang	The action of choline, adrenaline and ephedrine on gastric motility
1929	S. H. Li Jest Rand	The action ofpsedoephedrine Ⅰ. On the isolated uterus and bladder.
1929	Chub-Yung Pak, B. E. Read	The action ofpsedoephedrine Ⅱ. Its diuretic effects
1929	Tsan-Quo Chou	The alkaloids of Chinese Corydalisambigua, cham. Et sch (Yen-hu-so). Part Ⅲ. Corydalis Ⅰ and monomethyl ethers of Corydalis F and G

Time	Authors	Title
1930	Chub-Yung Pak, Tse King	The action of ephedrine andpsedoephedrine upon bronchial muscle
1931	Tsan-Quo Chou	The alkaloids of Chinesegelsemium, Kou Wen, Gelsemium elegans
1932	Hsiang-Ch'uan Hou	The pharmacological action ofgelsemicine Ⅲ. Action on circulation
1932	B. E. Read	The effect of benzyl-ephedrine on blood pressure
1932	Hsiang-Ch'uan Hou	Action of ephedrine and related substances on the bloodvesselsxx
1932	T. Q. Chou	The alkaloids of Chinese drug Pei-mu, fritillaria roylei Part Ⅰ. Peimine and peiminine
1932	Hsiang-Ch'uan Hou	The pharmacological action ofgelsemicine Ⅳ. Action on intestine, uterus and urinary bladder
1933	Chub-Yung Pak, B. E. Read	Action of ephedrine on the portal circulation
1933	Chub-Yung Pak, T. K. Tang	The mechanism of themydriatic antion of ephedrine
1935	C. H. Wang, M. P. Chen	Effect of scopolamine and atropine on the muscle tonus increased by passive movements in a post-encephalitic parkinsonism patient
1938	T. P. Feng	Further observations on the propagation ofveratrine contracture
1940	F. T. Dun, T. P. Feng	Studies on the neuromuscular junction XIX. Rereograde discharges from motor nerve endings in veratrinized muscle

Time	Authors	Title
1941	T. P. Feng, T. H. Li	Studies on the neuromuscular junction XXIV. the repetitive discharges of mammalian motor nerve endings after treatment withveratrine, barium and guanidine
1941	T. P. Feng	The production of prolonged after-discharge in nerve byveratrine

Of all the 88 research papers related to TCM published on " *Chinese Journal of Physiology* " in 1927 – 1948, 37 articles were contributed to by the researchers of the pharmacology department of PUMC, followed by two other institutions – National Academy of Peiping (北平研究院) and Institute of Materia Medica of Chinois-Franco University (中法大学药物研究所), as well as Henry Lester Institute of Medical Research in Shanghai, although primary researchers from these institutions all trained extensively within the pharmacology department of PUMC.

Stage 3: Experimental research into the chemistry of Chinese materia medica

T. Q. Chou was a pioneer in the study of chemical composition of TCM. T. Q. Chou, called himself Shimin, and was from Jiangyin County of Jiangsu Province. Born on December 11, 1885, he received a bachelor's degree from the University of Manchester in 1910 and a master's degree from the Swiss Institute of Technology in 1912. After graduation, Shimin was transferred to the university of Geneva, Switzerland, and continued studying under the guidance of Professor A. Pictet, a famous natural organic chemist at that time. In 1914, he defended his Ph. D thesis and became a lecturer shortly after graduation. In 1916, T. Q. Chou was employed in the research department of Roche pharmaceutical manufacturer in France, and was later promoted to director of the research department. Shimin's family owned a shop and sold natural remedies, and so he was familiar with TCM from an early age. This had a profound influence on his later study on Chinese herbal medicine. In 1925, T. Q. Chou was further promoted to professor of pharmacochemistry concurrently acting as the director of pharmacology department. There, he began his research into Chinese herbal drugs, and studied the chemical composition of ma huang, Chinese corydalis ambigua, illicium anisatum L., fritillaria and gelsmium elegans, and published a number of papers – the pioneer in chemical research of Chinese herbal medicine.

At the beginning of 20th century, although the organic chemistry had advanced, and chemists emphasized the study of phytochemistry, China at that time had not adopted the scientific method to systematically study the Chinese herbal medicine. Chou implemented modern chemical methods conducting systematic research into ancient Chinese herbal drugs, making outstanding contributions to the exploration and improvement of TCM treatments, as well as training a large number of academic leaders who formed the backbone of the modern TCM community.

T. Q. Chou attached great importance to laboratory work and rigorous experimental techniques. In his long-standing research in the laboratory, he accumulated rich experiences in the fractional crystallization of phytochemistry, especially of alkaloids. Chou also created a unique isolation method where toxins were first isolated from Rhododendron molle.[8] At that time, the classic method for isolating plants' active ingredient was done using ethanol, so that the composition of the crude extract was complex and not easily purified for the crystallization. Considering that the plants' active ingredients are mostly alkaloids, Chou used a method of alkaline leaching and benzene grinding according to the characteristics of alkaloids, so that the composition of the extracted was less complex which greatly reduced the degree of difficulty of further isolation of monomers.

Chou also designed different methods according to different research subjects. He and his students systematically studied the chemical composition of more than 30 kinds of Chinese herbal drugs, such as: Tripterygium wilfordii, herba asari, pseudo-ginseng, fritillaria, Radix Dichroae, Stephania tetrandra, Chinese Corydalis ambigua, Gelsmium elegans and Chinese ephedra, and obtained a lot of monomer crystallization of new alkaloids, making it possible for the pharmacology researchers to select the valuable ones to suggest for clinical trials for further development. In this way, they established a set of scientific methods for the country to assort the TCM systematically. At the same time, Chou and his students published a number of papers in the prestigious journals home and abroad, attracting great attention and appreciation by Chinese and foreign scholars.

Using the set of isolation and extraction method invented by himself, Chou was able to isolate a variety of crystals from one plant, making contributions to the phytochemistry. For example, he carried out a series of studies on Chinese Corydalis ambigua. He was the first one to isolate five kinds of alkaloids from plants,"From the tubers of Chinese Corydalis ambigua, Cham, et Sch. (Yen-hu-so) five alkaloids have up to now been isolated from the non-phenolic fraction which were provisionally named Corydalis A, Corydalis B, Corydalis C, Corydalis D and Corydalis E. One of which is identical with Corydaline and the other four were new."[9]By 1936, he isolated at total of 13 types of alkaloids of Chinese Corydalis ambigua.

In addition, Chou also isolated 7 kinds of crystalline alkaloids from different varieties of Gelsmium elegans and from Radix Dichroae he obtained 3 kinds of isomers that could be converted to each other under certain conditions. T. Q. Chou's extraction method played an important role in the international phytochemistry. He extracted the crystalline diosgenin of pseudo-ginseng and proved that it was the same with panoxadiol in terms of compound, 20 years ahead of the study made by the famous Japanese chemists who isolated panoxadiol from Panax ginseng.

T. Q. Chou also reinvestigated some of the studies into a few Chinese herbal drugs which had been studied before and succeeded in isolating new ingredients from them. For example, from Ma Huang he isolated the new alkaloid pseudoephedrine, from Datura stramonium he isolated the new alkaloids such as Mandarin celery and Mandala. Every time Chou obtained an alkaloid, he would do detailed pharmacological testing. For example, as for the Dichroine C isolated from the Radix Dichroae, its antimalarial effect was 148 times of that of quinine; and the Corydalis B isolated from the Chinese Corydalis ambigua was already been administered in clinical practice as analgesics and sedative. It became the new drug created in China and is included in the Pharmacopoeia of People's Republic of China

Concluding remarks

After 1932, due to a variety of factors, scholars from the pharmacology department of PUMC, who had made important contributions to the research of the TCM drugs left PUMC in succession. Invited by Li Shizeng（李石曾）, T. Q. Chou left to establish the Institute of Materia Medica of National Academy of Peiping. In 1927, the Kuomintang Central Political Conference decided to set up the Academia Sinica, at the same time under the proposal of Li Shizeng, a member of an ad hoc committee, to establish the National Academy of Peiping, resulting in two important national scientific research institutions, one in the south, and the other one in the north of China. Cai Yuanpei was the director of Academia Sinica, while Li Shizeng headed the National Academy of Peiping. Responding to Li Shizeng's warm invitation, Chou took up the offer and became the Director of the Institute of Materia Medica of National Academy of Peiping（国立北平研究院药物研究所所长）and continued research of TCM treatments, making important achievements in the study of in Chinese Corydalis ambigua, the pharmacological effects of pseudoephedrine, the analysis of the chemical composition of Datura stramonium, as well as of herba asari and Stephania tetrandra.

Invited by Shanghai Henry Lester Institute of Medical Research, B. E. Read became the director of the institution's department of physiology. Henry Lester Institute of Medical Research was the largest private medical research institution at that time in China, which was founded according to the will of Henry Lester (1840 – 1926), a real estate businessman and philanthropist in Shanghai. There were three department at the institute; department of physiology, department of pathology and clinical department. B. E. Read continued to conduct research into TCM drugs at the institute. For example, he and his colleagues studied the chemical composition of more than 80 types of medicinal herbs and animal drugs mentioned in the *Pen Ts'ao Kang Mu* that could treat the nyctalopia and analyzed the toxicity of Chinese eupatorium. E. chinense, Lan-t'sao has been studied. It differs from the American species, E. urticaefolium is not producing acetonuria or marked hyperglycemia. The amount of green plant readily consumed daily by rabbits or guinea pigs does not cause fatal effects but produces a chronic poisoning, showing necrotic degeneration of the liver and mainly tubular nephritis, as a result glycosuria invariably occurs without albuminuria or hyperglycemia. What is more, a number of Chinese plant remedies for beriberi have been analyzed for vitamin B1. Most of the seeds, especially that of plantain, contain significant quantities of the vitamin. The values for mulberry leaf, loquat leaf and carpenter weed are also high. The vitamin B1 content of their barks and stems is low.

Chen Ko-kuei left PUMC in 1925 and returned to the Medical School of the University Of Wisconsin to continue his medical education. In 1926, he was transferred to the Johns Hopkins University. In 1927 he obtained a MD there. Subsequently, as an assistant teacher at pharmacologist John J. Alber's lab and continued his scientific research. Although Chen Ko-kuei left China, his passion for the research of TCM drugs continued, and he maintained close contact with colleagues in China, cooperating with T. Q. Chou and continuing research into TCM drugs. In 1937, he and Chou coauthored and published "*The action and toxicity of menisine and menisidine*" on the *Chinese Journal of Physiology*. In 1939, he published "*The mode of action of gelsemicine*", "*The action of gelsemicine on the acid-base balance in rabbits*", and others.

Above all, the pharmacology department of PUMC has made important contributions to the promotion of pharmacology research into TCM drugs in recent history in China, and the research methods invented were also instrumental in the development of TCM drug research throughout the world.

Bibliography

1. W. Jefferys & J. Maxwell. *The diseases of China*. Philadelphia: P. Blakiston's Son & Co. 1911, p 17.

2. A. W. Douthwaite. *Notes on Chinese materia medic.* CMMJ. 1889. 3 (2): 53.

3. Jos. C. Thomson. *Chinese materia medica: its value to medical missionaries.* CMMJ. 1890. 4 (3): 117.

4. *A. W. Douthwaite. The use of native drugs by medical missionaries. CMMJ. 1890. 4 (3): 100.*

5. 宋大仁, 中西医报 (*Chinese and Western medicine*)

6. Carl F. Schmidt, B. E. Read, and K. K. Chen. *Experiments with Chinese drugs.* The China Medical Journal. 1924. 38 (5): 362 – 375.

7. K. K. Chen and Carl F. Schmidt. *Ephedrine and related substances.* London: The Williams & Wilkins Company, 1930. Pp. 76.

8. Tsan-Quo Chou. *Poisonous principles from Chinese rhododendron, Nao-yang-hua, rhododendron hunnewellianum.* Chinese Journal of Physiology. 1927 1 (2): 157.

9. Tsan-Quo Chou. *The alkaloids of Chinese corydalis ambigua, cham. Et sch. (yen-hu-so)* part 1. Chinese Journal of Physiology. 1928. 2 (2): 203.

斯乃博：二战时期在北京协和医学院的荷兰医生

阿瑞尔·波尔格浩特 (Arie Berghout)

阿瑞尔·波尔格浩特 (Arie Berghout)，医学顾问，内分泌专家，在荷兰鹿特丹的一所大型教学医院担任内科主任，并担任医学、护理和辅助医学学科研究生培训和教育部主任。他是荷兰医学协会成员及年度大会主席，荷兰教学医院教育质量管理委员会委员。2012 年退休后，他开始撰写内科医生斯乃博 (Isidore Snapper) (1889 – 1973) 的传记，将于 2017 年发表。他现任荷兰医学协会历史委员会主席，荷兰 Urk 荷兰医学史中心和医学史图书馆管理委员。

斯乃博 (Isidore Snapper) 来自阿姆斯特丹。1939 年至 1942 年，他在北京协和医学院（简称"协和"）担任内科教授。来中国前，斯乃博是阿姆斯特丹大学的内科学教授，阿姆斯特丹大学是当时荷兰最重要的医学中心。超过半数的荷兰医学生在阿姆斯特丹接受培养。1919 年，时年 30 岁的斯乃博成为医学教授。他在医学期刊上用荷兰语、德语、英语发表过 200 多篇论文，出版过骨科方面的书籍，还与人合著荷兰的医学教科书，在荷兰乃至整个欧洲享有很高的知名度。此外，他还是一名成功的足球裁判。

那么，为什么斯乃博要放弃自己在荷兰的辉煌事业，离开祖国和家人，不远万里来到中国呢？毕竟远在亚洲的中国与荷兰迥异，而且斯乃博并不会说一句中文；何况从 1937 年起中国动荡不安，包括他即将工作的协和医院所在地——北京在内的广大区域都被日军占领，旅程注定危险重重，恐怖与战乱将伴随其职业生涯；在中国当时的首都南京无数人被残杀，城市毁于一旦，饥荒、抢劫和瘟疫不时发生。他究竟是为何决定来中国呢？

北京协和医学院是坐落在北京的一所由纽约洛克菲勒基金会出资建立的美国医院，它并非一所普通的医学院，而是被视作洛克菲勒基金会"王冠上的明珠"。这所医学院不以培养普通的医生和护士为目的，而以培养中国未来的医学精英、培养能够解决中国健康问题的教师和领导者为目标。它致力于为中国引进"西方医学的精华"，希望能够与欧美顶尖大学相比肩。[1]因此，北京协和医学院以重视学生质量而非数量为原则，选拔非常严格，录取人数很少。预科学习包括中文、英语、法语或德语、生物、化学和物理。初步筛选后，学生们需参加随后的录取选拔考试。[2]对于斯乃博这样一个雄心勃勃的人，协和无疑是他的不二的选择。

被誉为"中国的约翰·霍普金斯大学"的北京协和医学院，以享有美国医学界盛誉的模范医学院为样板建立，难道这就是吸引斯乃博及其他先于他来到协和执教的美国教授的原因吗？在过去，协和吸引了许多医生来担任一年或更长时间的教授，甚至成为一名正式员工。许多知名学者，如来自哈佛医学院的生理学家凯恩农（Walter Cannon）［他继承克劳德·博纳德（Claude Bernard）的观点，在其代表作——《身体的智慧》（The Wisdom of the Body）一书中提出稳态的概念］和身兼细菌学家、免疫学家、作家为一身的辛瑟尔（Hans Zinsser）以及来自纽约康奈尔大学的欧匹（Eugene Opie）都曾担任过协和的客座教授。[3]

当然，还有一个重要因素吸引斯乃博来中国。斯乃博非常了解洛克菲勒基金会。洛克菲勒基金会的代表曾经在阿姆斯特丹拜访过斯乃博并资助了他的甲状腺研究；斯乃博在美国参观大学和医院时也曾经拜访过洛克菲勒基金会。任教于一所美国大学一直是斯乃博的心愿。此外，中国的工作似乎没有斯乃博在阿姆斯特丹的职位那么严格，因此他希望来到中国后有更多的时间做科研。

不过，斯乃博接受在中国职位还有个更加迫切的原因。他是犹太人。希特勒当权后，德国的反犹太人势力迅速发展，并如同瘟疫一般向整个欧洲蔓延。许多犹太人逃离德国和奥地利，其中有很多医生逃至荷兰。斯乃博是救助犹太流亡者的委员会成员。1938 年春天，他前往维也纳参加会议，亲身感受了 1938 年 3 月奥地利向纳粹德国投降、德奥合并后反犹太人的风潮。1938 年 3 月 20 日，斯乃博写了如下信件给洛克菲勒基金会驻巴黎代表丹尼尔·欧布瑞恩（Daniel O'Brien）：

> 您很可能体会近来欧洲发生的事件多么令我震惊，尤其我在维也纳的许多最好的同事所遭受的特别待遇。这些天发生的事情在我心头愈发沉重，以至于我想放弃我在这里的工作，逃离欧洲越远越好。尽管在荷兰还没有丝毫反犹太人的迹象。但这几年来，我已经开始考虑在美国或澳大利亚寻找一个全职的教学或研究岗位……[4]

欧布瑞恩将斯乃博的信件转交给了纽约洛克菲勒基金会的负责人："阿姆斯特丹的斯乃博希望得到一份内科学的全职工作，我猜测原因可能与反犹太人主义引起了其不安情绪。他是所有西欧国家中最有才干的内科学家之一。"

1938 年 5 月，斯乃博收到了北京的工作邀请，没过多久他便决定接受这个职位。他离开没多久，1938 年 6 月，由于纳粹的种族主义法律，与他相交甚厚的维也纳同事被永远禁止行医。1938 年 11 月 9 日晚，"水晶之夜"事件在德语国家爆发，大量犹太人的房屋和商店被损毁，无辜的犹太公民被袭击并被投入监狱。斯乃博离开欧洲的决定无比正确。

斯乃博和妻子海迪（Hetty）在离开荷兰之前，他们将自己三个子女中的 2 个送往美国。他们最小的女儿艾莉丝（Elisie）在纽约由斯乃博的同事照顾，他们的儿子厄恩斯特（Ernst）在普林斯顿学习数学，而他们最大的儿子福利兹（Frits）正在服兵役所以没有离开荷兰。

去中国的旅程

为抵达中国，斯乃博环球航行了 50 天。他们首先坐船到英国。他们已经订好票，本打算从英国南部港口城市南安普顿（Southampton）乘坐蒸汽轮船"罗斯福总统号"前往纽约。然而由于暴风雪阻隔，他们无法从伦敦抵达南安普顿，他们只得改乘下一班前往美国的英国皇家邮政船"法兰克尼亚号"（Franconia），该船于 1923 年在格拉斯哥（Glasgow）为观纳德航线公司（Gunard Line）建造的。在纽约，他们受到了洛克菲勒基金会负责基金会亚洲事务的机构——罗氏驻华医社（China Medical Board）的热情欢迎。纽约后的旅程是经由加拿大太平洋铁路抵达温哥华，接着从温哥华乘船到达亚洲。然而，他们又遇到暴风雪，行程不得不再次延期。1939 年 1 月 21 日，他们乘加拿大太平洋公司的"俄国女皇号"前往日本横滨，接着搭乘火车抵达神户，从神户乘船到中国北方的港口城市天津。最后，他们再次乘火车到达北京。他们本可以途径上海走较短的路线，但是由于霍乱暴发被劝阻了。

抵达北京时，这个城市热闹、肮脏、拥挤不堪。胡同里的北京居民生活极其穷苦，而在市区人民也拥挤在一起。斯乃博一家需要适应与荷兰截然不同的气候，另外当时正是战时，尽管日本军队尚未干扰协和医院的运转，但日本军队在大街小巷处处可见，总是让人感到祸患随时有可能发生。

斯乃博一家在北京无亲无故。在中国，作为犹太人又意味着什么呢？北京没有犹太人社区，在哈尔滨、香港和上海情况则不同。特别是在上海，成千上万的来自欧洲的犹太移民抵达上海并受到欢迎，没有受到任何限制也无需签证。[5]另外，斯乃博一家是否了解中国文化呢？事实上，斯乃博一家在北京受到了非常热烈的欢迎。协和举办了接待会，欢迎斯乃博以及同时到任的另外两位教授——来自芝加哥、曾在柏林和莱比锡学习的产科医生韦达科（Frank Whitacre）和来自密歇根的神经学家希尔（Theron Hill）。[6]协和给他们分配了一套公寓，坐落在邻近故宫的协和医学院的宿舍大院中，在协和工作的绝大多数外籍员工都住在这里。

北京协和医学院

协和并不是美国在中国建立的第一所医院，但却是当之无愧最好的医院。起初，西医通过多个教派的传教士传入中国。[7]法国和英国的医生早就来到中国，英国人在汉口教授医学，[8]美国教会在苏州和济南开办了医学校，[9]耶鲁大学在中国中部湖南的省会长沙建立了医学院和医院——"湘雅"。[10]

　　20世纪初，洛克菲勒基金会涉足中国医学领域。美国人的内心深处相信自己应当成为中国人的榜样，而中国人也希望在多年之后像美国人一样。美国人希望在这个过程中担任领导者，最终将中国变为基督教国家。而像洛克菲勒这样的富豪家族应该在其中起作用。[11]

　　协和成为全中国医疗健康体系的大计划的一部分，或者更确切地说，是要一劳永逸地建立中国医疗健康体系。当时，获得西方学位的医生与居民的比例大约为一比十五万。[12]事实上，中国一直只认同传统中医。美国人认为这种状况亟需改变，这不仅仅出于他们相信中国人就该改变，同时还夹杂着经济的原因。贫穷且欠发达的中国，医疗卫生欠缺，能成为好的贸易伙伴吗？同样，中国自身对于西医的接受也不仅是因为西医知识和研究的巨大发展，还因为西方的公共卫生与健康知识在中国根本就没有形成。[13]1940年斯乃博到中国时，中国的人均寿命只有30岁，而当时美国的人均寿命已经超过了60岁。[14]由于持续多年的内战、自然灾害、饥荒和糟糕的医疗体系，中国十分落后，被称为"东亚病夫"。传染病也四处肆虐，1930到1940年代流行的主要疾病是痢疾、霍乱、斑疹伤寒和天花。在大城市，肺结核、呼吸道感染和脑血管疾病则十分猖獗。那时的中国只有10%的人口有文化。[15]

　　北京协和医学院的医学课程是由福莱克斯纳（Simon Flexner）和韦尔奇（William Welch）设计的，前者是纽约洛克菲勒医学研究所的负责人，后者则是巴尔的摩约翰·霍普金斯医学院的微生物学家及教授。他们知道如何吸引美国知名大学的教授来协和任教。[16]除了斯乃博之外，还有两位荷兰人也到访了协和。1924年，荷兰脑科学研究院的凯普尔斯（C. U. Ariens Kappers）来到协和担任客座教授，解剖学教授福顿

（A. B. Droogleever Fortuyn）则在北京欢迎了斯乃博一行的到来。

科研与人员

北京协和医学院的科研条件十分出色，有最新的实验室和藏书丰富的图书馆。当时开展的科研项目与酸碱平衡、胃酸分泌、传染性疾病、蓖麻碱毒性及肾上腺分泌的应激激素肾上腺素有关，并在国际上发表了研究成果。有天赋的协和华人毕业生能够有机会去美国继续深造，并有机会在美国开始职业生涯，比如在纽约西奈山医院工作过的、以研究痛风与尿酸闻名的专家郁采蘩。刘士豪曾与斯乃博合作撰写过几篇论文，之后刘士豪成为维生素 D 缺乏和骨质软化症——当时中国的两种常见病的专家。最终，刘士豪成为了北京协和医学院的教授。无可置疑的是，正是在北京协和医学院，在中国殿堂里开展了西方医学。[17]

尽管一切听起来是那么完美，但也有一些批评的声音。北京协和医学院是精英主义者，其教育也太西化，学生选拔太严格，规模也太小。协和的教育并没有与中国社会接轨，培养的医生和护士也比较缺乏实践经验。[18]

协和的美国模式，令斯乃博并不需要学习中文。协和的语言环境为英文。重要的是把学生培养为一流的医生，而英语是国际科学界使用主要语言。协和的员工遵循洛克菲勒的理念——全职教职及与之相匹配的薪水，这使得他们无需也无法私下开业赚取外快补贴生活，他们能够将所有的时间和精力用于教学、照顾病人和做研究。医院每年接受大约六千人入院，门诊量两万余人。协和内科拥有近一百张床位：35 张接收男性患者，12 张接收女性患者，11 张用于代谢性疾病研究，20 张用于传染病研究，剩余 20 张为高级患者服务。

1940 年，北京协和医学院有 250 名医学生和 80 名护理学生，他们大多来自于北京和周边北方省份。由于处于战争状态下，中国南方与北京的联系很难维系。这就是斯乃博来到北京时的状况，在随后的几年里他们一直没有离开北京。

由于协和规定将逐渐聘用更多的华人医生加入到岗位中，医院的雇员主要由华人医生组成，而他们又都是协和培养的。在林宗杨的任期内，来自西方的医生大幅减少。在协和早期，西方医生与中国医生的比例为22∶9，斯乃博抵达时比例已经降为10∶109，在所有教授中有 7 名西方教授、7 名中国教授。[19]当然，北京协和医学院西方医生数量的减少与当时中国被日本占领、西方人来中国的兴趣减弱有关。

当时在协和工作的几个西方雇员有：校长胡恒德，他负责向位于纽约的洛克菲勒基金会负责中国工作的罗氏驻华医社报告，还有来自美国加利福尼亚的药理学家安迪生（Hamilton Anderson）。此外还有之后成为罗氏驻华医社负责人的外科医生娄克斯（Harold Loucks）、明尼苏达大学的儿科专家麦克库瑞（Irvine McQuarrie）、皮肤科医生傅瑞斯（Chester Frazier，后赴波士顿麻省总医院任职）以及来自瑞士的寄生虫学家何博礼（Reinhard Hoeppli）。[20]

在医院

斯乃博的前任狄瑞德（Francis Dieuaide）是一个和蔼谦逊、总是喜欢提问引发讨论而不直接给出临床解决方案的人。简言之，典型的美国自下而上的大学文化。斯乃博的个性则与他相反是一个老派的教授，标准的德国“枢密型教授”，他表现出极强的信心、权威、不容置疑，体现出欧洲自上而下的文化。斯乃博的风格很受中国学生的欢迎，他学识渊博，面对临床问题直接提供解决方案、作出诊断，作风坚决果断。[21]

斯乃博来到协和时，他脑子里在想些什么呢？他在《中国给西医的教材：北京协和医学院对地域医学的贡献》一书中记录了当时心境，如下：

显然，对于移植到中国北方的西方临床医生而言，要处理许多问题，这在他来东方之前是不会想到的。幸运的是，北平协和医学院内科为粗枝大叶的人做了许多细致的安排，以免初来乍到的人陷到诸多麻烦事里……

员工中有华人，他们有着丰富的医学临床经验。而且，只要您不过于傲慢或固执的话，很容易就能从他们温和礼貌的话语中捕捉到诊疗的线索……[22]

员工和住院医师一起努力工作，只要新手能够注意犯错时其他人的语调的变化及脸上细微的吃惊的表情，就足以让新手避免太离谱的错误……

斯乃博教授非常小心地不犯错误、不说蠢话，他惯于不暴露出自己的弱点。对此，他的策略是承认自己不是万事通，不狂妄自大，注意观察中国医生的表现，观察他们的语气和面部表情。他意识到自己孤零零一个人来到了中国，然而在中国，超然独立的人不能被当作一个真正的人，中国人只知道社会人，人类是社会动物。[23]

直面中医

斯乃博来到中国时，中医主要基于传统、教义和其适应性。与之相反，西医，特别是协和所开展的西医是建立在实验和革新基础之上。[24]中医的传统是："五行"、"阴阳"两极，运用针灸、艾叶，重视患者的病史和家族背景，把脉，观察患者的眼睛。从外部传入的佛教和草药也影响着中国。斯乃博对传统中医没有特别的好感，相反，中医的观点与他对于医学的看法甚至相左。例如，中医反对尸检，而在斯乃博看来，这是医学教育中不可或缺的组成，正如他早年在荷兰北部格罗宁根（Groningen）所接受的教育一样，这也是19世纪教学医院的法则。[25]此外，可以帮助做出最后诊断的放射性仪器也很受限。根据儒家哲学，身体发肤受之于父母，在去世后，尸体应该完整地入土为安。由于去世者的家属通常不会同意医院对去世者进行尸检，所以医生们大多会在患者入院时询问这个问题，只是备用。

尽管如此，斯乃博依然在中国找到了自己的位置，这是因为他关于人的法则承袭自他在格罗宁根的老师——西家门·凡·邓波尔（Hijamans van den Bergh），其与中医的人体是一个整体的观点十分接近。[26]

中医的望、闻、问、切对于做出最后的诊断十分重要。[27]斯乃博在这些技能上很高超，而且他不仅仅能够把脉，还非常仔细地检查患者身体的其他部分——整个身体。重要的是，斯乃博同样也会询问患者家庭的情况，作为他诊疗的重要考量。这在中国十分重要，因为在中国，患者的家人在决定患者的最终治疗方案上常常有很大的发言权。

此外，西医也有一些与传统中医共同的观点。从根本上讲，传统中医的本体论认为，由于一些本身并无大碍的微小生物从外界进入人体内，从而在功能理论上说，人体内的各种关系和进程被扰乱而导致了疾病。显而易见，这个观点与生化过程一致，与斯乃博生物化学的背景相吻合：他曾是《德国生物化学杂志》（Biochemische Zeitschrift）的编委，该期刊在生物化学领域享誉世界。

除了这些考虑外，西医和中医能够相处并在这个国家共存与发展——尽管20世纪初中国混乱不堪，[28]但还有另一个因素可以解释中国人对西医的接纳。1910年，在抗击东北鼠疫大暴发的过程中，西医发挥了重要作用。没有外来的帮助，中医很难对抗这次瘟疫。尽管与民意相左，但在隔离了大量感染者后，疫情的蔓延停止了。清朝皇帝甚至允许了尸体火化，这在当时的中国是闻所未闻的。[29]

斯乃博与学生

学生们对斯乃博在医院的各科病房教学热情很高。他在病房教学不同寻常，令人印象深刻。[30]与传统上对待老师的态度一样，学生们非常尊敬斯乃博。在中国，老师与学生的关系类似父子或君臣关系，这种关系建立在尊敬和服从基础之上。[31]在学生们看来，斯乃博是个真正的教授，秃顶——这说明他每天挑灯夜战；此外，他佩戴一副眼镜，这表明他阅读各种科学文献，连字体很小的脚注也不放过；最后，他大腹便便，这清晰地证明他常常受邀为富裕患者们诊治疾病。

1940 年，罗氏驻华医社的主席罗本斯丁（Edwin Lobenstine）访问北京，他写了一篇热情洋溢的报告给纽约总部：

> 医学院很欣赏斯乃博，他本身也对医学院怀有热情。他喜欢这里的工作，因为在这所学院教授是全职基础上给付薪水，不需要依赖在外执业补贴家用。他喜欢中国人也受到中国人的爱戴。每周他都要做讲座，讲述其在诊断某些疑难杂症上的方法，总是座无虚席，来听讲座的人甚至挤进了隔壁的房间，所有中国教师、医学生和许多护士都来旁听，他是一位杰出的讲者。[32]

1939 年 6 月 4 日星期天，很有纪念意义，斯乃博受邀在毕业典礼上向学生们致辞：

> 我的同胞——18 世纪荷兰莱顿（Lyden）著名的医学教授波尔哈福（Boerhaave）的座右铭是："简洁是所有真知灼见的标志。"这句箴言值得被我们所有人永远铭记。即使在这个专业分科的时代，观察病人仍然是诊断最重要的手段，简单的治疗方法可以治愈大多数可治疾病。首先，我想请各位铭记，应用简单方法甚至比使用现代的诊疗设备更加困难。奇妙的是，它比使用复杂的机器需要更多的技能和实践。比如，我们可以考虑使用心电图诊断冠状动脉血栓或使用 X 光诊断十二指肠溃疡。但实际操作中，我们通常只通过详细地询问病史、做体格检查，就能做出诊断；当然，少数情况下，使用更复杂的检查方法是有必要的，以便确保我们诊断的准确性。但是做心电图或拍 X 光总是比询问病史更加简单。为了获得完整的病史，有必要探寻患者的个性。要想做细致的体格检查，就需要有安静的环境以保证医生能够全神贯注。所有这些显然比使用现代化的仪器更加困难，需要比操作仪器更多的技能与能力。
>
> 我想要着重强调的是，理解患者的心理对于成功的医疗实践具有重要

意义。也许我们常常并没有意识到，生病入院并不仅仅是简单的医学问题，更代表一个人的悲剧经历。根据我个人的经验，与在医院围墙之外相比，我们在医院内部并不能够敏锐地感受到病人与疾病相伴的心理问题以及其心理的悲伤。只有我们身处患者家中，才能够深切地感受到家庭成员的疾病会给整个家庭带来怎样的不幸。

一位著名的医生曾说，医生不能总是如其所愿治愈病人，但常常能够减轻病人痛苦且总是能够去安慰病人。医生在治愈病人的英雄行为之外，也常常遇到不可治愈的病人，他们在去世之前不得不经历一段被病痛折磨的痛苦的时日。每一天，病人们都在期待医生的探望，作为医生，我们能够通过话语给予他们精神支持缓解他们的病痛

这说明在医学知识之外，要存在医学的艺术。不管男性或女性，只有好人才能够成为好医生，而医学技能本身是不够的。因此，高质量的学校内严谨的医学教育和传授是必不可少的。[33]

斯乃博十分享受他在中国的时光，"这是一种全新的体验，患者们的疾病在临床上的表现是如此不同寻常，这是一个另外的世界"。"这里的生活祥和、平静、放松"，他在给荷兰朋友的信中写道，"中国学生对于学习有很高的热情，教他们是一件很愉快的事。我们很少关注欧洲的战事，如果我没有阅读报纸，我甚至不会知道那里的局面多么糟糕。"[34]

斯乃博[35]：《中国给西医的教材：北京协和医学院对地域医学的贡献》[36]

斯乃博在中国的主要著作是《中国给西医的教材：北京协和医学院对地域医学的贡献》（*Chinese Lessons to Western Medicine：A Contribution to Geographical Medicine from the Clinics of Peiping Union Medical College*）。他只花了一年半的时间就写完了此书，于 1941 年末出版。从各个方面看，这本书都十分独特，不易分类。值得一提的是，在协和工作的西方医生中，只有斯乃博一人大量记录了在中国的经历，另一位出版了有关协和的书籍的是协和的秘书福梅龄（Mary Ferguson）。[37]

荷兰医生曾在印尼荷兰殖民地开展出色的科研工作,[38] 比如伊克曼（Eykman）和格瑞金（Grijns）对脚气病的研究、维生素 B1 的发现；詹森（Jansen）和多纳斯（Donath）对维生素 B1 的分离；斯卫伦格瑞贝尔（Swellengrebel）对疟疾的研究；克南（Kuenen）在痢疾的公共卫生工作；舒福乃尔（Schuffner）对钩端螺旋体的研究；凡·罗海穆（Van Loghem）对于虫害传播的地理性描述；欧腾（Otten）对抗虫害的疫苗的研发以及德郎根（De Langen）对于胆固醇和其与心血管疾病的关系的研究。[39]这些都使斯乃博备受启发。

《中国给西医的教材：北京协和医学院对地域医学的贡献》一书的前言里提到了诺贝尔奖得主乔治·迈瑙特（George Minot）关于恶性疟疾的工作。斯乃博在中国也面临着重大的医疗健康问题，比如营养和维生素缺乏、传染病、心血管疾病等。尽管他在阿姆斯特丹对大部分疾病都有处理的经验，但是他在中国的病人毕竟是不同人种，饮食习惯等都与荷兰不同。此外，营养不良是当时中国人的主要病因，这反映出当时中国的社会经济状况。另外，清洁设施与卫生对于人们的健康也有很大的影响。许多种不同疾病的临床表现都与阿姆斯特丹不同，这不仅归因于气候和营养不良，也由于患者们往往都处在疾病的终末阶段。换言之，正如斯乃博自己所言："显然，被移植到中国北方的西方临床医生要处理来东方之前没有在意过的问题。"

协和收治的大多数病人都十分穷苦。当时的北京有无数乞讨者，其中有许多俄罗斯人，他们是"白俄"，是革命后的流亡者。他们找不到工作。还有许多从乡下到城里的店铺和工厂学徒的年轻男孩也过着极其贫穷的生活，他们生活环境恶劣，工作十分辛苦。患者们步行来到医院就医，或者在警察的陪伴下用手推车送到医院来。

每一项医疗干预手段都需要得到患者家属的同意，然而由于迷信，治疗常常被拒绝。有时，由于患者居住在离城市很远的地方，无法很快得到其家属的同意，宝贵的治疗时间被耽误。在当时的中国有另一个严重问题是献血。[40]最明显的，在产科接生期间的失血必须要治疗，然而大多数的中国人都不愿意献血。只有很贫穷或者鸦片上瘾的人才会为了钱去献血，但是他们的血液中常常携带梅毒螺旋体或疟原虫。

食物供应

当时，协和的大多数病人都患有严重营养不良。此外，许多人还吸食鸦片上瘾。人们的饮食以素食为主，每天平均的能量摄入只有 2000 卡路里，无法满足大多数人从事重体力劳动的需求。尽管低卡路里的素食饮食对于防止心血管疾病有一定帮助，但也增加了得传染性疾病和严重维生素缺乏的风险。中国贫民大多吃白菜和菠菜度日，他们用油炒菜，大多数维生素都在加热中流失，蛋白质丰富的食物对于绝大多数人而言十分昂贵。

患病率最高的营养缺乏是维生素 D 缺乏，这是由于不良饮食、牛奶摄入不足、晒太阳不够导致的。同时缺维生素 D 和低钙会导致严重的骨骼异常：骨软化病。斯乃博在阿姆斯特丹时对此很了解。骨骼畸形、易骨折、病人行动不便和疼痛：这种疾病常见于孕妇，因为孕期时身体对于维生素 D 的需求增加，而且哺乳期间钙会从母亲那里传给孩子。新生儿常常因为缺钙而手足抽搐；许多女性由于骨盆畸形无法正常分娩。

维生素的缺乏则属于地方性流行症，会导致夜盲、眼睛干涩和皮肤发炎。斯乃博还遇到过维生素 C 缺乏导致的坏血病。斯乃博认为维生素 A、D 的缺乏的原因是因为中国人饮食中没有含有这些维生素的黄油。

传染病

斯乃博在华期间写了大量关于中国最常见传染病的文章。那时，除了磺胺吡啶外，还未有其他抗生素。[41]直到二战发生之后才逐渐研发了抗生素。为了避免医院内感染的蔓延，采取了卫生措施，患者们被隔离开来。

大多白喉患者都在疾病的晚期才来医院就诊，当时还没有白喉疫苗，患者只能用抗毒素治疗，但是疗效存疑。治疗的主要并发症是喉部堵塞，这可能导致窒息，需要急诊手术抢救。

肺炎常常是麻疹的并发症，是十分常见的致命疾病。大多数患者表现出并发症，如败血症和休克，出现脓肿和高热，这时再使用磺胺吡啶已经太迟。

腮腺炎和猩红热也大范围传播很广。斯乃博强调，在那时，腮腺炎通常继发于中枢神经系统感染、脑膜脑炎，但也有可能继发于多发性神经根炎和脊髓灰质炎。斯乃博记录了一例患有腮腺炎和胰腺炎的患者病例，这在现在十分罕见。

斑疹伤寒由立克次氏体导致，经由鼠类等啮齿动物身上的跳蚤传播给人类，在当时十分流行。这主要是由于当时卫生条件和居住环境比较差。斯乃博对于这种疾病的临床知识仅仅来源于第一次世界大战。这是一种高致死率的疾病，也被戏称为"医生杀手"。斯乃博警告斑疹伤寒也可能在人们乘坐当时北京人常常乘坐的交通工具——人力车时被感染。和莱姆病、梅毒一样，回归热也是一种由螺旋体导致的疾病，是大多数生活环境原始而不卫生的穷人高发的疾病。

斯乃博观察到许多患者由于感染副伤寒和痢疾而导致腹泻，夏季尤其常见。阿米巴痢疾则属于地方性疾病，常常导致肝和腹部的囊肿。霍乱则比较少见。

黑热病，又称利什曼病，经由白蛉从狗向人类传播，在中国北方十分常见。医生每每遇到发热的病人都需要考虑该病的可能性。该病由于会导致皮肤变黑，被称为黑热病。斯乃博在书中记录了一个患儿由黑热病发展成所谓"走马疳"的皮肤感染，这种感染会导致面部严重毁容。在中国，狗的数量很多。另一种由狗传染的疾病是狂犬病，患有狂犬病的病人会全部死亡。

斯乃博将北京结核高发的原因归咎为营养不良、维生素 D 缺乏、卫生条件差以及住房过于拥挤。许多人的居住环境十分狭小，一个房间里常常同时住很多人，这导致病传染给全家人。由于没有治疗方法，大多数结核病人都死亡了。斯乃博还观察到了一些罕见的未发生在西方国家的结核并发症，比如肠结核。

斯乃博反复强调，传染病在中国高发，最常见于家境贫穷、无法满足温饱的百姓。

心血管疾病

斯乃博在中国对心血管疾病开展了非常有趣的观察，观察其与饮食的关系、动脉粥样硬化以及血液中胆固醇的水平等。这实际上是他的朋友、前同事德郎根于 1915 年在印尼荷属殖民地所开展的原始研究工作的延续。德郎根观察到在欧洲多发的心血管疾病在印尼十分少见。因此他开始检测首都巴达维亚（Batavia）的爪哇人血液中的胆固醇水平，发现其浓度低得惊人。与之相反，在欧洲客轮上当乘务员的爪哇人的胆固醇水平则高，与爪哇原住民几乎全素的饮食相反，这些乘务员饮食中有较多的富含卡路里的动物蛋白。[42]

斯乃博在北京重复了这一研究，证实其前同事德郎根的观察结果。斯乃博在中国工作期间，只遇到了三例由于心脏血管狭窄引发胸痛的病例，其中一位病人发生了心肌梗死，这位病人吸烟，就像斯乃博本人和当时的大多数医生一样。而吸烟和动脉粥样硬化之间的关系在那时尚未被证实。

饮食中含有蔬菜、心血管疾病的低患病率（同样患病率低的还有胆结石）和较低的胆固醇水平之间的联系是独特的研究成果，其在国际上也是独一无二的、领先的成果。但是由于德郎根将研究成果发表在荷兰期刊（*Het Geneeskundig Tijdschrift voor Nederlandsch Indië*）上，他的贡献失去了得到国际的认可机会。斯乃博的眼界则更开阔，他在《美国心脏学杂志》（American Journal of Cardiology）发表了成果，并给文章起了一个抓人眼球的题目："饮食与动脉粥样硬化：真相与谎言"。[43]

斯乃博的论文吸引了广泛关注，吸引了医学界精英的注意力，因此斯乃博和德郎根的开创性工作最终得到了国际的承认。[44]他们被戏称为"医学界的马可波罗"。他们的研究为心血管疾病的流行病学研究以及揭示心血管疾病与饮食、吸烟、工作条件之间的关系打下了基础。[45]

鸦片成瘾

吸食鸦片在中国各阶层都十分普遍。与吸烟的轻微毒效相比，食用或注射鸦片的毒性更加危险。每年协和大约会收治 100～200 例鸦片中毒的患者。[46]一旦患者中毒昏迷，死亡率很可观，高达 75% 的人会死去。受害者吸食鸦片的剂量是用"鸦片价格是多少美元"表示。主要的并发症是呼吸抑制，进而导致支气管肺炎。当时并无解药。

昏迷的病人会被送入 *Drinker* 机器，该机器是一种人工呼吸器，又被称为"铁肺"，于 1929 年在美国由德瑞因科尔（Drinker en McKhann）设计。"铁肺"原用于治疗脊髓灰质炎。然而，人工呼吸并不是十分有效，通过洗胃将鸦片排出患者体内同样无效，反而常常会导致吸入胃液，引发肺部损伤和肺炎。

斯乃博使用可拉明治疗昏迷的病人，该药物能够刺激呼吸中枢。在与助手朱贵卿和郑德悦的共同努力下，治疗取得了惊人的成绩，患者死亡率降到了 20%。[47]此外，他还使用抗生素磺胺吡啶进行治疗，进一步取得了令人瞩目的效果。

《中国给西医的教材：北京协和医学院对地域医学的贡献》一书受到

包括《新英格兰医学杂志》（New England Journal of Medicine）[48]、《美国医学会杂志》（Journal of American Medical Association）[49]和《内科学年鉴》（The Annals of Internal Medicine）[50]的热议。《儿科学杂志》（The Journal of Pediatrics）建议军队阅读该书为在远东地区服役做准备。1965 年，该书第二版发行，被广为收藏。

困境

斯乃博与妻子海迪在 1940 年末前往美国休假。与此同时，政治形势恶化，日本对中国的侵略加剧，在中国的西南，国民党军队抵抗着日本的铁蹄，共产党的游击队则在北方展开了战斗。[51]1941 年 1 月，所有外国女性被建议尽快离开中国，尽管如此，海迪依然决定冒险和丈夫一起回到北京。

和斯乃博一起在 1939 年抵达中国的妇产科专家韦达科医生则决定回到美国。斯乃博听说后很吃惊，他向纽约的罗氏驻华医社发电报说："惊悉韦达科也要回美国，事情怎么变成了这样？"斯乃博为越来越多的医务人员离开忧心忡忡，最后他们会成为唯一留在北京的外国医生。交通阻断、物价飞涨、商品和食物供应紧缺。1941 年秋，所有美国人都被建议离开中国。1941 年末，只有 20 名美国人仍在协和工作，他们中的大多数都是单身，只有斯乃博、荷兰解剖学家福顿和美国外科医生娄克斯这三对夫妇一起留在北京。[52]一位在协和就医的美国人在信中提供了例证："除了著名的诊断学家斯乃博医生，其他工作人员都是中国人。"[53]

珍珠港事件

1941 年 12 月 7 日星期天的清晨，日本军队出其不意地袭击了美国海军在夏威夷的基地珍珠港，毁灭性的炮火袭击几乎摧毁了整个美军太平洋舰队。不可避免，美国对日宣战，太平洋战争真正爆发。

次日清晨，日军包围北京协和医学院并占领医院。门诊关闭，患者不得入院。[54]斯乃博在家中被逮捕，与协和校长胡恒德、总务博文（Trevor Bowen）、燕京大学校长司徒雷登（Leighton Stuart）以及人数未知的外国人被押送至日军司令部，最终被关押在美国大使馆海军陆战队的营房，不得探视。

1942年1月10日，斯乃博和胡恒德、博文、司徒雷登一起被转到协和校长官邸英宅（Ying House）囚禁，他们被8名日本士兵日夜看管。[55]其他人则被释放。

1月22日，北京协和医学院彻底关闭。虽然有日本人的承诺，但几个月后医院内部一片混乱。医院的家具被损坏，解剖标本的收藏丢失，中国医生逃离，藏在小医院和诊所中。所有外国员工必须离开家、从而离开这个国家。[56]

洛克菲勒基金会试图向美国政府施压，希望用日本俘虏交换被关押的美国人，但是由于斯乃博和妻子是荷兰人而非美国国籍，无法获得帮助。[57]而荷兰政府也没有能力或愿意帮助斯乃博，因为他们在中国为美国机构工作，荷兰政府没有兴趣营救他们。简而言之，斯乃博和妻子被困在中国了。

1942年5月8日，斯乃博等四人被迫搬家至空的办公场所，他们被完全隔离开来，禁止探视。只有一封封被打开检查过的信件不时地交给斯乃博。他们能够活动的空间只是一个6米见方的院子。在夏天，气温高达40度，卫生间也被破坏。[58]他们无法预知未来会怎样。

在监禁期间，斯乃博学习解剖学准备美国医生资格考试，努力使自己忙碌起来，他被要求定期在日本病房提供咨询，尽管这些活动能够使他的精神状态保持稳定，但渐渐地他愈发抑郁了。

重获自由

历经 8 个月的监禁，斯乃博于 1942 年 8 月 10 日获释，得以与妻子重新团圆。他被用于交换 6 名于战争之初开始在澳大利亚被关押的日本外交官。[59]这是战争期间最后几次关押人员交换之一。与他一起关押的其他三名人员则未被释放，这可能因为他们都是美国人，尤其受到日本人的仇视。斯乃博十分担心仍在囚禁的三个人的安危，[60]他努力说服美国政府尽一切可能营救他们。[61]然而，剩下三人直到三年后的 1945 年日本投降时才被释放。这场战争中，1200 万中国人丧命（原文如此。——译者注）。

斯乃博首先乘火车前往上海，从上海乘船到位于非洲东海岸的莫桑比克首都洛伦索马奎斯（Lourenco Marques），在那里他们被和日本外交官交换。从莫桑比克出发，他们前往英国，首先抵达利物浦，再到伦敦准备了需要的护照、邮票、文件和其他材料，寻找轮船前往美国。尽管是自由身，但斯乃博一家已经没有了祖国，他们不能回中国，也不能去荷属殖民地印尼，因为两处都被日本占领；他们更无法回到荷兰，因为荷兰被德国占领。由于没有英国的永久签证，他们也无法停留在莫桑比克。他们寄希望于美国。

终于，他们得到命运的眷顾，得到了去美国的许可。他们甚至受到了非常热情的欢迎，因为美国政府可以利用斯乃博在热带医学方面的专长帮助其在东方的美国军队。

最终，他们在 1942 年 10 月 25 日，他们乘坐伊丽莎白女王号（Queen Elizabeth）从格拉斯哥（Glasgow）前往纽约。

受邀五角大楼

抵达美国后，斯乃博被华盛顿五角大楼邀请担任总医官下属的预防医学部门的热带病专家。国防部需要专家指导太平洋战争中的医疗问题，以"保护人力资源"、"保存军队的战斗力"。当时美国的军事力量增长迅猛，截至 1944 年底，超过四百万美军在世界各地作战。因此，医疗队也从 1942 年的 1600 人增加到 1944 年的 4300 人。[62]包括大学教授、员工在内的各个领域的专业人士都被应征入伍。

美国所涉足到的各个国家的信息都被收集和整理成册，斯乃博撰写了被日本占领的荷属殖民地印尼的医疗卫生情况的详细报告。[63]特别地，他尤其呼吁关注痢疾和疟疾，这是困扰在东方作战的美军的两个主要健康问题。

荷兰的亲友

斯乃博的大儿子福利兹经历了一段险象环生的旅程从荷兰逃至意大利。在意大利北部山区，他参加了意大利游击队投入战斗。福利兹的妻子海伦娜·森德万（Helena Sondervan）在德国卑尔根－贝尔森（Bergen-Belsen）的集中营幸免于难。

1940 年 5 月，德国占领荷兰后，斯乃博曾从北京发电报给他唯一的姊妹贝齐（Betsy），强烈建议她尝试办理美国签证。然而，贝齐的努力没能成功，她命中注定留在了阿姆斯特丹。她是一家犹太女孩孤儿院的董事会成员。1942 年末，孤儿院中的所有女童被赶入集中营，大部分人不幸遇害。贝齐及其丈夫也被送往德国的一个集中营，不过有幸被用于交换巴勒斯坦的德国囚犯而存活下来。

海迪·斯乃博的母亲卡瑟琳娜·凡·布瑞恩杜墨石（Catharina van Buuren-du Mosch）在德国集中营中被杀害，同样的厄运也发生在斯乃博在阿姆斯特丹的姨妈和表姐妹身上。斯乃博在阿姆斯特丹大学医院的同事、来自敖德赛（Odessa）的化学家阿尔夫瑞德·格瑞鲍姆（Alfred Grünbaum）起初为逃避反犹太主义逃到俄国，最终也不幸遇害。斯乃博的好友、同事、药理学教授俄尔斯特·拉奎尔（Ernst Laqueur）在战争中活了下来。

斯乃博对于北京协和医学院的评价

斯乃博在 1940 年末的一次采访[64]和 1942 年的一份书面报告[65]中表达了对北京协和医学院的看法。在斯乃博看来，与世隔绝制约了学校的发展。他提醒读者，建立协和的初衷是将其办成医学研究中心，同时培养未来的医学教育者。然而，由于其与外界的隔绝，协和无法收到来自邻近大学的建设性意见以提高自己的工作水平。这对于科学研究有着负面的影响。协和的教学以各学系负责人的知识水平为基础，然而缺乏外界环境的影响，这种根基会越来越薄弱。在西方国家，科系的负责人从助手那里学到的东西要比其言传身教给助手得多。协和与外界的隔绝导致其在北京享受不到新鲜血液的注入。尽管学校中年轻员工被送往国外进行短期的访问进修，依然难以解决这个问题。协和的另一个问题与语言有关，教授们上课用英语、课本也是英文的，而中国学生用英文学医是十分困难的。

但是斯乃博的态度很积极。建校以来，洛克菲勒基金会与协和已经取得了显著的成就，四千万美元被用于提升中国医学教育的水平。在几乎所有中国大学中，协和的毕业生们都遥遥领先，他们培养未来医学领军人才的目标已然实现。此外，协和也为中国医学教育树立了榜样。

斯乃博建议，中国的医疗卫生事业应该是政府的任务，从中央层面组织。不过，这样做的风险在于，受到良好教育的专科医生拿着政府的薪水，却花费时间、精力在私人开业行医上。因此，根据法律，年轻医生应该在公立医院服务几年，此外，医生还必须接受定期的毕业后教育。因此，应该开设用于毕业后教育的医院。

在拥有六亿人口的庞大国家，公医制应该起到核心作用。显然，政府还需要展开预防医学和公共卫生项目，而人民自身也应该在这个组织中发挥作用。

斯乃博总结，将来北京协和医学院将发挥重要作用。在日本占领时期，中国医生与西方国家的联系被切断，因此在医学飞速发展的情况下处于落后地位。协和应该开办最新的课程和毕业后教育，与西方尤其是美国医生交换知识，协和的教职人员中应该既有东方血脉也有西方面孔。[66]

后来的事业发展

在为国防部的工作结束后，斯乃博成为纽约曼哈顿西奈山医院的教授，在西奈山，他得到了很高的认可和声誉。他的大查房和讲演都十分有名，并出版了一本关于骨科疾病的新书《骨科疾病的临床诊断》（Medical Clinics on Bone Diseases）。不过使他收获最多赞誉的是《床旁医学》（Bedside Medicine）一书，这本书非常好地记录了他在内科学领域的全部经验，不断重复着他的愿景：医学就在病人的床边。

参考书目

1. M. E. Ferguson，*China Medical Board and Peking Union Medical College：A chronicle of fruitful collaboration 1914 – 1951*（New York，1970），pp. 27 – 55

2. J. Z. Bowers，*Western Medicine in a Chinese Palace. Peking Union Medical College 1917 – 1951*（Philadelphia 1972），pp. 78 – 9

3. J. Z. Bowers，*Western Medicine in a Chinese Palace. Peking Union Medical College 1917 – 1951*（Philadelphia 1972）p. 79

4. I. Snapper，brief aan O. Brien，20 maart 1938，folder 1210，box 166，series 601，DGC 1938，Rockefeller Foundation Archives RAC

5. J. Goldstein，*Jews in China. Historical and Comparative Perspectives*（New York 1999）

6. Dossier Snapper，Archives PUMC，Beijing

7. P. U. Unschuld，*Medicine in China. A History of Ideas*（Berkeley Calif 1985）

8. P. Huard en M. Wong，*Geneeskunde in China*（Amsterdam 1967）

9. C. U. Ariens Kappers, *Reiziger in breinen. Herinneringen van een hersenonderzoeker* (Amsterdam 2001)

10. E. Hume, *Doctors East*, *Doctors West* (London 1949)

11. R. Mitter, *China's war with Japan 1937 – 1945* (London 2014) pp. 34 – 48

12. B. Andrews, M. Brown Bullock, *Medical Transitions in Twentieth-Century China* (Bloomington, USA 2014) pp. 185 – 190

13. P. U. Unschuld, *Medicine in China. A History of Ideas* (Berkeley USA, 1985)

14. B. Andrews, M. Brown Bullock, *Medical Transitions in Twentieth-Century China* (Bloomington, USA 2014) p. 19

15. Idem, p. 219

16. J. D. Wilson, 'Peking Union Medical College Hospital, a Palace of Endocrine Treasures' *J Clin Endo Metab* 76, 1993, pp. 815 – 6

17. J. Z. Bowers, *Western Medicine in a Chinese Palace. Peking Union Medical College 1917 – 1951* (Philadelphia 1972)

18. C. U. Lee, brief aan China Medical Board, 14 juni 1944, Collection CMB, Box 35, Criticism 1933 – 1944, Rockefeller Archives, RAC

19. Mary Brown Bullock, *An American Transplant*, *The Rockefeller Foundation and Peking Union Medical College*, (Los Angeles 1980) pp. 78 – 107

20. Report PUMC, folder 1314, box 182, series 601, RG 2 – 1939, Rockefeller Foundation Archives RAC

21. Idem, pp.

22. I. Snapper *Chinese lessons to western medicine* (New York 1941)

23. H. Schulte Nordholt, *China & de barbaren* (Amsterdam 2015) pp. 387 – 90

24. E. H. Hume, *The Chinese Way in Medicine* (Baltimore 1940) pp.

25. J. Le Fanu, *Rise and Fall of Modern Medicine* (London 1999) p. 201

26. R. Porter, *The greatest benefit to mankind. A medical history of humanity from antiquity to the present* (London 1997) pp. 147 – 62

27. E. H. Hume, *The Chinese Way in Medicine* (Baltimore 1940)

28. P. U. Unschuld, 'History of Chinese Medicine', In: K. F. Kiple, (red.) . *The Cambridge World History of Human Disease* (Cambridge 2008) pp. 20 – 6

29. C. F. Nathan, 'The acceptance of Western Medicine in early 20th century China: The story of the North Manchurian plague prevention service', In: J. Z. Bowers and E. F. Purcell (red.) *Medicine and Society in China* (Philadelphia 1974) pp. 55 – 81

30. Brief H. S. Houghton aan E. C. Lobenstine, August 9, 1939. folder 601, box 125,

series CMB, RG PUMC Snapper, Rockefeller Foundation Archives, RAC

31. H. Schulte Nordholt, *China & de barbaren* (Amsterdam 2015) pp. 58 – 63

32. Letter E. C. Lobenstine to the China Medical Board. Folder 601, box 125, series CMB, RG PUMC Snapper. Rockefeller Foundation Archives RAC

33. I. Snapper, 'The mile-stone of graduation', Archives J. Snapper, Charlottesville, NC

34. Stadsarchief Gemeente Amsterdam. College van Curatoren. Inventarisnummer 279, Ingekomen en uitgaande stukken, 1938, nummer 195.

35. 斯乃博的中文名。

36. I. Snapper, *Chinese Lessons to Western Medicine* (New York 1941)

37. Mary E. Ferguson, *China Medical Board and Peking Union Medical College: A chronicle of fruitful collaboration 1914 – 1951* (New York 1970)

38. I. Snapper, 'Medical contributions from the Netherlands Indies', *Science and Scientists in the Netherlands Indies, Surinam, and Curacao,* (New York 1945) pp. 309 – 20

39. J. L. Hydrick, *Intensive Rural Hygiene Work in The Netherlands east Indies* (New York 1944)

40. I. Snapper et al. , 'Anemia from blood donation. A haematological and clinical study of 101 professional donors' *Chin Med J* 56, 1939, pp. 400 – 423

41. I. Snapper et al. , 'Haematuria, renal colic and acetyl-sulfapyridine stone formation associated with sulfapyridine therapy' *Chin Med J* 56, 1939, pp. 1 – 10

42. C. D. de Langen, 'Cholesterol metabolism and racial pathology' *Gen Tijdschr Ned Indië* 56, 1916, pp. 1 – 34

43. I. Snapper, 'Diet and atherosclerosis: Truth and fiction' *Am J Cardiol* 11, 1963, pp. 283 – 9

44. James Le Fanu, *Rise and Fall of Modern Medicine* (London 1999) pp. 322 – 50

45. H. Blackburn, '20th-Century "Medical Marco Polos" in the origins of preventive cardiology and cardiovascular disease epidemiology' *Am J Cardiol* 109, 2012, pp. 756 – 67

46. Brief I. Snapper aan A. Gregg, 2 october 1941, Folder 1558, box 224, series 601, RG 2GC 1941, Rockefeller Foundation Archives RAC

47. I. Snapper, I. K. C. Chu, T. Y. Cheng, 'Treatment of acute opium poisoning. Beneficial effect of coramine' *Am J Med Sciences* 204, 1942, pp. 409 – 19

48. Anoniem, 'Book reviews' *N Engl J Med* 227, 1942, p. 498

49. Anoniem, 'Book notices' *JAMA* 118, 1942, p. 1262

50. Anoniem, 'Reviews' *Ann Int Med* 16, 1942, p. 1027

51. R. Mitter, *China's war with Japan 1937 – 1945* (London 2014) pp. 210 – 25

52. CMB inc, Box 119, Personnel 1919 – 1949, Rockefeller Archives RAC

53. Brief W. O. Inglis aan John D. Rockefeller Jr, 14 July 1939, folder 1314, box 182, series 601, RG 2 – 1939. Rockefeller Foundation Archives RAC

54. Idem, pp. 174 – 84

55. I. Snapper, brief aan A. E. Clattenburg, 30 october 1942, Record Group 59, CDF 1940 – 1944, 740. 00115a Pacific War/301, Box 2910, National Archives

56. R. Mitter, *China's war with Japan 1937 – 1945* (London 2014) pp. 239 – 63

57. Brief Board Rockefeller Foundation aan Nederlandse Ambassade Washington, 19 maart, 1942, folder 652, box 91, RG Medicine Staff, CMB, Rockefeller Foundation Archives, RAC

58. I. Snapper, brief aan A. E. Clattenburg, 30 october 1942, Record Group 59, CDF 1940 – 1944, 740. 00115a Pacific War/301, Box 2910, National Archives

59. M. J. van Lieburg, *Isidore Snapper's notes for memoirs 1889 – 1973*: *The autobiographical recollections of 'the Champion of bedside medicine'* (Rotterdam 2004) pp.

60. Interview met I. Snapper, 13 november 1942, folder 910, box 125, series CMB 1942 – 1948, RG Political Situation, Rockefeller Foundation Archives RAC

61. Brief A. E. Cohn aan Mr Justice Felix Frankfurter, Supreme Court of the United States, October 26, 1942, folder 910, box 125, series CMB 1942 – 1948, RG Political Situation, Rockefeller Foundation Archives RAC

62. Surgeon General Annual Reports 1939 – 1946, National Archives, Record Group 112, A1 – 46 – A, boxes 1 – 3

63. I. Snapper, 'Medical and sanitary data on the Netherlands East Indies', Medical Intelligence Branch, Preventive Medicine Division, Office of the Surgeon General, U. S. Army, National Archives, Record group 112, Medical and Sanitary Data, 1941 – 1958, box 2.

64. Interview with Dr I. Snapper, New York December 18, 1940.

65. I. Snapper, 'Comments on the Peiping Union Medical College', 1942, folder 652, box 91, RG Medicine Staff, China Medical Board, Rockefeller Foundation Archives, RAC

66. I. Snapper, 'Health Organization in China', Folder 652, box 91, RG Medicine Staff, China Medical Board, Rockefeller Foundation Archives, RAC

Isidore Snapper and PUMC
During the Second World War

Arie Berghout

Arie Berghout FRCP（1947）was a consultant of medicine,
specialized in endocrinology, head of the department of medicine, and
director of the department of postgraduate training and education for
the medical, nursing, and paramedical disciplines, in a large
teaching hospital in Rotterdam the Netherlands. He was member of the
board and chairman of the annual congress of the Dutch Society of
Medicine and member of the committee on quality control of educational
programs of teaching hospitals in The Netherlands. After his retirement
in 2012, he wrote a biography of Isidore Snapper（1889 – 1973）,
internist, which will be published fall 2017. He is presently chairman of
the historical committee of the Dutch Society of Medicine and
conservator at the Center and Library of the History of Medicine, at
Urk, The Netherlands.

Isidore Snapper, from Amsterdam, acted from 1939 until 1942 as a
professor of medicine at the Peiping Union Medical College, or PUMC, in
Beijing. Snapper was professor of medicine at the University of Amsterdam,
then the most important centre of medicine in the Netherlands. More than half of
all medical students in Holland followed their study in Amsterdam. Snapper
became professor of medicine in 1919, at the age of 30 and was quite famous,
at home as well as all over Europe. He had published already more than 200
articles in medical journals, in Dutch as well as German and English, and
published books on bone diseases and was the co-author of a Dutch textbook of

medicine. Besides that, he was also a successful football arbiter.

Why would someone like Snapper leave his country and his family, and interrupt his splendid career to come to China? It was very different from The Netherlands, far away in Asia, and he did not speak any Chinese. It was also dangerous to travel since from 1937 large parts of China were occupied by the Japanese, including Beijing, the city where the hospital was located and where he was going to work. That occupation was characterised by terror and chaos. Many in Nanjing, the former capital of the country were murdered, and the city destroyed. There was starvation, burglary and epidemics. Why had he agreed to come?

PUMC was an American college in Beijing, an initiative sponsored by the Rockefeller Foundation in New York. It was one of the 'jewels in the crown' of the Foundation, not just an ordinary college. The objectives of the college were to educate the future medical elite of China, to train teachers and leaders to solve the problems of diseases in China. It was not the intention to train just ordinary doctors and nurses. 'The best of the West in medical science' should be introduced in China, comparable with the best American and European universities. [1] Therefore, the students selection was rigorous and the numbers of admitted students low. Quality, not quantity, was the slogan. The preparatory study comprised Chinese, English, French or German, biology, chemistry and physics. After screening, an admission exam followed. [2] For an ambitious man like Snapper this was certainly a place to go.

Was this the reason why this American transplant the 'Johns Hopkins of China,' – modeled after the prestigious prototype of American medical faculty – was attractive to Snapper, and not only to him but also to those many American professors who went to China before him, to teach at PUMC? In the past, PUMC was quite a popular destination for doctors to spend a year or more as a professor or just to be a member of the staff. Celebrities like the physiologist Walter Cannon, who, followed the ideas of Claude Bernard, had introduced the concept of homeostasis in his opus magnum *The Wisdom of the Body* and Hans Zinsser, bacteriologist and immunologist as well as writer, both from Harvard Medical School in Boston, and Eugene Opie, pathologist at Cornell University in New York, had been visiting professors. [3]

Surely, that was an important factor. Snapper knew the Rockefeller Foundation very well. Representatives of the foundation had visited him in Amsterdam and had sponsored his thyroid research. Snapper had visited the foundation as well when he was in the United States on his tours around universities and hospitals. It had always been Snapper's ambition to teach at an American university. Moreover, Snapper looked forward to have time for research when in China, as it seemed to be a less demanding post compared to his present position in Amsterdam.

But there was another, more pressing reason why Snapper had accepted the post in China. Snapper was Jewish. After Hitler came to power, antisemitism developed rapidly in Germany. Now it was spreading all over Europe, like an epidemic. Many Jewish people had fled Germany and Austria. Among them were many physicians who had come to the Netherlands. Snapper was member of a committee to support these refugees. When he attended a congress in Vienna in spring 1938, he was personally confronted with the antisemitic effects of the *Anschluss*, the submission of Austria to Nazi-Germany in March 1938. On the 20th of March 1938, Snapper wrote the following letter to Daniel O'Brien, the representative of the Rockefeller Foundationin in Paris:

> *You will easily understand that I am intensely shocked by the recent events in Europe, specially by the treatment to which many of my best colleagues in Vienna have been submitted. These happenings are weighing upon my mind to such an extent that I am quite willing to give up my position here to put as many miles between*

Europe and myself. In Holland there are not the slightest traces of antisemitism. Since a few years I am already looking for a possibility of getting a full-time teaching or research job in America or Australia...[4]

O'Brien forwarded the letter to the head office of the Rockefeller Foundation in New York:

Snapper at Amsterdam is looking for a full time position in internal medicine. The reason, I surmise, a restlessness on the subject of antisemitism. He is one of the ablest men in internal medicine in any of the Western European countries.

In May 1938 Snapper was offered the post in Beijing and it didn't take long for him to make up his mind and come to a decision. Shortly thereafter, in June 1938, Viennese colleagues, with many of whom Snapper was acquainted very well, were – according to the Nazi race laws – forbidden to practice any longer. In the night of November 9, 1938, in the German speaking countries the *Reichskristallnacht* happened, many Jewish houses and shops were demolished, innocent Jewish citizens attacked and put into jail. Snapper had made the right decision to leave Europe.

Before leaving the Netherlands, Snapper and his wife Hetty, had sent two of their three children to the United States. Their youngest, daughter Elsie, was in New York, under the care of a colleague of Snapper. Their son Ernst studied mathematics in Princeton. The eldest son, Frits, was in military service and could not leave his country.

Travel to China

To arrive in Beijing, the Snappers traveled around the world in 50 days. They first sailed to England. They had booked for New York on board of the Steam Ship *President Roosevelt*, leaving Southampton, a harbor in the south of England. But due to snow storms traveling from London to Southampton was impossible. They had to take the next boat to America, the Royal Mail Ship *Franconia*, built in 1923 in Glasgow for the Cunard Line. In New York they were warmly received by the China Medical Board, the office of the Rockefeller foundation that served the activities of the Foundation in Asia. From New York, further traveling was planned by the Canadian Pacific Railroad, to Vancouver. From there, ships left for Asian destinations. However, there were snow storms again, so the trip again had to be postponed. On January 21, 1939, they could sail from Vancouver to Yokohama in Japan, on board of the *Empress of Russia*, of the Canadian Pacific Line. From Yokohama, the Snappers went by train to Kobe, and from Kobe by boat to the Northern Chinese harbor of Tientsin. Again by train, they finally arrived in Beijing. A shorter trip was possible, by Shanghai, but an outbreak of cholera had been advised against.

At the time they arrived, the city of Beijing was busy, dirty and overcrowded. People lived in extreme poverty in *hutongs*, in urban areas where people were packed together. The Snappers needed to adapt to the climate, so different from Holland. And it was war time. Although the Japanese military did not occupy the hospital then, their presence was overly visible with the permanent imminence that something could happen at any moment.

The Snappers did not know anybody in Beijing. What did it mean to be Jewish in China? There was no Jewish community in Beijing, in contrast to Harbin, Hong Kong and notably Shanghai where thousands of Jewish immigrants from Europe had arrived and had been welcomed, without any limitation, without the need to have visas. [5] Furthermore, what did they know of Chinese culture? On the other hand, the Snappers were more than welcome in Beijing. A reception was organized for Snapper and two other new professors, the obstetrician Frank Whitacre from Chicago, who had studied in Leipzig and Berlin, and the neurologist Theron Hill from Michigan. [6] They got an appartement in the area of PUMC, near the 'forbidden city', in a compound where most foreign staff members of the hospital were lodged.

PUMC

PUMC was not the first American medical institution in China. But certainly the best. In the beginning, Western medicine had entered China following missionaries of different denominations. [7] Doctors from France and England had long before been active in China. The British mission taught medicine in Hangkow. [8] The American mission had started a medical school in Soochow and in Tsinan. [9] Yale University had established a medical faculty and hospital in Changsha, the capital of Hunan, in Central China, a 'Yale-in-China'. [10]

At the beginning of the 20th century the Rockefeller Foundation had entered the field of medicine in China. Deep in their heart, the Americans believed that they acted as a role model for the Chinese people, and that in the long run the Chinese wanted to be like Americans. They wanted to be in the lead in this process. Eventually China would turn into a Christian nation. Rich families like the Rockefellers had to play a role in this process. [11]

PUMC was part of a grand program to reform health care in the whole of China, or more properly stated, once and for all to set it up. The number of doctors with a Western diploma was about 1 to 150,000 inhabitants. [12] In fact, China knew only traditional medicine. That should be changed according to the Americans, not only because they believed it should, but also for economic reasons. Was not a poor, underdeveloped China with an insufficient health care system, a poor trading partner? China on its turn, not only welcomed Western medicine because of the enormous development of Western medical knowledge and science, but also because of Western knowhow of public health and hygiene that was not developed in China at all. [13] Life expectancy in China in

1940, the time of Snappers arrival, was just 30 years, whereas in the USA it was over 60. [14] This enormous lag of China – *the sick man of Asia* – was due to civil wars that lasted for years, natural disasters, famine, and the bad health care system. Infectious diseases were epidemic, in the period 1930-1940 notably dysentery, cholera, typhus, smallpox. In the big cities tuberculosis, airway infections and cerebrovascular diseases were rampant. Only 10 percent of the population could read or write. [15]

The curriculum of the medical education of PUMC was designed by Simon Flexner, director of the Rockefeller Research Institute in New York, and by William Welch, microbiologist and teacher by profession, at the Johns Hopkins university in Baltimore. They knew to attract professors for PUMC from the big American universities. [16] Two other Dutchmen also visited PUMC. In 1924 C. U. Ariens Kappers, the director of the Netherlands Institute for Brain Research was visiting professor. A. B. Droogleever Fortuyn, professor of anatomy, was present in Beijing to welcome the Snappers.

Program and staff

The research program of the PUMC was excellent, the laboratory up-to-date, and there was a big library. Research was done in the field of acid-base equilibrium, the secretion of gastric juice, infectious diseases, ricine toxicity, and adrenalin, the stress hormone, produced by the adrenal glands. International publications had followed. Talented Chinese graduates got the opportunity to continue their studies in the USA and possibly start a career over there like Yu Ts'ai-fan who became well known as a gout and uric acid expert and professor at the Mount Sinai Hospital in New York. Liu Shih-hao co-authored with Snapper some articles and became an expert in vitamin D deficiency and the sequelae for the skeleton that was frequent at that time in China. Eventually he became professor at PUMC. There could be no doubt about it: in PUMC *Western Medicine in a Chinese Palace* was performed. [17]

Although all this sounds perfect, criticisms were ventilated. PUMC was elitist, the educational program too Western, the student group too small, too selective. The education did not find connection to Chinese society, the graduated doctors and nurses lacked practical skills. [18]

In consequence of the American model, Snapper did not need to learn Chinese: PUMC was an English spoken environment. It was essential to train the students as first class doctors, and English was the main language of the international scientific community. The staff at PUMC had - following the Rocke-feller ideology - full time positions and were paid accordingly, making it not necessary and even impossible to run a private practice to supplement the university salary. They could give all their time and energy to education, patient care and research. About 6,000 patients were admitted to the hospital yearly and more than two hundred thousand seen at the outpatient clinics. The department of medicine of PUMC had nearly hundred beds: 35 for males, 12 females, 11 for metabolic research, 20 for infectious diseases, and 20 beds for private patients.

In 1940 PUMC had 250 medical and 80 nurse students, most from Beijing and the northern provinces. Contact with southern China was nearly nonexistent due to the war. This was the situation in Beijing when the Snappers arrived, and in the coming years they would not leave the city.

As a result of the sinification policy, which was to appoint gradually more Chinese doctors in staff positions, the staff was primarily made up of Chinese, trained in PUMC. The Dean was Dr. C. E. Lim (Lim Chong-eang) Consequently, the number of Western doctors had greatly dwindled. In the early years of PUMC the ratio of Western versus Chinese doctors had been 22: 9, at the time of Snappers arrival it was 10: 109. Of all professors 7 were of Western and 7 of Chinese origin. [19] However, the low number of Western doctors working for PUMC was also the result of the Japanese occupation as interest to go to China had decreased considerably.

The director was Dr. Henry Houghton who reported to the China Medical Board in New York, the office for China of the Rockefeller Foundation. The Americans Hamilton Anderson, pharmacologist from California, Harold Loucks, surgeon and later director of the China Medical Board, Irvine McQuarrie, paediatrician from the University of Minnesota, and Chester Frazier, dermatologist, who went from Beijing to Massachusetts General Hospital in Boston, as well as Reinhard Hoeppli, parasitologist, from Switzerland, were among the few Western staff members. [20]

In the hospital

Snapper was the opposite of his predecessor, Francis Dieuaide who was a kind, modest person, who always posed questions, never offered direct solutions to clinical problems and always wanted to stimulate discussion. In brief, the prototype of the bottom-up culture of American universities. Snapper, on the contrary, was the old fashioned professor, the typical German ' Geheimrat Professor. ' He showed confidence, was an authority, a stronghold, the prototype of European top-down culture. Snapper was popular among the Chinese students: one learned very much, he definitely offered solutions, made diagnoses, supplied assurance. [21]

What was in Snappers mind when he entered PUMC? In the foreword to his book *Chinese Lessons to Western Medicine* he tells us the following:

> *It is evident that a Western clinician, transplanted into North China, has to cope with many problems which did not come to his attention before he moved to the Orient. Fortunately, the Department of Medicine of the Peiping Union Medical College is so carefully organized that it helps the unwary to avoid most of the traps*

which are awaiting the newcomer…

The staff consists of Chinese clinicians with wide experience in medicine, and, if one is not conceited or stubborn, it is quite easy to take one's diagnostic and therapeutic cue from their gentle and polite remarks…

The combined efforts of the staff and resident are more than sufficient to prevent a greenhorn from making too ridiculous mistakes, at least, if the newcomer remembers that he must heed even the gentlest vocal inflection and the slightest expression of polite surprise…[22]

The professor was anxious not to make mistakes, not to make stupid remarks! Snapper was not used to showing weaknesses. His solution was - don't think you know everything, don't be conceited, take notion of the reactions of the Chinese staff, their voice, their facial expression. He realized that he came as an individualist. But here in China alone standing human being is not a real human being. The Chinese only know social persons, man is a social being.[23]

Confrontation with Chinese Medicine

At the time Snapper arrived in China, Chinese medicine was based on tradition, beliefs and adaptation. On the contrary, Western medicine, especially as it was done in PUMC, was based on experiments and renewal.[24] Tradition: the "five elements" or "phases", the "Yin Yang" dualism, acupuncture, moxa burning, and the emphasis on the story of the patient and his family, the palpation of the pulse, the inspection of the eyes. From outside, Buddhistic and herbal medicine had influenced China. Snapper had no particular affinity with traditional Chinese medicine. On the contrary, it sometimes contradicted his ideas about the practice of medicine. For example, Chinese tradition was against the post-mortem examination, in Snappers opinion an essential part of medical education, just as it was when he was in training in

Groningen, in the north of the Netherlands, similar to what was the rule in the teaching hospital of the 19th century. [25] Moreover, radiological facilities that could help to make a final diagnosis, were limited. According to Confucianistic philosophy, however, the body that was regarded as a present from the parents, should after death be returned to the gods, intact. As the family of the deceased usually did not give consent to the post-mortem examination, it was a custom to pose the question to the patient at admission to hospital, just in case.

But Snapper wonderfully found his place in China. This is because his ideas about the human constitution as he had learned from his teacher in Groningen, Hijmans van den Bergh, were closely connected to the holistic approach of Chinese medical thinking. [26]

For the Chinese physicians the sequence of inspection, listening, interview, and finally the investigation of the pulse, was very important to reach a diagnosis. [27] Snapper was a master in these skills, and moreover, he not only investigated the pulse, but also and very thoroughly the other parts of the human body, the whole body. Importantly, Snapper took also the story of the patient's family which was told him very seriously into account. That was important, as in China the family plays a major role in the decisions that have to be taken in the final treatment of the patient.

Furthermore, Western medicine has some common ideas with the traditional background of Chinese medicine. That had its basis, among other things, in the ontological approach that holds that disease follows after the entering from outside into the body of microorganisms that are *per se* innocent and in the functional idea that processes and relations within the body are disturbed. Notably that last mentioned line of thought was in accordance with the idea of biochemical processes. That connected with Snapper's background in biochemistry as he had been in the editorial board of *Biochemische Zeitschrift*, one of the first and most prestigious biochemical journals of the world.

Apart from these considerations, where Western and Chinese medicine touched and could grow on one and the same matrix-notwithstanding the chaotic situation of China in the beginning of 20th century - there was another explanation of the Chinese acceptation of Western medicine. [28] Western medics had played to halt the dramatic bubonic epidemic in Manchuria in 1910. Without external assistance, traditional medicine could not stop the plague. Only after the isolation of the numerous victims, against the will of the population, the epidemic had come to a standstill. The Chinese emperor had even permitted mass cremations, something unheard of in that time in China. [29]

Snapper and the students

The students were very enthusiastic about Snapper's teaching rounds in the hospital. His way of doing ward rounds were unusual, everybody was deeply impressed. [30] Traditionally, the students regarded Snapper with great respect. The relation between teacher and student was in China similar to the relation of a father to his son, or of the emperor to the citizen, based on respect and obedience. [31] They regarded him as a true professor because he was bald, which meant that he was reading every night under a lamp; secondly, he wore spectacles which indicated that he was used to read even the footnotes in small print of the scientific articles; lastly, he had a round belly which clearly proved that he had been invited for consultations by many rich patients.

Edwin Lobenstine, chairman of the China Medical Board paid a visit to Beijing in 1940. He reported enthusiastically to New York:

Snapper's presence is greatly appreciated in the college. He, on his part, is also enthusiastic. He likes it because he is working in an institution in which the professors are engaged on full time pay and not dependent on outside assistance. He likes the Chinese and he is liked by them. His weekly lectures, when he explains the way in which he has reached his diagnosis of some difficult case, are crowded to the doors and even overflow into an adjoining room. The whole Chinese faculty and students, and many of the nurses, turn out to hear him. He is a brilliant lecturer. [32]

Snapper was asked to address the students at the mile-stone of graduation ceremony, Sunday June 4, 1939:

My famous compatriot Boerhaave, professor of medicine in Leyden, Holland, about 1700, had the motto that simplicity is the stamp of all true things. These golden words should forever be present in our minds. Even now in this time of specialisation, observation of the patient is still the greatest diagnostic help and simple remedies still cure the greater part of curable diseases. First of all, I want to impress upon you that the application of simple methods is even more difficult than the handling of modern diagnostic and therapeutic apparatus. Remarkably enough - the simpler methods require more skill and more application than the complicated machines. For example, let us consider the diagnosis of coronary thrombosis by an electocardiogram or of duodenal ulcer by a roentgenogram. In actual practice we nearly always diagnose these diseases only by taking a complete history and by making a careful physical examination; in a minority of cases are the more complicated methods necessary even if we use them not seldom in order to make certain that we are not mistaken. It is, however, often easier to make an electrocardiogram or a roentgenogram than to take a careful history. In order to obtain a complete history, it is necessary to penetrate the personality of the patient. A careful physical examination requires quiet surroundings where intense mental concentration is possible. All this is much more difficult and asks for more ability and skill than the application of modern devices.

I want to emphasize especially the importance of the understanding of the psychology of the patient for the successful practice of medicine. Perhaps we are not always aware of the fact that an occupied hospital bed means not only a medical problem but may also represent a human tragedy. I know from personal experience that within the walls of the hospital the psychological problems and much of the human sadness which accompany disease are less poignant than in practice outside the hospital. Only if one has to go to the home of a patient can one fully understand how often sickness of one member of the family leads to disaster for the entire household.

A famous physician has stated that even if a physician does not bring healing as often as he wishes, he usually brings alleviation of suffering and always brings consolation. But apart from the heroic part of medicine the doctor has also to take care of the incurable patient who has to live through the difficult months of suffering until the end is reached. Every day the patient will be waiting for the visit of his doctor, and the words which you will give to him will be the moral support which will ease his suffering.

This is, apart from medical knowledge, the art of medicine. Only good men and good women can be good physicians-technical skill alone is not sufficient. Therefore a careful medical education and teaching in a highly qualified school is necessary. [33]

Snapper enjoyed his stay in China tremendously.

A complete new experience, patients with unusual clinical presentations, an other world. " *"Life is quiet here, peaceful, and relaxed,"* he wrote to a friend in Holland. *"Students are very eager to learn, it is pleasure to teach them. We are only minimally aware of the war in Europe. If we did not read the newspapers, I would not even know about the terrible events that happen over there.* [34]

Snapper[35], Chinese Lessons to Western Medicine[36]

Snapper's major publication in China was *Chinese Lessons to Western Medicine: A Contribution to Geographical Medicine from the Clinics of Peiping Union Medical College*. He wrote the book in the very short time of one and a half year and it was published at the end of 1941. It was a unique book in all respects, not easily falling in a category. Remarkably, Snapper was the only western physician who worked in PUMC who reported extensively about his experiences in China. Mary Ferguson, also published about her work as secretary at PUMC. [37]

Snapper was inspired by Dutch physicians who had performed excellent scientific research in the Dutch Indies. [38] For instance, the elucidation of the beri-beri problem, the detection of vitamin B1, *thiamine*, by Eykman and Grijns; the isolation of vitamine B1 by Jansen and Donath; the malaria research by Swellengrebel; public health work on dysentery by Kuenen; the *leptospira* research by Schuffner; the geographic description of the spread of the pest by Van Loghem; the development of vaccins against the pest by Otten; the fascinating cholesterol research and its relation with cardiovascular disorders by De Langen. [39]

"*A contribution to Geographical Medicine from the clinics of Peiping Union Medical College*" wrote George Minot, Nobel prize winner for his work on pernicious anemia. In the introduction, Snapper was confronted in China with immensely important health care problems, such as nutrition and vitamin deficiencies, infectious diseases and cardiovascular disorders. Obviously, he had experience with most diseases in Amsterdam, but circumstances like diets and habits were different, and the patients were people from another race. Foremost, nutrition was one of the major determinants of disease in China, reflecting the social and economic situation. On top of that, sanitary facilities and hygiene had great effect on health care. That the clinical presentation of various diseases was different from Amsterdam, not only due to climate and malnutrition, but also due to the fact that patients presented at a later stage of disease. In his own words, Snapper stated that:

It is evident that a Western clinician, transplanted into North China, has to

cope with many problems which do not come to his attention before he moved to the
Orient.

Most patients who were admitted to PUMC were extremely poor. In Beijing, at that time, unlimited numbers of beggars could be found, among them many Russians. They were "White Russians", refugees after the revolution. They were unable to find work. Also in extreme poverty lived many apprentices, young boys from the countryside who had come to the city to work in shops and factories. They lived in extreme circumstances and had to work very hard. Patients came walking to hospital or were transported by handcart, accompanied by a policeman.

For every medical intervention, permission of the family needed to be obtained. More often than not, treatment was refused because of superstition. Sometimes valuable time was wasted because permission had to be obtained from family living miles outside the city. A great problem in those days in China were the blood donations. [40] Notably at the department of obstetrics blood loss during delivery had to be treated, but most Chinese people were unwilling to donate blood. An exception was formed that the poor and the opium adddicts who wanted to donate for money, but their blood was often contaminated with syfilis or malaria.

Food supply

Most patients in PUMC in those days suffered from severe malnutrition. On top of that, many were addicted to opium. The main diet was vegetable and contained only 2,000 calories, insufficient for most adults – the majority of whom had to perform heavy bodily labour. Although the low calory, vegetarian diet might be good for the prevention of cardiovascular disorders, it increased the risk to develope infectious diseases and serious vitamin deficiencies.

The diet of the poor Chinese people consisted mostly of cabbage and spinach. As they baked the vegetables in oil, most vitamins were destroyed by the heat of the cooking. Protein food for most people was too expensive.

One of the most prevalent deficiency disorders was vitamin D deficiency. That was due to the poor diet, the low milk intake, and the lack of exposition to sunlight. The combination of a low vitamin D and low calcium could lead to severe disturbances of the skeleton: *osteomalacia*. Snapper knew this well from Amsterdam. Bones were deformed, fractured, and the patient got immobilized and suffered from pains. Notably pregnant women suffered because of the increased need of vitamin D during pregnancy. On top of that, calcium went from mother to child during breastfeeding. The newborns often presented with tetany due to low calcium. Deformation of the pelvic bones made normal delivery impossible for many women.

Vitamin A deficiency was endemic. It resulted in night blindness, dry eyes, and inflammation of the skin. Snapper also observed scurvy, due to vitamin C deficiency. Snapper ascribed the deficiencies of the vitamins A and D to the lack of butter that contains these vitamins in the Chinese diet.

Infectious diseases

Snapper wrote extensively about infectious diseases, the most prevalent disorders in China during his time. Antibiotics were not yet available – they would in majority be developed during and after the war – with the exception of sulfapyridine. [41] To prevent spread of infections in hospital, hygienic measures were taken and patients were isolated.

Most of the diphteria patients came to hospital late in the course of the disease. They were treated with antitoxin-vaccination was not yet available-but the effect was questionable. The main complication was laryngeal obstruction, that could result in asphyxia. In such cases an emergency operation was necessary.

Pneumonia, often a complication of measles, was a frequent, lethal disorder. Most patients presented with complications, like abcesses and high fever with sepsis and shock. The treatment with sulfapyridine was often too late.

Mumps and scarlet fever were widely spread. In those days, Snapper emphasized, mumps was often followed by inflammation of the central nervous system, meningo-encefalitis, but also polyradiculitis and myelitis. Snapper gave a case history of a young patient with mumps and pancreatitis, nowadays rare.

Typhus fever, caused by a rickettsia and transmitted by fleas from rodents like rats and mice to humans, was very prevalent. That was due to poor hygiene and bad housing conditions. Snapper knew the clinical picture only from stories from the time of World War I. It was a disease with a high mortality rate, also called by the nickname "the doctors' murderer." Snapper warned that an infection also could occur during transport in a ricksha, a popular means of transport in Beijing. Remitting fever, caused by a spirochaete just like Lyme's disease and syphilis, was also a disease for most poor people living in primitive and unhygienic circumstances.

Snapper observed many patients with diarrhea due to infection with paratyphus and dysentery, notably during the summer. Dysentery by infection of amoebes was endemic and often caused abscesses in liver and abdomen. Cholera was rare.

Kala-azar, leishmaniasis, or black fever, transmitted by sandfly from dogs to humans, was so frequent in north China that one had to consider this diagnosis in every patient with fever. It was called black fever because the skin could become dark coloured. Snapper gave a description of children who had developed an infection of the skin due to kala-azar, the so-called "noma". [10] This could result in horrible disfigurement of the face. Another disease that was transmitted by dogs - and there were many of them in China - was rabies or hydrofobia. All patients died, there was no remedy.

The high prevalence of tuberculosis in Beijing was ascribed by Snapper to malnutrition, vitamin D deficiency, poor hygiene and overcrowding of the houses. As most people lived in small houses, many slept in one single room resulting in infection of whole families. Most people died: there was no treatment available. Snapper observed rare complications of tuberculosis, not seen in the West, like intestinal tuberculosis.

Time and again, Snapper emphasized that infectious diseases were highly prevalent and occurred mostly in the poor and underfed patient.

Cardiovascular disorders

Snapper made in China a series of interesting observations on diseases of the heart and bloodvessels: the coherence of diet, atherosclerosis, and blood cholesterol levels. It was in fact follow-up studies after the original work of his friend and former colleague De Langen, in the Dutch Indies, in 1915. De Langen had observed that cardiovascular disorders that were prevalent in Europe, were not seen in the Dutch Indies. Consequently, he started measuring cholesterol in the blood of the Javanese living in Batavia, the capital. This turned out to be remarkably low. On the contrary, cholesterol was high in Javanese who worked as servants on the European passenger steamers. These servants used in contrast to the native population who were almost vegetarian, a high calory diet rich of animal fat. [42]

Snapper repeated this research in Beijing and could confirm the observations of his former colleague. During his stay in China, Snapper came across only three presentations of chest pain due to narrowing of the heart vessels. One patient had a cardiac infarction, but that was smoker just like Snapper himself and like most doctors in those days. The relationship between smoking of cigarettes and arteriosclerosis had not yet been demonstrated.

The combination of a vegetarian diet, the low prevalence of cardiovascular disorders (and also of gallstones) and a low cholesterol was a unique finding, the first in its kind, in fact a world primary. But De Langen missed international recognition because he published his findings in *Het Geneeskundig Tijdschrift voor Nederlandsch Indië*, a journal in Dutch. Snapper had a broader view and had his article in the *American Journal of Cardiology*, with the attractive title: "*Diet and atherosclerosis: truth and fiction*". [43]

Snapper reached a large audience and attracted the attention of the medical elite. In this way the pioneering work of Snapper and De Langen eventually got international recognition. [44] They were nicknamed "medical Marco Polo's". It formed the basis of epidemiological studies of cardiovascular disorders and their link with diet, smoking and working conditions. [45]

Opium addiction

The smoking of opium was widely spread in China, in all layers of society. In contrast to the mild toxic effects of smoking, it was a far more dangerous poison when taken by mouth or by injection. Yearly, about 100 – 200 cases of opium intoxication were admitted to PUMC. [46] Once comatose, the mortality rate was considerable: 75% of the patients died. The amount of opium taken by the victim was expressed as "number of dollars' worth of opium". Major complications were suppression of the respiration and consequently bronchpneumonia. An antidote was not available.

The comatose patient was placed in a *Drinker*-machine, an artificial respirator or 'iron lung', designed in the USA in 1929 by Drinker en McKhann for the treatment of patients with poliomyelitis. However, artificial respiration was not very effective. Neither was washing the content of the stomach in order to remove the opium. On the contrary, this more often than not resulted in aspiration of stomach fluid; causing damage to the lungs and pneumonia.

Snapper treated the comatose patients with coramine, a stimulant of the respiratory center. Together with his assistants Irving Chu and Teh-yueh Cheng he got remarkable results, the mortality dropped to 20%. [47] But he also gave his poor patients the antibiotic sulfapyridine, a further explanation for his spectacular results.

Chinese Lessons to Western Medicine was well received by journals like the *New England Journal of Medicine*, [48] the *Journal of the American Medical Association*, [49] and *The Annals of Internal Medicine* [50]. The *Journal of Pediatrics* advised the military to take the book for preparation of service in the Far East. In 1965 a second edition was published. Thereafter it became *collector's item*.

Troubles

Snapper and his wife Hetty went on furlough to the USA at the end of 1940. In the meantime the political situation became worse. The Japanese occupation intensified, in the South West Nationalist troups tried to stop the Japanese, and in the North communist guerilla warfare had started. [51] In January 1941, all foreign women were advised to leave China as soon as possible. Nevertheless, Hetty decided, on her own risk, to return together with her husband to Beijing. Dr. Whitacre, gynaecologist, who had arrived in 1939 together with Snapper, had, however, decided to return to the US. Alarmed by this news, Snapper sent a cable to the China Medical Board in New York:

SHOCKED BY NEWS THAT WHITACRE ALSO RETURNS. HOW CAN THINGS GO ON IN THIS WAY? Snapper was very worried by the situation if more members of the medical staff would leave. Eventually, they would be the only foreign physicians in Beijing. Travelling was no longer possible, life was increasingly expensive and shortages of supply of goods and food were imminent. In fall 1941, all Americans were advised to leave China. By the end of 1941, only twenty Americans still worked in PUMC, mostly singles. Snapper, the Dutch anatomist Droogleeever Fortuyn and the American surgeon Harold Loucks were the only couples with their wives. [52] This citation from a letter from an American who stayed in PUMC as a patient is exemplary: *"All were Chinese, with the sole exception of Doctor Snapper, noted diagnostician."* [53]

Pearl Harbor

Sunday morning December 7, 1941, by surprise, Japan attacked the American naval base at Pearl Harbor, Hawaii. It was a devastating barrage destroying nearly the whole Pacific marine fleet. Unavoidably, the United States declared war on Japan. World War II was a fact.

Early the following morning, Japanese military surrounded PUMC and occupied the hospital. Patients could no longer be admitted, the outpatient's clinic closed. [54] Snapper was arrested at home and together with Henry Houghton, the director of PUMC, Trevor Bowen, the administrator, and Leighton Stuart, president of the Yenching University in Beijing, plus an unknown number of foreigners transported to the military headquarters and eventually confined in the marine quarters on the terrain of the American embassy. Visitors were not allowed.

January 10, 1942, Snapper, Houghton, Bowen and Stuart were transferred to the Ying house, home of the director of PUMC. They were being watched day and night by eight Japanese soldiers. [55] The others were released.

January 22, PUMC was closed down completely. Several months later, despite Japanese promise, the interior of the hospital was a complete mess. The furniture was damaged and the anatomical collections were missed. The Chinese physicians had fled and hid in smaller hospitals and clinics. All foreigners had to leave their homes and thereupon the country. [56]

The Rockefeller Foundation tried to influence the American government to exchange the American prisoners, but could not do anything for Dr. Snapper and his wife because they were Dutch, not American. [57] On the other hand, the Dutch government could or was not willing to do much for the Snappers because they were in China to work for an American organization. It was simply not in their interest. In brief, the Snappers were entrapped in Beijing.

May 8, 1942, the four men were moved to empty office spaces. They were completely isolated, no visitors were allowed. A single letter, opened, reached Snapper from time to time. A courtyard of 6 by 6 meter was the only space for movement. In the summer temperatures rose to 40℃ the bathroom was broken. [58] They had no idea about their future.

During custody, Snapper tried to keep himself busy with the preparation for the American medical qualifying examination by studying anatomy books. At regular times he was asked for consultation by the Japanese wards. Although all that kept him mentally stable, gradually he became more and more depressive.

Free at last

After eight months of confinement, Snapper was released on the 10th of August 1942 and could see his wife again. He was exchanged against six

Japanese diplomats who were imprisoned in Australia since the beginning of the war. [59] It was one of the last exchanges of prisoners. His three fellow prisoners, were, however, not released, probably because the Japanese bore even more resentment against all Americans. As Snapper was extremely worried about their wellbeing, [60] he made efforts to persuade the American government to do everything in order to liberate them. [61] However, they would only be set free three years later, in 1945, after the Japanese capitulation. The war had taken the life of 12 million Chinese people.

First, the Snappers went by train to Shanghai. From there, they sailed to Lourenco Marques, the capital of Mozambique at the African east coast where the exchange with the Japanese diplomats would take place. From there they went to England and arrived at Liverpool. From Liverpool they went to London to get all the necessary passports, stamps, documents and other papers and to find shipment to the USA. Although free, the Snappers had in fact become people without a country. They could not remain in China, they could not go to Dutch Indies because occupied by the Japanese, they could not return to Holland because of the German occupation, they had no permanent visa for England, they could not stay in Mozambique. They had set their hope on the United States.

Now, luck was on their side. They got permission to travel to the United States. They were even more than welcome, because the American government could make use of Snapper's expertise on tropical medicine on behalf of the American army at war in the Orient.

Finally, on October 25 1942, they could travel from Glasgow to New York, on board of the *Queen Elizabeth*.

Invited by the Pentagon

After arrival in the US, Snapper was invited by the Pentagon in

Washington to act as an expert on tropical disease for the department of preventive medicine, acting under the Surgeon General. The war department was in need of experts to advise on medical issues for the Pacific war, for "the conservation of manpower" and "the preservation of the strength of the military forces". At that time the US had increased its forces tremendously: by the end of 1944 more than 4 million military were in combat somewhere on the globe. Consequently, the medical corps had increased from 16, 00 in 1942 to 43, 00 in 1944. [62] Doctors from all specialties were drafted, including staff and professors form the universities.

Information was collected and documents were produced about all countries the American army came in contact with. Snapper wrote a detailed report about the health care situation in the Dutch Indies-then occupied by Japan. [63] Notably, he called attention to malaria and dysentery, the major health care problems that opposed American troops in the East.

Family and friends in Holland

Snapper's eldest son Frits had succeeded in escaping Holland and had arrived in Italy after an adventurous journey through Europe. There he, as a soldier fought on the side of Italian partizans in the mountains of Northern Italy. His wife, Helena Sondervan survived the nazi concentration camp Bergen-Belsen in Germany.

May 1940, just after the German occupation of The Netherlands, Snapper had sent a telegram from Beijing to his only sister, Betsy, with the strong advice to try to get a visa for the USA. Her efforts were without any success and it was her destiny to remain in Amsterdam. She was on the board of the Jewish girls orphanage. At the end of 1942 all girls were deported to concentration camps and most of them were killed. Betsy and her husband were also sent to a concentration camp in Germany, but survived and were eventually exchanged with German prisoners in Palestinia.

Hetty Snapper's mother, Catharina van Buuren-du Mosch was murdered in a German concentration camp, as well as Snapper's aunts and sisters who had lived in Amsterdam. Alfred Grünbaum, from Odessa, chemical scientist, Snapper's co-worker and colleague in the university hospital in Amsterdam, who first had escaped antisemitism in Russia, was also murdered. Ernst Laqueur, Snapper's friend and colleague, professor of farmacology, managed to survive the war.

Snappers view of PUMC

Snapper expressed his ideas about PUMC during an interview, at the end of 1940,[64] and also in a written report in 1942.[65] According to Snapper's opinion, the development of the school was hampered by its isolation. He reminded the reader that the school was once designated as a center of scientific research where also future teachers of medicine should be educated. Due to its isolation, however, there was no constructive criticism of neighbouring universities that could increase the standard of the work. That had a negative influence on the scientific work. Teaching was based on the knowledge of the chief of the department, and when there are no influences from outside, the basis becomes gradually smaller and smaller. In the western part of the world the chief learns more from his assistants than he teaches them. The isolation of PUMC is the reason why in Beijing, this rejuvenating process was conspicuous by its absence. The sending of junior staff for short visiting fellowships abroad did not solve this problem. Another problem was the language issue. It was difficult for the Chinese students to learn medicine from English speaking professors and textbooks in the English language.

But he was also positive. The Rockefeller Foundation and PUMC had since the start made remarkable accomplishments. 40 million dollars was spent to increase the level of medical education in China. The aim-to train future leaders of medicine had been reached as among nearly all Chines universities former students of PUMC were in the lead. The medical school was an example for other medical education in China.

Health care in China should be a task of the government and be organized at a central level, advised Snapper. The danger was that specialists, well educated with money from government, would set up private practices and spend their effort and time. According to law, young doctors should be obliged to work during several years in state hospitals. Further, postgraduate training should be obligatory at a regular basis. Therefore, special postgraduate hospitals should be set up.

State medicine should play a central role in the care of the 600 million inhabitants of the enormous country. Notably preventive medicine and public health programmes were a task for the government. The population itself should play a role in the organization.

Snapper concluded that PUMC could play an important role in the future. During the Japanese occupation, Chinese physicians had been cut off from communication with the West and therefore lagged behind in the rapid development of medicine. PUMC could organize up-to-date courses, postgraduate trainings, and exchange of knowledge with physicians from the West, notably the USA. The staff should be mixture of East and West. [66]

Later career

After his work for the war department, Snapper became professor of medicine at the Mount Sinai Hospital, Manhattan, New York. There he gained wide recognition and popularity. His grand rounds and presentations were famous. He published a new book on diseases of the skeleton, *Medical Clinicis on Bone Diseases*. But he would become most famous for *Bedside Medicine*, a remarkable book about internal medicine where he reported about all his experience and repeated his vision: medicine is at the bedside where the patient is.

Bibliography

1. M. E. Ferguson, *China Medical Board and Peking Union Medical College: A chronicle of fruitful collaboration 1914 – 1951* (New York, 1970), pp. 27 – 55

2. J. Z. Bowers, *Western Medicine in a Chinese Palace. Peking Union Medical College 1917 – 1951* (Philadelphia 1972), pp. 78 – 9

3. J. Z. Bowers, *Western Medicine in a Chinese Palace. Peking Union Medical College 1917 – 1951* (Philadelphia 1972) p. 79

4. I. Snapper, brief aan O. Brien, 20 maart 1938, folder 1210, box 166, series 601, DGC 1938, Rockefeller Foundation Archives RAC

5. J. Goldstein, *Jews in China. Historical and Comparative Perspectives* (New York 1999)

6. Dossier Snapper, Archives PUMC, Beijing

7. P. U. Unschuld, *Medicine in China. A History of Ideas* (Berkeley Calif 1985)

8. P. Huard en M. Wong, *Geneeskunde in China* (Amsterdam 1967)

9. C. U. Ariens Kappers, *Reiziger in breinen. Herinneringen van een hersenonderzoeker* (Amsterdam 2001)

10. E. Hume, *Doctors East*, *Doctors West* (London 1949)

11. R. Mitter, *China's war with Japan 1937 – 1945* (London 2014) pp. 34 – 48

12. B. Andrews, M. Brown Bullock, *Medical Transitions in Twentieth-Century China* (Bloomington, USA 2014) pp. 185 – 190

13. P. U. Unschuld, *Medicine in China. A History of Ideas* (Berkeley USA, 1985)

14. B. Andrews, M. Brown Bullock, *Medical Transitions in Twentieth-Century China* (Bloomington, USA 2014) p. 19

15. Idem, p. 219

16. J. D. Wilson, ' Peking Union Medical College Hospital, a Palace of Endocrine Trea-

sures' *J Clin Endo Metab* 76, 1993, pp. 815 – 6

17. J. Z. Bowers, *Western Medicine in a Chinese Palace. Peking Union Medical College 1917 – 1951* (Philadelphia 1972)

18. C. U. Lee, brief aan China Medical Board, 14 juni 1944, Collection CMB, Box 35, Criticism 1933 – 1944, Rockefeller Archives, RAC

19. Mary Brown Bullock, *An American Transplant*, *The Rockefeller Foundation and Peking Union Medical College*, (Los Angeles 1980) pp. 78 – 107

20. Report PUMC, folder 1314, box 182, series 601, RG 2 – 1939, Rockefeller Foundation Archives RAC

21. Idem, pp.

22. I. Snapper *Chinese lessons to western medicine* (New York 1941)

23. H. Schulte Nordholt, *China & de barbaren* (Amsterdam 2015) pp. 387 – 90

24. E. H. Hume, *The Chinese Way in Medicine* (Baltimore 1940) pp.

25. J. Le Fanu, *Rise and Fall of Modern Medicine* (London 1999) p. 201

26. R. Porter, *The greatest benefit to mankind. A medical history of humanity from antiquity to the present* (London 1997) pp. 147 – 62

27. E. H. Hume, *The Chinese Way in Medicine* (Baltimore 1940)

28. P. U. Unschuld, 'History of Chinese Medicine', In: K. F. Kiple, (red.) . *The Cambridge World History of Human Disease* (Cambridge 2008) pp. 20 – 6

29. C. F. Nathan, 'The acceptance of Western Medicine in early 20th century China: The story of the North Manchurian plague prevention service', In: J. Z. Bowers and E. F. Purcell (red.) *Medicine and Society in China* (Philadelphia 1974) pp. 55 – 81

30. Brief H. S. Houghton aan E. C. Lobenstine, August 9, 1939. folder 601, box 125, series CMB, RG PUMC Snapper, Rockefeller Foundation Archives, RAC

31. H. Schulte Nordholt, *China & de barbaren* (Amsterdam 2015) pp. 58 – 63

32. Letter E. C. Lobenstine to the China Medical Board. Folder 601, box 125, series CMB, RG PUMC Snapper. Rockefeller Foundation Archives RAC

33. I. Snapper, 'The mile-stone of graduation', Archives J. Snapper, Charlottesville, NC

34. Stadsarchief Gemeente Amsterdam. College van Curatoren. Inventarisnummer 279, Ingekomen en uitgaande stukken, 1938, nummer 195.

35. Snappers name in Chinese characters

36. I. Snapper, *Chinese Lessons to Western Medicine* (New York 1941)

37. Mary E. Ferguson, *China Medical Board and Peking Union Medical College: A chronicle of fruitful collaboration 1914 – 1951* (New York 1970)

38. I. Snapper, 'Medical contributions from the Netherlands Indies', *Science and Scientists in the Netherlands Indies, Surinam, and Curacao*, (New York 1945) pp. 309 – 20

39. J. L. Hydrick, *Intensive Rural Hygiene Work in The Netherlands east Indies* (New York 1944)

40. I. Snapper et al. , 'Anemia from blood donation. A haematological and clinical study of 101 professional donors' *Chin Med J* 56, 1939, pp. 400 – 423

41. I. Snapper et al. , 'Haematuria, renal colic and acetyl-sulfapyridine stone formation associated with sulfapyridine therapy' *Chin Med J* 56, 1939, pp. 1 – 10

42. C. D. de Langen, 'Cholesterol metabolism and racial pathology' *Gen Tijdschr Ned Indië* 56, 1916, pp. 1 – 34

43. I. Snapper, 'Diet and atherosclerosis: Truth and fiction' *Am J Cardiol* 11, 1963, pp. 283 – 9

44. James Le Fanu, *Rise and Fall of Modern Medicine* (London 1999) pp. 322 – 50

45. H. Blackburn, '20th-Century "Medical Marco Polos" in the origins of preventive cardiology and cardiovascular disease epidemiology' *Am J Cardiol* 109, 2012, pp. 756 – 67

46. Brief I. Snapper aan A. Gregg, 2 october 1941, Folder 1558, box 224, series 601, RG 2GC 1941, Rockefeller Foundation Archives RAC

47. I. Snapper, I. K. C. Chu, T. Y. Cheng, 'Treatment of acute opium poisoning. Beneficial effect of coramine' *Am J Med Sciences* 204, 1942, pp. 409 – 19

48. Anoniem, 'Book reviews' *N Engl J Med* 227, 1942, p. 498

49. Anoniem, 'Book notices' *JAMA* 118, 1942, p. 1262

50. Anoniem, 'Reviews' *Ann Int Med* 16, 1942, p. 1027

51. R. Mitter, *China's war with Japan 1937 – 1945* (London 2014) pp. 210 – 25

52. CMB inc, Box 119, Personnel 1919 – 1949, Rockefeller Archives RAC

53. Brief W. O. Inglis aan John D. Rockefeller Jr, 14 July 1939, folder 1314, box 182, series 601, RG 2 – 1939. Rockefeller Foundation Archives RAC

54. Idem, pp. 174 – 84

55. I. Snapper, brief aan A. E. Clattenburg, 30 october 1942, Record Group 59, CDF 1940 – 1944, 740. 00115a Pacific War/301, Box 2910, National Archives

56. R. Mitter, *China's war with Japan 1937 – 1945* (London 2014) pp. 239 – 63

57. Brief Board Rockefeller Foundation aan Nederlandse Ambassade Washington, 19 maart, 1942, folder 652, box 91, RG Medicine Staff, CMB, Rockefeller Foundation Archives, RAC

58. I. Snapper, brief aan A. E. Clattenburg, 30 october 1942, Record Group 59, CDF

1940 – 1944, 740. 00115a Pacific War/301, Box 2910, National Archives

59. M. J. van Lieburg, *Isidore Snapper's notes for memoirs 1889 – 1973: The autobiographical recollections of 'the Champion of bedside medicine'* (Rotterdam 2004) pp.

60. Interview met I. Snapper, 13 november 1942, folder 910, box 125, series CMB 1942 – 1948, RG Political Situation, Rockefeller Foundation Archives RAC

61. Brief A. E. Cohn aan Mr Justice Felix Frankfurter, Supreme Court of the United States, October 26, 1942, folder 910, box 125, series CMB 1942 – 1948, RG Political Situation, Rockefeller Foundation Archives RAC

62. Surgeon General Annual Reports 1939 – 1946, National Archives, Record Group 112, A1 – 46 – A, boxes 1 – 3

63. I. Snapper, 'Medical and sanitary data on the Netherlands East Indies', Medical Intelligence Branch, Preventive Medicine Division, Office of the Surgeon General, U. S. Army, National Archives, Record group 112, Medical and Sanitary Data, 1941 – 1958, box 2.

64. Interview with Dr I. Snapper, New York December 18, 1940.

65. I. Snapper, 'Comments on the Peiping Union Medical College', 1942, folder 652, box 91, RG Medicine Staff, China Medical Board, Rockefeller Foundation Archives, RAC

66. I. Snapper, 'Health Organization in China', Folder 652, box 91, RG Medicine Staff, China Medical Board, Rockefeller Foundation Archives, RAC

第二部分　传承 Transition

"老协和"的回忆[1]

玛丽·布朗·布洛克

玛丽·布朗·布洛克（MARY BROWN BULLOCK），杜克昆山大学第一任美国执行副校长，曾担任美国中华医学基金会（CMB）董事会主席。她的出版物包括：《洛克菲勒基金会与协和模式》（An American Transplant：The Rockefeller Foundation and Peking Union Medical College）（1980）及《油王：洛克菲勒在中国》（The Oil Prince's Legacy：Rockefeller Philanthropy in China）（2011）。她也曾经担任过艾格尼丝·斯科特学院（Agnes Scott College）的前校长，也担任过埃莫瑞大学（Emory University）的杰出客座教授。

1984 年 5 月 14 日，协和 1933 届毕业生、长期担任中国医学科学院和首都医科大学校长一职的黄家驷博士，因心脏病发作在老协和医院的院落中去世。遗憾的是，他没有活到 1987 年，亲眼目睹协和的七十周年庆典与中国医学科学院三十周年庆典。[2]因为那时，首都医科大学[3]已经恢复了其原来的带"协和"的名字——中国协和医科大学（PUMC，以下简称"协和"）。二十世纪走过其第一个四分之一（1925），协和迎来了它的第一次毕业庆典。在毕业典礼上，毕业生穿着华丽的长袍（以协和最初的毕业生长袍为模型）接受了毕业文凭，并在协和的大理石庭院里欢声笑语、载歌载舞。

黄家驷博士去世前一周之时，我很荣幸对他进行了一次长时间的访谈，那次他分享了他的生活故事：[4]

> 1924 年时我还是南开中学的高年级医学预科生。碰巧那时我去探望在

北京的哥哥，并经过了协和的校园。当时我就想，这是多么美丽的学习的
地方啊……但我那时觉得，我不可能通过考试的。

他在协和所受的培养与"老"协和的其他毕业生一脉相承：长学制
的预科、临床前教育与临床培养、由协和一位重要的西方教授来作
导师——这对于黄家驷来说，他的导师是娄克斯（Harold Louks）。接着
他在协和医院进行集中住院医师培养，然后去国外留学。黄家驷在美国
工作四年，期间师从密歇根大学的胸外科医生约翰·亚历山大（John
Alexander），二战后返回中国。他很出色地融入了国际的、世界范围的医
学圈，在本书第一章中达尔文·斯塔普顿（Darwin Stapleton）对此做了很
出色的描述。后来他与苏联的医学顾问一起工作了一段时间，并观察到：

> 协和的医学培养模式（和苏联）不同。在临床上，我们得心应手与他
> 们一样的出色，甚至或许我们比苏联顾问更加优秀，这就造成了一些困难。
> 但他们在基础研究方面更强。因为他们相当教条主义，所以有时也会有一
> 些矛盾，但我们还是成了好朋友：我们的私人关系相当好。

黄家驷最为自豪的是，他在中国医学科学院伊始所发挥的作用，以
及后来在20世纪50年代末和20世纪70年代末重组北京协和医学院时的
付出。因为协和的名字变来变去，很让人困惑，并且我也想知道这是否
意味着其性质的变化，于是我问他："首都医科大学是老协和一脉相承的
继承者吗？"他的回答很明确：

> 是的，很多教师、很多规定以及课程方面都是。我们有一个八年制的
> 医学课程，其中两年半的基础课程（预科课程）在北大，后五年半则在首
> 都医科大学……同老协和一样，我们是小班授课，并鼓励学生开展自己的
> 研究。……中国不可能让所有学校都像首都医科大学这样办学。人们一直
> 指责我们建设的是"象牙塔尖"，但是你没有建到象牙塔顶部的水平的话，
> 你也就无法建起来象牙塔了。

马超在其讨论协和百年历史的教学模式的章节里证实了黄家驷所确
认的内容。虽然他详细说明了在民国时期和毛泽东时代协和多次停办、

教授的教学风格的差异以及遭到的严厉批判，但马超得出结论：八年制的课程几乎奉若神明，一直没有大的变化——医学预科课程（两年半）；医学基础课程（三年）；临床课程（两年半）。毫无疑问，"八年制课程"已经成为协和的象征标志。虽然"八年制"常常被用来泛指培养一名顶尖医生所需的年限，但"八年制"不仅仅只意味着完成学业的时间。"八年制课程"寓意这一种根植于科学与临床医疗的医学精英教育。它引起过争议，因为在协和的历史上曾经有过一场全国性的辩论，探讨在中国究竟需要多长时间来培养一名医生。有很长一段时间，同时存在三年制课程、五年制课程和六年制课程，而协和的八年制课程是时间最长的。对八年制课程的存亡的威胁，也被视为对协和教员以及其毕业生的存在的威胁；由于这些原因，协和的领导层顽强地坚持他们所特有的八年制课程模式。

纵观整个世纪，对于被称为"约翰·霍普金斯模式"的坚持，肯定是协和最独特的属性之一。1991 年，协和内科老教授邓家栋（协和，1933 届）所写的文章中，不仅赞扬了约翰·霍普金斯的传统，还强调了其在北京的适应性：

> 协和从来都不是约翰·霍普金斯（以下简称"霍普金斯"）的原封不动的复制品，尽管在很多方面我们吸收了霍普金斯的经验。我们的课程与霍普金斯的课程不是一模一样的。第三和第四学年的临床见习和第五学年的实习与霍普金斯大学并不完全一样。公共卫生课程（由兰安生教授发起的课程）是协和原创的。但是，和霍普金斯一样，我们强调的也是学生的素质而不是数量。我们重视基本科学（知识）的良好基础。我们看重实验室和实践学习，而不是照本宣科的教学。我们努力培养创造性思维，避免填鸭式教育，诸如此类等等。[5]

十多年后的 2007 年，在协和 90 周年庆典之际，讴歌在其书中高度赞扬了这一教育模式及其对协和的影响：

> 约翰·霍普金斯大学强调学生自己的实践而不是课堂讲学……年轻的

医学生不再是被动的观察者，而是参与者。他们获取知识的方法，从聆听
讲座和观摩展示变为在实验室里进行的实际操作，还有临床教学，以及在
实习中对患者的责任……协和深受霍普金斯的影响……极其重视实践与技
能的培养。[6]

与此同时，协和公共卫生学院教授黄建始也写到他称之为的"协和
现象"，并悉数其背后的理由，即：表述清晰的使命；世界认可的模式；
独一无二的文化与传统；持续的改革与创造精神。[7]

到 1951 年，当美国撤回其资助时，协和已经成为一所机构设置完整、
专业自主和自我存续的机构。其每个特征都对协和的永久存续非常重要。
即使有时遭到批判，但是其模式极其清晰连贯、众所周知。无论是在医
院实践还是在教育中，协和共同体制定了自己的标准和规范。后辈由他
们的前辈培养。在对三个不同时期——即 1984 届、1987 届和 2007 届的
协和毕业生所进行的大量访谈显示出，不管是从专业上还是从情感上，
他们都对原来的模式有着非同寻常的认同。这一模式被协和的领导者们
成功保持了下来，即使有二十年甚至更长的时间停止了教学工作，协和
的核心特征以一种明确的理念坚持下来。

学术共同体的概念有助于理解这些记忆的作用以及为保存协和的特
有文化所做的努力。学术共同体，就是有共同价值观和规范的知识共同
体，在专业认同上往往超越了国界。这样的共同体就是专业人士的一个
网络，这些专业人士具备"在一个特定领域被认可的专门知识和能
力……拥有一套共同的规范性和原则性信念……还有一套与一系列问题
相关的针对这些问题的共同做法，其出发点大概是基于这样的信念：即
人类福祉将因此而得到增强。"[8]协和的医学共同体，无论是在北京还是在
其他地区，都符合这些属性当中的许多条。几乎就其最深层的本质而言，
这是一个专家共同体，这些专家共享规范的价值观，致力于人类福祉。
但在这里，其亲密关系超越了同类，而成为一个非常具体的专业共同体，
根源于一所单个的机构，却也依然享誉国际。而且，正如白玛丽（Mary
Brazelton）所指出的，科学医学的功效是一个王牌，使得 1950 年代让解

放军军管部门将协和核心身份保留下来。反讽的是，协和的小规模和许多次中断可能增强了他们对母体机构的忠诚度。对过往的回忆，一次又一次地反反复复，将协和文化传递给后代。

1984 年对五座城市（北京、天津、上海、广州和成都）的"老"协和毕业生的采访揭示了"文化大革命"结束后得以解放的一个高龄共同体，他们渴望改革开放时期的专业开放和机遇。从 1927 届（诸福棠）到 1942 届（吴阶平）的 30 名协和毕业生（其中有 10% 毕业于 1942 年之前），有许多相似之处：无可挑剔的英语、重要的国际经验、领导角色、对其学生时代鲜活的回忆、八年制长学制的共同经历——以及对协和再次被认可为中国杰出医疗机构的渴望。[9]

这第一代协和人，通常是由于家人罹患疾病而促使他们选择了医疗职业生涯，但也反映了他们对独立的职业生涯的渴望。陈志潜（协和，1929届）与郁知非（协和，1940 届）二人的母亲早就过世；而林飞卿（协和，1932 届）作为一个女人则"想独立，不希望依靠别人"。她为自己感到自豪，因为她所在的班级中女性比男性完成学业的比例更高，在毕业时最终达到 11 人。总的来说，一些是获得奖学金资助的学生，其他人则来自于工程技术、军事或专业学术的家庭。所有人都铭记他们在协和的那些岁月的细节——比如，每个人都能有自己的显微镜，还有人记得美丽的协和校园。吴阶平详细地讲述了协和宿舍生活的儒雅，而有些人会把其描述为奢华。所有的人都谈及了漫长而艰苦的学业以及对独立思考的强调。

然而，最鲜明的是这些毕业生们在学科和机构中发挥的领导作用，及领导力是如何在中国其他地区（包括台湾）造就了类似协和的医学共同体。在这本书中，巴德年的章节提供了协和毕业生成为各医学院校长的细节。天津是协和之影响力的一个很好例证。第二次世界大战时期，协和被关闭，一些协和毕业生移居到附近的天津。这些人领导的几个机构常被称为"小协和"。朱宪彝（协和，1930 届）担任天津医学院的院长，金显宅（协和，1931 届）是天津肿瘤医院创始人和院长。施锡恩

（协和，1929 届）创办天津第一家泌尿学实验室，其中包括中国首批血液透析实验室之一。回忆起天津的早年生涯，朱宪彝回忆说，在 1940 年代初，天津还没有协和毕业生，但最终有 30 名甚至更多的人留在天津 12 所不同的医疗机构。朝鲜裔金显宅开始在原来的马大夫纪念医院（后来的天津肿瘤医院）工作，随着时间的推移，它后来成为中国最重要的癌症研究中心之一。金显宅所感慨的失去的十年，指的是 1940 年代和抗日战争时期。他还感慨创办医疗机构的挑战：白手起家、争取设备和训练有素的人员的艰辛。由于没有协和的实验室和医院，天津毕业生不得不适应当地条件。在他们试图将自己所接受到的卓越的医学培养带到一个新的环境期间，他们感到了彼此的友情。

相比之下，上海共同体则聚集在上海第一医学院，即今天的复旦大学医学院。上海第一医学院的早期领导人中包括颜福庆，他曾短暂担任协和的副校长，后由在协和学过药物学的朱恒璧接替。在去北京之前，黄家驷曾是第一位成功完成开胸手术并担任医学院校长的外科医生。其他仍然活跃在上海的协和毕业生非常兴致勃勃地要创造一个"小协和"——一个 30 名学生的班级，如同在原来的协和一样进行全英文教学。早在 1984 年，全英文教学得以实现，因为在上海第一医学院担任教师的老协和们，其英语水平很高，且政治氛围也可行——因为中国再次决定派遣学生出国接受培训。

广州的协和毕业生们多年来在陈国桢（协和，1933 届）领导下，对他们在今天的中山医科大学的作用感到自豪。让他们更引以为豪的是当时由何天琪（协和，1941 届）领导下建起的一所教学医院，正好坐落在 19 世纪初伯驾（Peter Parker）的眼科诊所之处。孙中山先生也曾于这所医学院就读过。虽然远离北京，广州却是不少协和最优秀的学生的来源地——许多人返回家乡为家乡服务。在那里的七人共同回忆起他们的协和教授林可胜（Robert Lim）的"严厉"、吴宪"讽刺的尖锐"、斯乃博（Isodore Snapper）及其他西方教授的令人无法忘怀的讲座。这些教授"创立了专业课程，并协助在美国选修"。当我在 1984 年见到陈国桢时，他谈起一年前举行的 1933 届五十年聚会。所有还在世的成员都算上了，还包括去世的同学的亲属。这次在人民大会堂举办了晚宴，活动很大，在政治上标志着对包括黄家驷在内的这个杰出班级的感谢。

在成都，我屡次遇见时常被称为中国公共卫生之父的陈志潜（协和，1929 届）。他是最早规划多级医疗人员培训项目者之一，后来被称作赤脚医生运动。他对协和忠心耿耿，但他对协和曾经强大的公共卫生专业的消亡及协和不再要求学生必须到农村或城市的卫生中心实习一段时间进行了批判。对他的采访中，最令人印象深刻的是他对中国公共卫生工作的热情。在他九十多岁时，还在继续倡导在农村地区培养医生。在他去世前两年，他给我写的最后一封信中，写道：

> 正如我 1975 年同你说过，我从一个苏联司机那里学到，要时常保持耐心。这有一个例子：1996 年 11 月，北京的最高领导讨论了中国的卫生问题……并提议：要求年轻医生必须在农村地区服务 6～12 个月。因此，很可能这所大学（四川医科大学）会考虑将毕业班的医学生送到农村中心进行实地培训。在卫生方面又恢复了过去的做法，这可以帮助我们数百万的贫困农民。[10]

当然，大多数的老协和毕业生仍然留在北京，留在协和工作。几个被采访的协和毕业生在新机构担任领导职务：北京友谊医院的钟惠澜（协和，1929 届）和北京儿童医院的院长诸福棠（协和，1927 届）。有些毕业生则担任中国医学科学院（CAMS）的下属研究机构的领导，如北京市心肺血管疾病研究所的吴英恺和病毒研究所的黄祯祥（协和，1934 届）。正如巴德年和白玛丽在随后章节中所讨论的，协和的毕业生还在北京医科大学、解放军 301 医院等地担任领导职务。

直到 2007 年，我才有机会采访了年轻些的共 18 名毕业生，他们在 20 世纪 40 年代末和 60 年代中期考入协和。[11]正是这些第二代和第三代的协和毕业生们，用非常不同的方式继承了协和的精神。他们没有被送往国外接受毕业后培训，而是被派到宁夏和西藏的乡村和远郊。然而，他们的经历有些类似于那些在天津、上海和广州的毕业生，在战争时期饱经风霜却依然对协和忠心耿耿。个人和专业上的困难反而加剧并理想化了其对于协和近乎神话的记忆。

那些于 20 世纪 40 年代末进入协和并于 50 年代毕业的一代协和人，将"老"协和与1960～70 年代间风云变幻的协和衔接起来。这种链接与回忆在 1980 年代变得至关重要：因为他们担负起恢复协和医学教育的责任。这些人先在燕京大学生物系接受预科教育，而后在 50 年代初燕京大学转变成北京大学时又转到了北大。长期担任燕京大学生物学教授的博爱理（Alice Boring）令学生们难忘，并常常提起：她将孟德尔的遗传学介绍至中国而获得人们的赞誉。当学生们回到协和学习基础医学课程和临床训练时，他们的老师是那些在老协和上学并代替了之前的外国教师成为各学科的带头人：诸福棠、林巧稚、张锡钧、吴英恺、吴蔚然、刘士豪、张孝骞等人。这些"老"协和毕业生在其教学与临床的地位，如同 50 年代和60 年代的医学明星，复制了自己学生时代所经历的专业和规范价值。协和文化既是对这些教授的挑战，也孕育了他们，在各种情形中都延伸到了其学生身上。从这个时代过来的受访者清晰地记着当时为延续苏格拉底的教学方法所做的努力、导师制、严格的实验室培训、暗地里去图书馆——甚至在协和被军管之时。正如神经病学系的汤晓芙（协和，1956 届）所记得的一样："他们教我们如何学习、如何思考、如何想象。"

当然，政治运动也影响了这中间一代——无论是抗美援朝、反"右"运动还是"文化大革命"。前协和医院院长方圻（1946 届）记得，"有许多政治运动干扰我们，没有时间读书"。他的同事罗慰慈（1953 届）记得，在"文化大革命"期间，协和闭校了十年，而且共有 500 个协和家庭在此期间搬迁到西北。虽然一些人对这期间的重重困难记忆犹新，但令人最强烈的感觉是，在 2008 年时，这一代人大多把记忆聚焦在 20 世纪80 年代，在此期间他们成为协和真正承上启下的一代人。

与 20 世纪 50 年代之前出国接受博士后培训的年轻协和人不一样，这个时期许多被送到国外的协和人，是作为 50 年代至 60 年代的年长的访问学者。他们在原始的协和文化中磨炼出医疗实践，之后20世纪50年代和60年代的风风雨雨干扰了其发展。朱元珏是最早的这批人之一。她1976年去了哈佛大学医学院附属麻省总医院交流两年。她回忆说，那是"很美好的经历"，她的英语水平是一大优势，而且有一种成就感："协和文化的一部分是：你需要出国留学。"对国际化经验的要求一直在不断强调。罗慰慈于1983年去约翰·霍普金斯研究肺病。他还与其他协和成员一起考察了美国医学的最新发展 —— 例如哈佛医学院的临床路径课程。汤晓芙则前往丹麦学习神经生理学。

戴玉华（协和，1954届）属于协和的这一代人，她还是协和复校之后的教务长。她特别记得张孝骞，是他教会他们如何真正关注各类病人，让他们学会独立学习。1987年，在协和70周年庆典之际，她评论说，协和的栋梁是这第二代的毕业生。

这一代人的第二批，是那些在1959～1966年这一短暂的宽松年代考入协和的学生，他们对其协和时光的回忆尤为心酸——部分原因是它如此之短。没有人能够完成常规的八年制课程。那些在20世纪50年代末在北京大学开始预科课程的，以及那些在1960年代初已经开始在协和学习医学课程的，还能够完成所有的预科课程及部分临床培养。而之后几年（1963年和1964年）才开始在北大读预科的人，则几乎立刻被卷入了红卫兵运动的政治混乱当中。几乎所有人都在20世纪70年代被送往偏远地区。

受访者记得最清楚的是他们在农村地区行医的经历：试图跟上医学发展，而最终能回到协和 —— 要么完成医学学业，要么成为医院或研究机构的合格的员工。协和这一时期的教务长章央芬，尽一切努力联络散落各地的学生，并试图与他们保持联系。20世纪70年代初，黄家驷则说服了周恩来，把180名学生调回协和。大约一年后，有些人不得不重新返回农村地区。1978年邓小平宣布所有希望继续学业的人员都可以参加考试。不是所有的人都可以重新进入协和，但是在1979年返回的人完成了三年的硕士研究生课程。对于那些最年轻的人来说，这就是他们所接受的唯一的不间断的正规医学培养。正是"文革"这一代最终填补了这一断层，并在 20 世纪 90 年代和 21 世纪初为中国的医学院和医疗机构提供了领导力量。

像他们的前辈们一样，"文革"这一代也被送到国外学习。药理学教授及主任张德昌于 1985 年获得药理学博士学位。协和医院前副院长马遂（协和，1963 届）去了波士顿的布里格姆妇女医院（Brigham Women's Hospital）。中国医学科学院肿瘤医院的头颈外科主任唐平章则去了英国以及（美国）北卡罗来纳大学（University of North Carolina）。中国预防医学科学院（Chinese Academy of Preventive Medicine）前副院长王克安在加拿大麦吉尔大学学习。协和医院前院长陆召麟在英国和加拿大学习。

这些文革时期的协和毕业生反映了同时期的其他很多学生的情况。尽管他们的教育被延误和中断，然而他们的职业生涯仿效了"老协和"人。强调给这些学业被削减而又年长些的访问学者提供国际化教育是中国国家总体战略的一部分。与早些年代的毕业生相比，那些在协和与中国医学科学院工作的人则能够复制出更为广泛的国际联系。协和再次成为一所国际化的学校。

在过去三十年，有关"老协和"的回忆在许多场合出现——在多本著作与回忆录、纪念出版物中。特别重要的是 1987 年开始的周年纪念庆祝活动。这是在中华人民共和国时期举办的第一个协和校庆，特别感谢了"老协和"的领导者们。参加者包括政治领域和医学领域的杰出人士，几乎每次发言都特别向林巧稚和黄家驷致敬，这两位在那时刚去世不久。卫生部部长陈敏章的贺词在其中很有代表性：

> 医科院与协和承担着满足全国需要和为全国服务的光荣历史使命。在过去的几十年中，医科院与协和为我们国家培养了一大批医学和卫生界的杰出人才，我国科学专业领域的卓越先驱。在国内外的许多地方都可以看到他们的身影。他们为发展、繁荣祖国的医学科学事业所做出的贡献，给我们留下了深刻的印象。[12]

十年后的 1997 年，中华人民共和国主席江泽民为协和题词："严谨、博精、勤奋、奉献。" 2007 年，协和的九十周年庆典通过举行约翰·D. 洛克菲勒的半身塑像揭幕仪式，溯源到美国人所开办的历史，洛克菲勒家族成员也出席了典礼。《九十周年纪念相册》把豫亲王原来的亭台楼阁与协和校园元素放在一起：大理石栏杆、绿色的雕刻屋顶、花园长廊、传统门厅和迎客石狮。协和医学院党委书记刘谦在该书的序言中说，难以言表的"永恒鲜明的协和精神"体现在协和建筑的每一处细节之中。他提出职业与抱负的精髓：

> 这些建筑不正具体体现协和高标准、高起点、高水平、精雕细刻的办学理念吗？当你徜徉于绿瓦灰墙、长廊甬道之时，你不觉得恰似穿越时光隧道，宛若先贤们就在你的身旁与你同行吗？

虽然这些先驱们深深爱着并铭记协和，但是他们亦不羞于呼吁其母校在新中国发挥更强有力的领导力。在协和 90 周年庆典上陈元方（协和，1957 届）提出问题："协和医学院的传统过时了吗？应该把协和医学院送进博物馆吗？"新的挑战包括知识爆炸、课程改革的需求、公共卫生问题的全球化、慢性病和医学伦理的要求。陈元方的讲话几乎就是对老协和的颂歌。对于她来说，"协和精神"就是长期附着在学院上的文化的结果，在那里"协和人……认真细致、尽职尽责、无私奉献，热爱科学、追求卓越、坚持真理、敢于直言、蔑视随波逐流。"[13] 同样在 90 周年校庆时，拥有协和医学院博士学位的校长刘德培，肯定了协和传统的延续，协和还没有束之高阁。他的愿景超越了八年制本科教育，还包括重视医学科学与研究；一所高端的医学教育机构，把中国医学科学院十八家研究机构以及北京协和医院整合在一起。[14]

"老协和"的理想化记忆有助于该机构的保持和永久存续。协和恐怕是唯一一个成立于民国时期并延续百年的美国或是外国的学校，得以保留其核心身份，并最终保留其名字的学校。后毛泽东时代的协和领导人——黄家驷、吴阶平、顾方舟、巴德年和刘德培，他们努力寻求创新与开创一个新的时代，但仍然感到对老协和强大回忆的压力。每个访谈人都显示了对于精英医学教育的深信不易，并提出了同等重要的标杆作用的价值观以及适应新时代的艰巨任务。随着协和百年华诞，这一挑战将得以持续：如何保存和保护"老协和"的最佳价值及如何适应第二个百年。

参考书目

1. 本章基于以下著作并引用了其中部分材料：《油王：洛克菲勒在中国》第四章（斯坦福大学出版社，2011 年）。

2. 这实际上是中国医学科学院的 31 周年庆典，因其成立于 1956 年。直到 2016 年协和才和中国医学科学院一起庆祝他们的周年纪念。

3. 关于协和十几个不同的名称的细节，请参见马超的章节。

4. 对黄家驷的采访，1984 年 5 月 9 日，北京。

5. 邓家栋致作者，1991 年 6 月 13 日。

6. 讴歌：《协和医事》；（北京：生活·读书·新知三联书店，2007 年），第 98 页。

7. Huang， "An Analysis of the 'PUMC Phenomenon' in Medical Education Development in China," in China Medical Board， 75th Anniversary Celebration， （New York：China Medical Board，2004，23.

8. Peter M. Haas， "Introduction：Epistemic Communities and International Policy Coordination," International Organization 46（Winter 1992）：3

9. 1984 年访谈的协和师生包括：北京 — 黄家驷，吴阶平，程贤秋，王季午，钟惠澜，王正仪，黄桢祥，吴英恺，严仁英，诸福棠，黄翠庭，叶恭绍，邓家栋。上海—荣独山，张主宾，熊汝成，林飞卿。天津 — 朱宪彝，施锡恩，金显宅，虞颂庭。广州 — 陈国桢，何天琪，唐紫光，许天禄，张峨，黄爱廉，黄淑云。成都 — 陈志潜。

10. 陈志潜致作者，1998 年 1 月 12 日。

11. 2007 年在北京访谈的协和毕业生包括：刘德培，王克安，潘孟昭，黄人健，吴明江，唐平章，马遂，汤晓芙，方圻，朱预，罗慰慈，高友鹤，张德昌，戴玉华，朱元珏，陈元方，陆召麟，吕式媛，倪超，胡天圣，吴蔚然，李学旺。

12. 来自协和七十周年纪念庆祝典礼的出版物。作者参加了这一庆典。

13. 陈元芳在协和九十周年庆典上的报告：《北京协和医学院：回顾与展望》，2007 年 10 月 14 日，此报告未曾出版过。

14. 刘德培在协和九十周年庆典上的报告：《协和的过去、现在和未来》，2007 年 10 月 14 日，此报告未曾出版过。

Memories of Old PUMC[1]

Mary Brown Bullock

Mary Brown Bullock was the first executive Vice Chancellor of Duke Kunshan University and was chair of the China Medical Board from 2005 to 2014. Her publications include An American Transplant: The Rockefeller Foundation and Peking Union Medical College (1980) and The Oil Prince's Legacy: Rockefeller Philanthropy in China (2011). She was the former president of Agnes Scott College and visiting distinguished Professor of Chinese history at Emory University.

On May 14, 1984 Dr. Huang Jiasi, PUMC class of 1933 and long-time president of the Chinese Academy of Medical Science and Capital Medical College, died of a heart-attack within the walls of the old PUMC. Regrettably he did not live to see the 1987 seventieth anniversary celebration of PUMC and the thirtieth anniversary of the Chinese Academy of Medical Sciences. [2] For it was on that occasion that the Capital Medical College [3] was returned to its original English name, Peking Union Medical College. And PUMC celebrated its first graduating class in a quarter of a century. The graduates wore resplendent robes (modeled on the original PUMC gowns), received their diplomas and there was singing and dancing in the marble PUMC courtyard.

I was privileged when Dr. Huang shared his life story in a long interview just a week before he died: [4]

I was a senior in medical school in 1924, at Nankai Middle School. I happened to visit my elder brother who was in Beijing, and passed by the PUMC complex. I thought what a beautiful place to study...but I thought I would never pass the examination.

His training echoed that of other graduates of the "old" PUMC: long pre-med and clinical program, training by a key western PUMC professor, in his case Harold Loucks, intense residency at PUMC hospital, and then study abroad. Huang spent four years in the United States working under John Alexander, thoracic surgeon, at the University of Michigan, returning to China after World War II. He was well-integrated into the international, cosmopolitan medical circles so well described by Darwin Stapleton in the first chapter of this volume. He later spent time working with Soviet medical advisors observing that

> *PUMC trained differently. In clinical work we were easily as good, perhaps better than our Soviet advisors, and this caused some difficulties. But they were stronger in basic research. There was some tension because they were quite dogmatic. But we became good friends: our personal relations were reasonably good.*

Huang was most proud of the role he had played in the beginning years of the Chinese Academy of Medical Science and subsequent efforts in the late 1950s and late 1970s to reconstitute Peking Union Medical College. Confused by the many name changes and wondering whether this signaled a change in identity I asked him: "Is Capital Medical College a direct descendent of the old PUMC?" His response was unequivocal:

> *Yes, in terms of many of the faculty and many of the policies and curriculum. We have an 8 year medical curriculum with $2\frac{1}{2}$ year premed at Beida: $5\frac{1}{2}$ years at Capital Medical College. ...we still have small classes and encourage the students to do their own research. ...China cannot afford to have all schools like*

Capitol Medical College and we have always been accused of "building the top of the pyramid. But you cannot level the top of the pyramid: then you will not have a pyramid."

Ma Chao's chapter on PUMC's academic program across its hundred year history echoes Huang Jiasi's affirmation. Although he details the multiple institutional closures, differences in teaching style of professors and heavy criticism during both the Republican and Maoist periods, Ma concludes that the almost sacrosanct 8 year curriculum, remained more or less the same-premed ($2\frac{1}{2}$ years); pre-clinical (3 years); clinical ($2\frac{1}{2}$ years). There is no question but that the "8 year curriculum" became the symbolic icon for PUMC. Although often reduced to merely the length of time required to train top physicians the "8 year curriculum" symbolized more than just time to graduate. The "8 year curriculum" became a metaphor for elite medicine grounded in both science and clinical care. It became controversial because throughout PUMC's history there was a national debate on how much education was required to train physicians for China. Three-year, five-year, and six-year programs co-existed for many years with PUMC's 8 years at the apex. Threats against it were seen as existential threats by PUMC faculty and graduates: for these reasons PUMC leaders clung tenaciously to their privileged 8 year model.

The persistence of what was known as "the Johns Hopkins model" across the century is surely one of PUMC's most distinct attributes. Writing in 1991 long time PUMC professor of medicine Deng Jiatung '33 celebrated the Johns Hopkins legacy but also emphasized the adaptations made in Beijing:

PUMC was never an exact replica of Johns Hopkins, but, in many ways we absorbed J. H.'s experiences. Our curriculum was never exactly the same as J. H.'s. The 3rd and 4th year clerkships and 5th year internships are not the same as in J. H. The public health course (a teaching program initiated by

Prof. J. B. Grant) was original here. But, like J. H. we emphasized quality and not quantity of students. We emphasized good foundation of basic sciences. We emphasized laboratory and practical studies instead of didactic teaching. We tried to cultivate creative thinking and avoid spoon-feeding, etc. [5]

Writing more than a decade later, in 2007 at the time of PUMC's 90th anniversary Ou Ge extolled this educational model and its influence on PUMC:

Johns Hopkins University emphasized students' own practice rather than lectures... Young medical students were no longer passive observers, but participants. The way they acquired knowledge had changed from listening to lectures and observing demonstrations to actual operation in labs, bedside teaching and intern's responsibility for patients .... The PUMC which was greatly influenced by Johns Hopkins.... emphasized practice and the cultivation of skills. [6]

Writing about the same time, Huang Jianshi, PUMC Professor of Public Health, explicated reasons writing for what he called "the PUMC phenomena:" a clearly stated mission; a world recognized model; a unique culture and tradition and a continuous spirit of reform and creativity. [7]

By 1951, when American support was withdrawn, PUMC had become an institutionally coherent, professionally autonomous and self-perpetuating institution. Each of these characteristics is important to the perpetuation of PUMC's identity. If sometimes criticized, the model was clear, coherent and well-known. The PUMC community, both in hospital practice and in education set its own standards and norms. And successive generations were trained by their predecessors. Scores of interviews with PUMC graduates at three different times - 1984, 1987 and 2007 - revealed an extraordinary professional and emotional identification with the original model, a model that was successfully perpetuated by PUMC's leaders. Even during the twenty or more years when education ceased, a clear conception of PUMC's core identity persisted.

The concept of epistemic communities is helpful in understanding the role of these memories and the efforts to preserve PUMC's distinct culture. An epistemic community is a knowledge community with a shared sense of values and norms, which is often transnational in its professional identity. Such a community is a network of professionals with "recognized expertise and competence in a particular domain … with a shared set of normative and principled beliefs … and a set of common practices associated with a set of problems to which their competence is directed, presumably out of the conviction that human welfare will be enhanced as a consequence. "[8] The PUMC medical community, both in Beijing and beyond, fits many of these attributes. Almost by its very nature a medical community is a community of experts who share normative values and are dedicated to human welfare. But here the affinity goes beyond the generic to the very specific, a professional community with roots in a single institution yet also with an international reputation. And, as demonstrated in Mary Brazelton's chapter, the efficacy of scientific medicine was the trump card which convinced the PLA in the 1950s to retain PUMC's core identity. Ironically, PUMC's small size and many interruptions also may have intensified loyalty to the parent institution. Memories, repeated over and over again, transmitted the PUMC culture to subsequent generations.

Interviews of the "old" PUMC graduates in five cities (Beijing, Tianjin, Shanghai, Guangzhou and Chengdu) in 1984 revealed an elderly community relieved by the end of the Cultural Revolution and relishing the professional openness and opportunities of the Reform and Opening period. Across a cohort of thirty graduates (10% of the pre-1942 graduates) from 1927 (Zhu Futang) to 1942 (Wu Jieping) many similarities were evident: impeccable English, significant international experience, leadership roles, vibrant memories of their student years and the shared experience of the long 8 year curriculumand a longing for PUMC to once again be recognized as China's preeminent medical institution. [9]

In this first PUMC generation the selection of a medical career often emerged from a family illness but also reflected a desire for an independent professional career. The mothers of both Chen Zhiqian' 29 and Yu Tsefei ' 40 mothers had died, while Lin Feiqing '32, as a woman " wanted to be independent, didn't want to depend on others. " She was proud that women had a better rate of persistence in her class than men, ending up with 11 each at graduation. Overall, some were scholarship students, others had families in engineering, military, academic professions. All remembered details of their PUMC years-that each had their own microscope, for example. Others remembered the beautiful PUMC spaces. Wu Jieping recounted details of a very civilized, some would say luxurious, dormitory life. All referenced the long, hard study, the emphasis upon independent thinking.

What was most distinct, however, was the leadership roles that they had played in disciplines and in institutions, and how that had led to the creation of PUMC-like medical communities in other parts of China, including Taiwan. Ba Denian's chapter in this volume provides details about the PUMC graduates who became presidents of medical colleges. Tianjin is a good example of PUMC's influence. With the closure of PUMC in WWII, a group of graduates migrated to nearby Tianjin. The cluster of institutions for which they provided leadership was often called "the little PUMC. " Zhu Xianyi ' 30, served as president of Tianjin Medical College and Jin Xianzhai ' 31, was founder and director of Tianjin Cancer Hospital. Shi Xien ' 29 developed the first urology laboratory in Tianjin which included one of the first hemodialysis labs in China. Remembering the early years in Tianjin Zhu recalled there were no PUMC graduates in Tianjin in the early 1940s but eventually 30 or more were based in 12 different medical institutions. Jin, of Korean origin, began his work in the original MacKenzie Medical School, but over time transformed this into one of China's foremost cancer research centers. Jin lamented the lost ten years, by which he meant the 1940s and the Sino-Japanese War, and the challenge of beginning medical institutions from scratch, of struggling for equipment and trained personnel.

Without the PUMC labs and hospital the Tianjin graduates had to adapt to local conditions. In doing so they felt a camaraderie with each other as they sought to bring the medical excellence of their training to a new environment.

In contrast, the Shanghai community had clustered around Shanghai First Medical College, today's Medical Center of Fudan University. The early leaders of Shanghai First included Yan Fuqing, who had served briefly as vice-director of PUMC, followed by Zhu Hengbi, who had studied pharmacology at PUMC. Before going to Beijing Huang Jiasi had both been the first surgeon to complete open lung surgery and to serve as the medical college's president. Other PUMC graduates still active in Shanghai were most excited about creating a "mini-PUMC" - a class of 30 students with all instruction in English, as in the original PUMC. As early as 1984 this had become possible because of the high English level of the old PUMC faculty at Shanghai 1st and politically feasible because China had decided, once again, to send students abroad for training.

The PUMC Guangzhou community was proud of their role at what is today Zhongshan Medical University, led for many years by Chen Guozhen '33, prouder still that one of its teaching hospitals, then led by He Dianji '41 is located on the site of Peter Parker's original early 19th century eye clinic. Sun Yat-sen also attended this medical school. Although far from Beijing, Guangzhou had been the source of some of PUMC's strongest students - many of whom returned to serve their native city. A group of seven remembered together their PUMC professors-Robert Lim's "toughness," Hsien Wu's "biting sarcasm, the unforgettable lectures of Isodore Snapper and other western professors. These professors were credited with "shaping their course of specialties and also helped in gaining post-docs with good people in the United States. " When I met with him in 1984, Chen Guozhen talked about the fiftieth reunion of the class of 1933 a year earlier. All living members were accounted for and relatives from those who had died also attended. The big event was a dinner at the Great

Hall of the People, signaling a new political appreciation for this distinguished class which also included Huang Jiasi.

In Chengdu I met on several occasions with Chen Zhiqian '29, sometimes called the father of China's public health. He was one of the first to design a multi-tiered medical training program for what became known in later years as the barefoot doctors. While devoted to PUMC he deplored the demise of its previous strong public health specialty, the diminished requirements for PUMC students to spend some time in a rural or urban health center. What was striking about his interviews was his passion for his continuing work in China's public health. Already in his nineties, Chen continued to advocate for the training of physicians in rural areas. In his last letter to me, just two years before his death, he wrote:

> As I told you in 1975 I learned from a Soviet driver to always be patient. Here is a case. In November 1996 the highest officials at Beijing discussed the health problems of this country…. it was proposed that young doctors be required to serve in rural areas for 6 – 12 months. It is therefore probable that this University (Sichuan Medical University) will consider sending senior medical students to rural centers for field training this year. This is a renewed health effort to help millions of our underprivileged farmers. [10]

Of course the majority of the old PUMC graduates remained in Beijing and at PUMC. Several who were interviewed played leading roles at newer institutions: Chong Huilan '29 at Beijing Friendship Hospital and Zhu Futang, '27 head of Beijing Children's Hospital. Others led institutes of the Chinese Academy of Medical Sciences, for example Wu Yingkai at Beijing Heart, Lung and Blood Research Institute, Huang Zhenxiang '34 at the Institute of Virology. As discussed by Ba Denian and Mary Braselton, in subsequent chapters, still others played leading roles at Beijing Medical University, at the PLA Hospital 301 and so on.

It was not until 2007 that I had the opportunity to interview 18 members of a younger cohort who had entered PUMC in the late 1940s and the mid-1960s. [11] It is this second and third generation that inherited the ethos of PUMC in much different ways. They were not sent abroad for post-doctoral training but rather to the countryside and far Ningxia and Tibet. Yet their experience was somewhat analogous to those in Tianjin, Shanghai, and Guangzhou who weathered wartime conditions and remained fiercely loyal to PUMC. Personal and professional hardship intensified and idealized the memories of what became an almost mythic PUMC.

The PUMC contingent that entered the institution in the late 1940s and graduated in the 1950s provided linkages from the "old" PUMC to the ever-changing institution during the 1960s and 1970s. These linkages and memories became critical in the 1980s: they became responsible for the re-generation of the PUMC medical education program. The pre-med training of this group was first in Yenching University's biology department which transferred into Peking University in the early 1950s. Alice Boring, long-time professor of biology at Yenching, was frequently cited as a memorable professor: she is credited by many for introducing Mendelian genetics to China. When they transferred to PUMC for pre-clinical and clinical training the PUMC faculty who taught them were those trained in the old PUMC who had replaced foreign faculty as leaders of their respective departments: Zhu Futang, Lin Qianzhi, Zhang Xijun, Wu Yingkai, Wu Weiran, Liu Shihao, Zhang Xiaoqian and others. In their faculty and clinical roles these "old" PUMC graduates were the medical stars of the 1950s and 1960s, replicating the professional and normative values of their own student years. The PUMC culture which had both challenged and nurtured these professors was extended to their students whenever possible. Those interviewed from this era remembered in great detail the efforts to continue Socratic teaching method, tutorials, rigorous laboratory training, clandestine trips to the library- even as PUMC was occupied by the PLA. As Tang Xiaofu '56 in neurology remembered: "they taught us how to learn, how to think, how to imagine."

Of course political movements also affected this middle generation-whether "resist America, aid Korea," the anti-rightist campaign, or the Cultural Revolution. Fang Qi, former PUMCH director, remembered that "there were many political movements that bothered us with no time to read." His colleague Luo Weici (Class 1953) remembered the closing of PUMC for ten years during the Cultural Revolution and the fact that altogether 500 PUMC families were relocated to the northwest during that period. While some recounted severe hardships what was most striking was that by 2008 this transitional generation preferred to focus on the 1980s, the decade in which they came into their own as true descendants of the original PUMC.

Many were sent abroad – not as the young post-docs in the pre-1950 period, but as older visiting scholars in their 50's and 60's, individuals whose medical practice had been honed in the original PUMC culture and truncated by the vicissitudes of the later 1950s and 1960s. One of the first, Zhu Yuanjue, went to Massachusetts General in 1976 for two years. She remembered "the wonderful experience, her English was a big plus, and a sense of fulfillment, "part of the culture of PUMC is that you need to study abroad." The claim of cosmopolitan experience was continually reasserted. Luo Weici went to Johns Hopkins in 1983 to study pulmonary disease. He also traveled with other PUMC faculty to study newest developments in American medical pedagogy-the Harvard Medical Pathways curriculum, for example, Tang Xiaofu went to Denmark to study neurophysiology.

Dai Yuhua, '54, herself a member of this generation and dean of PUMC during the years in which it re-opened, remembered especially Zhang Xiaoqian who taught them how to really pay attention to patients of all kind and made them learn independently. In 1987, at the time of PUMC's 70th anniversary, she commented that the mainstay of PUMC were the graduates from this second cohort.

The second wave of this cohort, those who entered PUMC during a brief period of relaxation, 1959 – 1966, had especially poignant memories of their time in the institution - in part because it was so short. None were able to complete a regular eight-year curriculum. Those who began their pre-medical program at Peking University in the late 1950s and their medical program at PUMC by the early 1960s were able to complete all their premedical education and some of their clinical work. Those who began just a few years later, in 1963 and 1964 were almost immediately plunged into the political chaos of the Red Guard movement. Nearly all were sent to remote areas in the 1970s.

What interviewees remembered most clearly were the various ways in which they practiced medicine in rural areas, tried to keep abreast of medical studies, and eventually were returned to PUMC - either to finish their medical training or to become full-fledged members of the hospital or research institutes staff. Zhang Yangfen, PUMC dean during this period, kept track of dispersed students and tried to stay in touch with them. Huang Jiasi lobbied Zhou Enlai to bring 180 students back to PUMC in the early 1970s. Some had to return to rural areas after a year or so. In 1978 Deng Xiaoping announced exams for all who wished to continue their studies. Not all were readmitted but those who returned in 1979 completed a three-year master program. For the youngest, this was their only sustained medical training. It is this Cultural Revolution generation that eventually filled the gap and provided medical and institutional leadership during the 1990s and early 21st century.

Like their predecessors this Cultural Revolution generation also were sent to study abroad. Zhang Dechang (graduate in 1972), Professor and Chairman of Pharmacology, received a Ph. D. in pharmacology in 1985. Ma Sui '63, former vice-president of PUMCH, went to Boston to Brigham Women's Hospital. Tang Pingzhang (class 1965 – 1970, returned to PUMC for graduate study 1978 – 1981) , chair, head and neck surgery, CAMS, went to the United Kingdom and also to the University of North Carolina. Wang Kean, former director

Chinese Academy of Preventive Medicine, studied at McGill University in Canada. Lu Zhaoling, former director of PUMCH studied in both the United Kingdom and Canada.

These Cultural Revolution era PUMC graduates are illustrative of many of their classmates. Despite delayed and interrupted education their careers came to emulate those of the "old PUMC." The emphasis on international education for an older generation of visiting scholars whose education had been truncated was part of China's overall national strategy. Those at PUMC and CAMS were able to replicate the extensive international connections of an earlier era. PUMC once again became a cosmopolitan institution.

During the last thirty years, memories of "old PUMC' were evoked on many occasions - in multiple books and memoirs, the commemorative publications. Especially important have been the anniversary celebrations beginning in 1987. This first anniversary celebrated under the People's Republic of China paid particular tribute to leaders of the "old PUMC." Attended by political and medical luminaries nearly each speech paid tribute to Lin Qiaozhi and Huang Jiasi, both of whom had only recently passed away. Minister of Health Chen Minzhang's congratulatory message was typical of those presented:

> The Academy and the College assume the glorious historical mission of being geared to the needs of the whole country and serving for the whole country. In the past decade the Academy and the College have trained a great number of excellent talents in medicine and health circles and some outstanding pioneers of specialties of sciences for our country. They can be found in many places both at home and abroad. Their contributions to developing and prospering the country's medical science cause has made a deep impression on us. [12]

Ten years later, in 1997, Jiang Zemin, president of the PRC, inscribed a special message of congratulations: "Rigorousness, Erudition & Expertise,

Creation, Devotion." And in 2007, on the occasion of the 90th PUMC anniversary, the American origins of PUMC were honored with the dedication of a bust of John D. Rockefeller and the attendance of members of the Rockefeller family. A commemorative album blends pictures of the original Prince Yu's pavilions with near-matching elements of PUMC - marble balustrades, green carved roofs, long garden corridors, traditional doorways, and welcoming Fu dogs. In his preface, PUMC Party Secretary Liu Qian evokes the ineffable "long-lasting and distinctive PUMC spirit" embodied in each of the buildings. He calls on their ethical and aspirational essence:

> Aren't these buildings the concrete reflection of PUMC's mission to deliver education at high standard, high starting point, and high level, and in fine craftsmanship? When you walk alongside the green sticks (columns), gray walls, and long corridors, don't you feel that you are running through the space-time channel with the former pioneers accompanying you?

Although these former pioneers remembered PUMC with great fondness, they were not shy in calling their alma mater to strong leadership in a new China. At the 90th anniversary, Chen Yuanfang '57 asked the question: "Are PUMC's traditions outdated? Should PUMC be sent to the museum?" The new challenges include the explosion of knowledge, the need for curricular reform, the globalization of public health issues, chronic health diseases and the need to emphasize medical ethics. Chen's talk is almost a eulogy for the old PUMC. For her, the "PUMC spirit" was the result of a long-vested institutional culture, where the "PUMC man ... works conscientiously, meticulously and dedicatedly, who loves science and pursues excellence, who sticks to the truth, dares to speak out and despise drifting with the tide."[13] At the same occasion, PUMC president Liu Depei, with a Ph. D. from PUMC, affirmed the continuing relevance of PUMC, that it is not ready to be sent to a museum. His vision expanded beyond the undergraduate education program to include an emphasis on medical science and research, an institution of advanced medical education well integrated with the eighteen research institutes of the Chinese Academy of Sciences and Peking Union Medical College. [14]

Idealistic memories of "old PUMC' helped to preserve and perpetuate the institution. It is the only American, and perhaps the only foreign institution, founded during the Republican era to celebrate its centennial - retaining its core identity and, ultimately, its name. The leaders of PUMC during the post-Mao period - Huang Jiasi, Wu Jieping, Gu Fangzhou, Ba Denian and Liu Depei were challenged by powerful memories of "old PUMC" even as they sought to innovate and expand for a new era. Interviews with each revealed dedication to the values of an elite medical education and exemplary service with the commensurate, and not easy, task of adapting it to a new era. As PUMC celebrates its centennial, the challenge will continue: how to preserve and protect the best values of the "old PUMC," and adapt it to its second century.

Bibliography

1. This chapter is based on, and cites material from, chapter 4 of my *The Oil Prince's Legacy*: *Rockefeller Philanthropy in China* (Stanford University Press, 2011).

2. This was actually the 31st anniversary of CAMS which was founded in 1956 but until 2016 PUMC and CAMS celebrated their anniversaries together.

3. For details on the dozen different PUMC names see Ma Chao's chapter. the

4. Interview with Huang Jiasi, May 9, 1984, Beijing.

5. Deng Jiadong to the author, June 13, 1991.

6. Ge Ou, *Xiehe Yishi* (Memories of Peking Union Medical College); Beijing: Shenghuo, Dushu Xinzhi Santian Shudian, 2007), 98.

7. Huang, "An Analysis of the 'PUMC Phenomenon' in Medical Education Development in China," in *China Medical Board*, *75th Anniversary Celebration* (New York: China Medical Board, 2004, 23.

8. Peter M. Haas, "Introduction: Epistemic Communities and International Policy Coordination," *International Organization* 46 (Winter 1992): 3

9. PUMC faculty and graduates interviewed in 1984 include: Beijing – Huang Jiasi, Wu

Jieping, Cheng Xianqiu, Wang Jiwu, Zhong Huilan, Wang Zhengyi, Huang Zhenxiang, Wu Yingkai, Yan Renying, Zhu Futang, Huang Cuiding, Ye Gongshao, and Deng Jiadong. Shanghai – Rong Dushan, Zhang Zhubin, Xiong Rucheng, and Lin Feiqing. Tianjin – Zhu Xianyi, Shi Xien, Jin Xianzhai, and Yu Songding. Guangzhou – Chen Guozhen, He Dianji, Tang Zeguang, Xu Tianlu, Zhang E, Huang Ailian, and Huang Shuyuan. Chengdu – Chen Zhiqian.

10. C. C. Chen to the author, January 12, 1998.

11. PUMC graduates interviewed in Beijing in 2007 include: Liu Depei, Wang Kean, Peng Mengzhao, Huang Renjian, Wu Mingjiang, Tang Pingzhang, Ma Sui, Tang Xiaofu, Fang Yi, Zhu Yu, Luo Weici, Gao Youhe, Zhang Dechang, Liu Zimin, Dai Yuhua, Zhu Yuanjue, Chen Yuanfang, Lu Zhaoling, Lu Shiyuan, Chao Ni, Hu Tiansheng, Wu Weiran, Li Xuewang.

12. This is from a PUMC seventieth anniversary publications. I attended this ceremony.

13. Chen Yuanfeng, "A Glance Back," presentation at PUMC's ninetieth-anniversary celebration, October 14, 2007, unpublished speech.

14. Liu Depei, "PUMC; s Past, Present and Future, presentation at PUMC's ninetieth-anniversary celebration, October 14, 2007, unpublished speech.

北京协和医学院的两代内分泌宗师——刘士豪和史轶蘩

李乃适

李乃适，中国协和医科大学医学系（八年制）毕业，医学博士、理学博士，2012～2013 年就读于荷兰格罗宁根大学医学中心分子遗传学系，获理学博士学位，现任北京协和医院内分泌科副主任医师，硕士生导师。北京医学会内科学分会青年委员会副主任委员，中国科学技术史学会医学史专业委员会常务委员，《中华健康管理学杂志》编委，《中国医学人文》编委。

协和在我国乃至国际内分泌学领域均有着卓越的贡献，长期执国内内分泌学界之牛耳，一度在国际上也享有盛名；即使在当前群雄逐鹿的时代，协和依旧在国内顶级学界占有一席之地。北京协和医学院毕业生中，先后有刘士豪、朱宪彝、王叔咸、周寿恺、史轶蘩、曾正陪、李光伟、向红丁、戴为信等从事内分泌工作，对我国内分泌学的发展起着巨大的作用。本章拟简单介绍刘士豪和史轶蘩这两位不同时代的内分泌学泰斗的成长历程，并对不同时代北京协和医学院医学教育的影响作一简要思考。

刘士豪（1900～1974）

从湘雅到协和——刘士豪求学经历简述

刘士豪，湖北武昌人，出生于一个家道中落的木材商家庭，于 1913 年进入武昌文华中学就读，用 4 年的时间学完了 6 年的课程而提前毕业，于 1917 年考入湖南湘雅医学专门学校预科。两年后，刘士豪从预科学校毕业，并未按常规途径进入湘雅医学院就读，而是考入了北京协和医学院，于 1919～1920 年在协和预科学校继续读第 3 年课程，此后方进入医本部学习。在医学生阶段，刘士豪的成绩就极为优异，在第一学年结束时，他和另一名同学并列第一，平分了"理事奖学金"；但此后 4 个学年，均是刘士豪 1 人囊括了学年成绩第一，因而毕业时以总成绩第一而获得"文海奖学金"。不仅如此，刘士豪的科研能力在医学生时代已经初现端倪。1924 年，刘士豪在哈罗普（George Harrop，肾上腺内分泌学专家）的指导下，对两名因抽搐而住院的佝偻病女童进行了详细的观察，并且用代谢平衡法证明了用鱼肝油治疗的疗效。刘士豪将这两例研究写成论文，于 1925 年在《中华医学杂志》上发表，成为了他的处女作"The influence of cod liver oil on the calcium and phosphorus metabolism in tetany（鱼肝油对搐搦症钙磷代谢的影响）"。因此，刘士豪的临床科研，实际上在医学生时期已经起步了。

从住院医师到教授——与"老协和"一起成长

刘士豪于 1925 年进入协和内科工作时，协和在国际上尚未达到声名鹊起的阶段。1926 年，刘士豪继张孝骞之后任内科第二任总住院医师。1928 年受聘主治医师后，刘士豪赴美国洛克菲勒医学研究所进修，师从著名生物化学家范斯莱克（D. D. van Slyke），于 1930 年回国；其间他对生物化学这一新兴学科进行了系统的学习，并在范斯莱克指导下对血气分析的方法进行了改进。而范斯莱克正是这一领域中和福林（Folin）齐名的顶级生物化学家；这段经历对刘士豪日后领导协和生物化学系帮助极大。三十年代开始，协和医学院在各方面的积累逐渐开始在国际上显露头角。而刘士豪也于这时回国，此后即主要从事内分泌代谢领域的临床和研究，在美国教授韩诺恩（R. R. Hannon）离开协和后成为协和内分泌代谢研究的领导者，长期主管代谢实验室和代谢病房的临床和研究工作。他所领导的团队，着力最多的是钙磷代谢研究，对各种相关疾病用代谢平衡法来评价钙磷在体内的分布如何改变，积累了大量的资料，为全世界这一领域的学者所瞩目。这一系列研究的巅峰之作是"肾性骨营养不良"的疾病命名，由刘士豪和朱宪彝共同署名，首先发表于 1942 年的《科学》杂志，后来又以全文的形式发表于 1943 年的《Medicine》。这项研究依然是用代谢平衡法在探讨肾衰继发骨软化的患者的钙磷代谢，从而发现这类患者的独特特征，并且发现用双氢速变固醇治疗有效；这一命名将"肾性骨营养不良"从维生素 D 缺乏性疾病中分离出来，此后对其机制研究和临床诊治均有大幅度推动作用。在内分泌领域的其他方面，刘士豪领导的团队也取得了长足的进展。他和娄克斯、周寿恺等在 1936 年于《临床研究杂志》《Journal of Clinical Investigation》发表了中国首例胰岛素瘤研究，成功切除了肿瘤并且对肿瘤标本提取物进行了胰岛素的生物测定。1938～1939 年，刘士豪赴英国伦敦进修，对去垂体大鼠进行了垂体 – 性腺轴的研究和水代谢的研究。这是模式动物用于生物学研究的开始阶段，当时也属非常先进的研究。1941 年 10 月，刘士豪晋升为内科学教授，这是协和毕业生中第 1 位协和教授。然而好景不长，1941 年底珍珠港事件爆发，日本对美宣战，日军迅速占领协和，将外国人悉数软禁，而中国人被全部驱逐。刘士豪遂于北京万历桥胡同开业行医。

身兼数职的生物化学系主任和《生物化学与临床医学的联系》

1947 年协和复校，刘士豪回到协和，继续担任内科教授；同时于 1948 开始兼任北京同仁医院院长，直至 1957 年。

1951 年初，协和被解放军接管，美国国籍的协和员工均被驱逐，其中就包括生物化学系主任窦威廉（A. William）。刘士豪被任命为系主任，直至 1958 年卸任。生物化学系主任兼任内科学教授，这也反映了刘士豪在基础和临床医学两方面的造诣均得到协和管理层的推崇。在生物化学系主任任期内，刘士豪在国内率先创建了多种内分泌激素测定及功能检测方法；这与他后来坚持创建胰岛素的放射免疫测定法的思想是一脉相承的，体现了他对学科发展的认识。

在任生物化学系期间，他还主持办过 4 届全国性的生物化学学习班，为全国各医学院培养生物化学人才。在反复授课的基础上，1957 年，一本经典著作《生物化学与临床医学的联系》由人民卫生出版社出版，很快引起了内科学界的轰动。当时京城各大医院内科据说均是人手一册。1954 届协和毕业生、著名血液病学专家张之南教授后来在撰写教学文章时也多次提及这本影响深远的书。他在《老协和临床教学》一文中这样写道："代谢病及生物化学专家刘士豪教授曾结合自己的工作撰写了《生物化学与临床医学的联系》一书，不只内容实用，而且树立了基础研究与临床结合的典范。"现在看来，这本书的思想确实高屋建瓴，可以说是转化医学思想的先行者。刘士豪在序言里这样写道："如果能引起生物化学工作者深入临床，临床工作者深入生化，使二者更密切地结合起来向医学进军，则本书抛砖引玉的目的即已达到。"这本书共 20 章，30 万字，但其对临床医生思考问题方式的影响是非常大的。同时，在生物化学界，这本书被认为是我国第一部临床化学的专著。刘士豪本人也非常重视这本书，曾经在六十年代初作了仔细修订，拟出该书的第二版，却因"文化大革命"到来而未能出版，成为医学界一大遗憾。

北京协和医院内分泌科的成立

1958 年，卫生部拟将原德国医院（现北京医院）改造为内分泌研究所，由刘士豪负责。刘士豪将生物化学系的激素测定组和协和医院内科内分泌专业的两组人员合并，于 8 月成立内分泌科，并准备向原德国医院旧址搬迁。这是我国第一个内分泌专科，刘士豪任科主任。然而，人员全部搬到位以后，又接到新通知，原德国医院拟改建为干部医院，刘士豪团队只能于同年 10 月搬回协和医院，重新成为内科的一个学组，直至 1961 年底重新挂牌。此后北京协和医院内分泌科招收了 4 届内分泌高级研修班，每届仅 4 人，此后均成为了我国各地内分泌学界的栋梁之才。

胰岛素放射免疫测定法的建立和首钢的糖尿病流行病学调查

1959 年，亚洛（Yalow）和伯森（Berson）成功建立了胰岛素的放射免疫测定法，并于 1960 年发表。刘士豪敏锐地发现了这篇重要文献，立即明白了这一方法的重要性。蛋白类的激素从此将可能通过放射免疫测定法来定量测定，临床内分泌学必将出现革命性的发展。于是在 1962 年，研究生制度重新开始实施时，刘士豪立即招收了研究生陈智周，课题就是建立胰岛素的放射免疫测定法。当时实验所用牛血清白蛋白全部需要进口，价格昂贵，而国家经济仍处于相对困难时期；刘士豪为此也遭到不少非议，但他硬是顶着巨大的压力坚持将课题进行下去，终于在 1965 年成功，陈智周顺利通过答辩毕业。答辩委员会成员有张孝骞、王世真、谢少文等鼎鼎有名的学术泰斗，对该成果的应用一致看好。

在同一时期，刘士豪还进行了另一尝试：调查首都钢铁厂职工的糖尿病流行情况。于是，从 1964 年开始，史轶蘩、潘孝仁等临床医生和邓洁英、孙梅励等科研人员均投入了这一工作，收集了大量资料。本来，以横断面调查为契机，建立糖尿病队列，并结合胰岛素的精确测定，必将取得丰硕成果。然而，1966 年 "文化大革命" 爆发，这些资料未及整理就不知所终，非常可惜。但由此培养的人才仍然得到了很好的科学训练。池芝盛教授在八十年代初领导的酒仙桥研究，潘孝仁教授领导的大庆研究，不能不认为在一定程度上受到刘士豪影响吧。

对应激学说的介绍和 "应激" 译名的确定

应激（stress）学说的提出始于 1936 年韩思·塞里发表于《自然》（Nature）的一篇论文。五十年代，苏联学者就这一概念展开了广泛讨论，从而在我国学术界也引起了巨大的反响。1962 年夏，天津市生理学会举办了塞里应激学说的讲座。而讨论过程中，刘士豪建议将 "stress" 译名由 "应力" 改为 "应激"，与会者均同意，从此 "应激" 这一译名被学术界广泛接受。1962 年刘士豪编《塞里应激学说概要》出版，较为系统介绍了应激学说，对这一学说在国内的推广起到了重要作用。

纵观刘士豪教授的一生，前半生异常顺利。除了过人的天分以外，老协和的医学教育也在他的生涯中起到不可忽视的作用。后期尽管在政治上饱受责难，但在学术上仍然受到极大的尊敬，在多方面均推动了我国内分泌学的进步。

史轶蘩（1928～2013）

第一次复校后的协和人

史轶蘩祖籍江苏溧阳，为著名"溧阳史氏"的后裔。上小学期间，日军全面侵华爆发，史轶蘩和兄弟姐妹均辗转来到在青岛的父母身边，此后进入著名的青岛圣功女中就读。她成绩出色，每年均能够获得全年级第一。1946 年考入燕京大学理学院医预系，1949 年正式考入北平协和医学院，1950 年夏和同班张之南、孙瑞龙、刘丽笙一起获得国际菲陶菲（φτφ）荣誉学会颁发的金钥匙奖（整个燕京大学理学院仅 10 人获奖），于 1954 年毕业时和张之南、孙瑞龙一起获得优秀毕业生的荣誉。

史轶蘩上大学的年代，是抗日战争刚刚结束后。当时燕京大学和协和医学院都在 1941 年 12 月 8 日珍珠港事件爆发后立即被日军占领，几乎洗劫一空。燕大校长司徒雷登和协和校长胡恒德均被日军监禁至抗战结束。燕大在满目疮痍的情况下，于 1945 年 9 月艰难复校。而协和的校园被借用为国共谈判的"军调处"，直至 1947 年才真正复校。而 1947 年后内战又全面爆发，至 1949 年初北平已经被解放军包围，学习环境实际上远非理想。虽然燕京大学当时属于城郊，不在炮火笼罩之中；但其对于师资和学习氛围的影响仍是不容小觑的。

史轶蘩于 1949 年秋进入协和医本部之时，北平已经解放。协和的教授们也已经以中国教授为主，但仍然实力雄厚，其中绝大多数都是早期老协和的毕业生。因此，无论是课程还是教学方法均和以前类似，依然是"精英教育"的思路。但是，到 1951 年 1 月，协和医学院收归国有，协和成了美帝国主义对中国进行文化侵略的反面典型，各种类型的政治运动纷至沓来，对当时的学习也造成了不小的冲击。1950 年燕大招收的医预班全部转系，自 1951 年起不再招收新的学生，"淘汰制"也作为糟粕被摒弃。虽然总体的教学体系尚存，但许多课程也相应出现了不同程度的改动。例如，原先最后一年实习是全科轮转，但史轶蘩所在年级就改成了专科实习，史轶蘩就是轮转了一年内科病房，以至于她后来始终觉得未能在实习时轮转外科、妇产科是一大遗憾。总之，尽管有着种种干扰，史轶蘩仍然系统接受了协和八年制医学教育，为后来的成长打下了良好的基础。

"文革"经历

史轶蘩毕业后即分配入北京协和医院内科工作。在担任内科住院医师期间，史轶蘩就以工作出色而著称。她不仅在医疗工作上尽职尽责，在教学工作上也是不遗余力。晚年时，她曾经对学生说起当年的做法：每天晚上都要想一想第二天的教学内容和教学方法，并且查阅参考书以达到最佳准备效果。比她低 2 届的师妹吴宁（后来北京协和医院心内科著名教授）曾经回忆说，他们班实习时史轶蘩在病房就问实习大夫怎样简单地鉴别心衰治疗后的疗效，最后仅仅通过抽掉病人平躺时常规垫着的两个枕头来观察病情变化就反映了情况，让在场的医学生都受用终生。

1958 年北京协和医院内分泌科作为国内第一个内分泌专科成立之时，刘士豪教授就让史轶蘩做了代理主治医师，主管病房工作。由于当时的政治运动应接不暇，导致晋升变成了一件很不确定的事情，史轶蘩直至 1963 年才真正成为主治医师。但史轶蘩一直是刘士豪教授所器重的主治医，这一点是公认的；当时在内分泌高级研修班进修的林丽香在多年以后仍然记得非常清楚，刘士豪教授让她到病房去学习临床，由史轶蘩负责。而当时的内分泌高级研修班，每年仅仅招收 4 名学员，是受到高度重视的，后来也都成为全国各地的内分泌学科带头人。因此史轶蘩作为内分泌科病房的主要业务骨干之一，长期受到刘士豪教授的指点和器重。

从 1955 年参与脑膜炎的临床研究开始，史轶蘩就一直在参加临床病例的总结工作。到了内分泌科成立以后，史轶蘩的临床研究工作就集中于各种内分泌疾病的临床总结了。1964 年，第一届全国内分泌与肾脏病大会在广州召开；史轶蘩虽然并未参加，但投稿 3 篇，分别为：《柯兴氏综合征的诊断和分型》（史轶蘩、刘士豪）；《柯兴氏综合征的转归》（史轶蘩刘士豪）；《原发性卵巢发育不全 12 例的临床表现和细胞系检查》（史轶蘩、吴旻等）。根据后来的档案资料，史轶蘩每次填写履历时都会在学术著作中填上这三篇论文，可以看出她对这 3 篇文献相关工作的重视程度。

刘士豪教授在创建内分泌科以后，以其超前的眼光在国内率先建立了胰岛素的放射免疫测定法，大约同时于 1964 年在首钢（首都钢铁厂）进行糖尿病的筛查。这两项工作的结合，如果没有"文化大革命"的干扰，本可以使我国产出一批达到国际先进学术水准的有关糖尿病的研究。史轶蘩参加了首钢的调查工作，但并未深层次地接触放射免疫测定法，但这项重要工作极有可能给她造成了深远影响；她日后一直在强调建立激素测定方法的重要性，也在身体力行地进行实践。

综上所述，史轶蘩在"文革"前阶段医教研工作均很出色，一方面是自身的天赋和努力，另一方面应该和名师指点以及当时内分泌科的学术氛围是分不开的。

"文革"期间的临床磨炼和相关科研

1966 年开始的"文化大革命"对于科学界是一场巨大的灾难，医学界也不能幸免。协和作为美帝国主义文化侵略的反面典型，自然成为重灾区；张孝骞、刘士豪、黄家驷等老教授均被作为白专典型批判，不但不能再教书育人，而且还要被批斗、关牛棚、打扫厕所……

然而医院毕竟是特殊机构，医疗秩序还是需要有最低限度的保证的。除去被批斗的"老专家"无法工作，积极参与运动的医生们也无法兼顾临床太多，就只剩下史轶蘩这样一批年轻医生在病房超负荷工作来满足病人的需要。各种疑难杂症摆在面前，在没有上级医师指导的情况下，史轶蘩需要自力更生对病人进行决策。有时候，史轶蘩也会悄悄去找正在打扫厕所的刘士豪教授请教解决方案。经过长年的积累，史轶蘩的临床水平得到了很大的提高。1970年云南通海大地震，北京协和医院派去救援队，最后在救援的事迹中，最成功的两个病例一个是朱预教授为首的外科团队治好了一位全身多处骨折的病人；另一个病人就是1型糖尿病，史轶蘩在当时根本没有胰岛素的条件下仅用补液便能够将患者脱离险境。尽管"文革"10年带来了无数负面影响，但史轶蘩在这种艰难的条件下练就了高超的临床能力，为以后开展临床研究打下了基础。

"文革"后期，在可能的条件下，史轶蘩也对一些新的治疗手段进行了尝试，其中最为突出的是嗜铬细胞瘤的药物准备。该病是肾上腺部位产生一个分泌儿茶酚胺的肿瘤，间断或持续释放儿茶酚胺导致患者出现阵发性或持续性高血压（或持续性高血压阵发性加重）；该病首选手术治疗，但在 α 受体拮抗剂进行药物准备以前，手术死亡率是很高的。北京协和医院最早怀疑嗜铬细胞瘤的病例记载于1939年，当时尚无手段明确诊断。到五十年代开始，已有成功切除嗜铬细胞瘤的案例，但当时负责主刀的吴阶平大夫的体会就是手术必须非常迅速，尽快切除瘤体，否则患者风险明显增加。七十年代，史轶蘩在国内首先用 α 受体拮抗剂对嗜铬细胞瘤患者进行了术前准备，把这一方案逐渐规范化并在全国推广，使嗜铬细胞瘤从一种风险很高的疾病逐渐成为了一种可以常规处理的疾病。

"文革"结束后，史轶蘩已经年逾半百，但她对重振协和内分泌科的豪情不减。一方面，她对协和医院诊治的多种内分泌疾病进行了系统的总结，其中最突出的当属发现国人的原发性甲旁亢常常伴有骨软化、对甲亢危象的诊治提出了"危象前期"的概念，对临床治疗均有重要的指导作用。另一方面，内分泌科为进一步提高诊疗水平进行了分组；作为刚刚成立的垂体组组长，史轶蘩对建立各种垂体激素的测定方法高度重视，首先是建立生长激素的放射免疫测定法。从那时开始，她牵头进行了一系列垂体疾病相关的临床与基础研究，最终获得国家科技进步一等奖。

美国国立卫生研究院（NIH）生涯

1981 年 1 月，史轶蘩飞赴 NIH，开始了为期两年的进修生涯。她的导师舍瑞（R. Sherins）是一位在男性生殖内分泌学领域卓有成就的医生兼科学家。一方面，史轶蘩参加舍瑞教授的男性生殖内分泌临床工作和基础研究；另一方面，她还积极参与其他病房各种内分泌疾病的各种形式的讨论。史轶蘩在 NIH 的具体工作最终发表为两篇原创性论文《Long-term stability of aqueous solutions of luteinizing hormone-releasing hormone assessed by an in vitro bioassay and liquid chromatography》和《Increased plasma and pituitary prolactin concentrations in adult male rats with selective elevation of FSH levels may be explained by reduced testosterone and increased estradiol production》。这两篇论文得到了舍瑞教授的高度评价，认为是那一时代对男性性腺内分泌疾病的病理生理机制认识的重要补充。

但是，比具体工作可能更为重要的是学术思想的提高。史轶蘩愈来愈认识到如何评价下丘脑－垂体－靶腺轴功能是研究垂体疾病的核心。其中首当其冲的是各种垂体激素的测定；对于波动过大而导致测定值不能完全说明问题的激素，功能试验就十分重要。这在史轶蘩回国后的研究中占了非常重要的比例。

另一方面，史轶蘩在 NIH 的原创性研究主要属于动物实验范畴。她也非常强烈地意识到动物研究和临床研究的互补性。她后来一直在强调临床和基础结合的研究方式，并且身体力行，显然受 NIH 的这段经历影响非常之大。

激素分泌性垂体瘤的临床与基础研究

激素分泌性垂体瘤的研究工作始于 1979 年。此前已经建立了生长激素的测定方法，但如何评价患者生长激素过多或过少尚未进行详细研究。史轶蘩成为垂体组组长以后，将建立其他各种垂体激素的放射免疫测定法并建立激素的正常值和病理值范围作为重要研究方向；在从 NIH 归来以后，这一方向就得到了进一步强化，并对于激素测定不能明确诊断的疾病，建立了相应的功能试验来协助临床诊断。例如，对于生长激素缺乏症的儿童，仅靠单纯测定血清生长激素水平并不能诊断生长激素缺乏症；因为正常儿童在基础状态时测定血清生长激素水平也非常低，与生长激素缺乏症患儿无异。因此必须建立生长激素兴奋试验，在合适的刺激下，正常儿童的血清生长激素水平就能够被兴奋起来，而患儿则不能；这样才能从正常儿童中区分出生长激素缺乏症患儿，避免漏诊和误诊。在激素分泌性垂体瘤进行报奖时，6 种激素测定方法的建立和 8 种功能试验方法的确立是作为对提高诊断水平的重要依据。当然，引入 CT 协助定位诊断、视野检查和病理诊断的价值也是不言而喻的。除了诊断以外，史轶蘩团队也在推动着治疗的进展，手术治疗、放射治疗和药物治疗，均成为垂体瘤治疗的重要选择；其中通过对生长抑素治疗副作用的细致观察，史轶蘩团队在国际上首次发现了生长抑素对于胆囊收缩的抑制作用。对于进一步的机制研究，史轶蘩又设计了动物试验进一步阐明。因此，协和内分泌的研究再次受到国际上学术同行的重视，美国西南医学中心的内分泌学教授在《美国临床内分泌代谢杂志》上撰写特稿介绍北京协和医院内分泌科。

垂体瘤研究的重要意义还在于它所带来的社会效益。在 1979 年，国内诊断垂体瘤几乎全靠经验，而到了 1992 年史轶蘩团队申报国家科技进步奖时，几乎所有类型的垂体瘤都能够得到和国际诊疗水平相当的恰当处理，实在是垂体瘤患者的福音。

由于垂体瘤及其他方面的贡献，史轶蘩于 1996 年当选为中国工程院院士，同年获"何梁何利"科学与技术进步奖。

青春发育研究、肥胖研究及其他

在垂体瘤研究圆满完成之后，史轶蘩晚年将研究方向转向青春发育和肥胖领域。首先仍然是建立正常值，史轶蘩在 70 多岁时仍带领研究生去大庆进行儿童青少年的青春发育调查，力图建立中国北方儿童青少年的青春发育启动的正常年龄范围，以便对我国青少年的性早熟和青春发育延迟等青春期疾病做出更为精确的诊断；她还参与制定了中国人肥胖和超重的现行诊断标准，并试图从传统草药中筛选有效成分。在史轶蘩主持下，卫生部内分泌重点实验室于 1988 年在北京协和医院成立，这是第一个在医院成立的卫生部级的内分泌实验室。

此外，史轶蘩对于我国的临床药理工作有着重要的贡献。早在 1983 年，史轶蘩出任内分泌科主任不久，北京协和医院内分泌科就被定为卫生部临床药理基地。此后对于各种内分泌新药如溴隐亭等，都在这里完成了临床试验。1995 年，史轶蘩创立北京协和医院临床药理中心并兼任主任，同时她还曾参与起草 GCP 的工作，对我国临床药理的规范化功不可没。

史轶蘩教授的一生，在学习阶段就受到了一定程度的干扰，但仍然以优异成绩毕业。在北京协和医院内分泌科成立以后，史轶蘩的主要时间都在临床工作上，尤其是"文革"期间；但繁重的工作也使她的临床能力在当时条件下达到炉火纯青。改革开放后，NIH 的进修经历让史轶蘩的科研思想和科研能力得到了迅速提高，回国后对垂体瘤的研究紧密联系了基础和临床，最终获得国家科技进步一等奖，并当选为中国工程院院士。

两代内分泌宗师的学术成长轨迹及教育体系思考

刘士豪和史轶蘩作为我国两代内分泌学术泰斗，也是协和内分泌领域的两代领军人物，成就斐然是无可争议的，也意味着北京协和医学院医学教育的成功。虽然他们经历的年代有近 30 年的差别，但作为校友，作为师生，他们学术成长轨迹仍然有惊人的相似之处，所经历的医学教育体系有传承也有相当的改变。那时的先进医学教育体系到现在是否仍然是最先进的，对培养医学界的领军人物是否仍然有着重要作用，实际上是一个非常值得协和人认真思考的课题。

"老协和"的医学教育体系在当年是弗莱克斯勒报告发表后所形成的最先进的医学教育体系。强调预科，强调床边教学，强调实践，强调自学……从1924年到1943年毕业的20届医学生可以说完全是这一教育体系在中国的实践。刘士豪是第二届毕业生，尽管当时协和的教育体系还未达到最佳状态，如预科是自办而不像后来在燕京大学，但完全是依照美国新式教育体系的思想而开展的。因此刘士豪教授可以算是这一教育体系的最佳代言人之一，在毕业后也一直受到医学院和医院高层的高度重视，在毕业后的学术生涯里，得到继续教育的机会也非常顺利。加上他刻苦努力和才华过人，41岁即在协和被聘为教授。他受到的八年制医学教育，实际上是预科教育——基础医学教育——临床医学教育，然后毕业工作。工作以后，首先是经历住院医师阶段，然后因为工作出色当选总住院医师，结束后开始当主治医师。刘士豪在当主治医师后不久就有了出国学习的机会，去当时非常先进的纽约洛克菲勒医学研究所跟随生物化学大师范斯莱克学习，从此奠定他在生物化学研究方面的基础。此前他也发表了若干论文，但基本上是病例报道和临床总结；美国归来以后，他的基础医学研究能力就大为提高，为后来胜任生物化学系主任打下了基础。而在受聘襄教授以后，刘士豪再次得到机会出国进修，赴英国的医院米德尔塞克斯郡（Middlesex），学到了当时非常先进的实验动物研究技术。因此，刘士豪的两次出国经历，可以说是他在科研上的两次飞跃，因而他后来的学术水平在生物化学界和内分泌学界都得到公认。如果不是建国后屡次受各种"运动"冲击，刘士豪教授的成就还会远超我们现在耳熟能详的部分。

考察史轶蘩教授的学术成长轨迹，实际上要比刘士豪教授复杂得多。但史轶蘩同样也就读于北京协和医学院，只不过时间在第一次复校以后。燕京大学的医预科阶段，虽然有国共内战的一定干扰，但仍然是沿袭着以前的教育体系。进入医本科阶段，北京已经解放，但开始时协和作为美国的资产，并未受到太多影响；但朝鲜战争的爆发是一个转折点，1951年1月，中国人民解放军接管了北京协和医学院和医院，并宣布收归国有。因此史轶蘩在临床医学阶段的学习是在协和收归国有以后进行的，协和医学院已经不再继续招生。有关史轶蘩在这一学习阶段的具体情况，目前资料十分缺乏，但可以想象各种政治运动对医学生的冲击。另一方面，虽然学习环境发生了较大的变化，但是协和强大的教学传统料想并未因此而改变，因为教师的状况并未发生本质变化。尽管抗美援朝调用了一大批手术科室的医生，但留在协和医院继续工作的医生同样能够保证小班授课的质量；而重视床边教学和重视自学的传统，又在一定程度上使教学质量更主要靠学生的素质而不是老师的授课经验。因此，我们有理由推测，当时的"老协和"教育体系仍然在第一次复校后的医学生中起着核心作用，1945 级至 1949 级这 5 届协和医学生仍然是在"老协和"教育理念中成长起来的。

但不同于刘士豪在毕业后的一帆风顺，史轶蘩在毕业进入内科及内分泌科工作后，基本上完全在从事临床工作，能够进行系统临床科研的机会都非常少，更遑论出国进修了。只因刘士豪教授是基础与临床兼擅的全才，所以在内分泌科还是有一些机会（如查房等）学习科研思想。而十年"文革"间，史轶蘩几乎只能将全部精力用于临床工作，并在超高强度的实践中锻炼出了过人的临床能力。而她科研能力的飞跃得力于NIH 的进修生涯：一方面是体验了动物研究和临床研究可以互为补充，另一方面则是直接参与了激素测定的工作。因此，史轶蘩回国以后以垂体相关激素的定量测定为首要任务，围绕着激素测定对临床的作用进行了系列研究，最终使我国垂体疾病的诊断和治疗水平和国际接轨，并在这些研究过程中做出了一部分独创性的发现；也因此最终获得了国家科技进步一等奖。另外，史轶蘩在 NIH 接触到了当时最先进的临床科研，这也部分影响了她对临床药理工作的高度重视，日后组建了北京协和医院临床药理中心并任第一任主任。

刘士豪和史轶蘩的学术成长轨迹在本质上有相当多的共性：医预科阶段广泛接受通识教育并具备理学院学生的思维模式；基础医学的学习阶段经过科学实验的磨炼；临床学习阶段通过高质量的床边教学培养出了较强的自学能力，为成为临床医学家打下了基础。在经历高强度的住院医阶段后，择期出国学习国际上最先进的科研思想与科研方法，回国后与自己的领域相结合，在高质量临床工作的基础上，做出了独创性的学术贡献。也就是说，协和八年制培养了他们良好的科学素养和临床基本功；经过住院医师阶段后将临床水平提升到一个新的高度；出国到国际领先的科研平台进修学习，将前沿的科研方法带回协和，与临床工作相结合，在厚积薄发的基础上获得突破性进展。尽管刘士豪早在 29 岁就赴美进修而史轶蘩晚至 52 岁才走出国门，但留美经历对他俩科研能力的提升却是有目共睹的。

二十世纪的后半叶是生命科学蓬勃发展的时代。分子生物学的兴起带动了一系列新的学科出现，使基础医学在深度和广度上都与"老协和"时代不可同日而语，也使刘士豪这样同时精通生物化学和临床医学的医学家越来越不可能出现。新兴的统计学深深渗入了临床医学的几乎每一个领域，临床研究对于统计学的依赖在循证医学兴起后达到了前所未有的境界。这样的结果导致了基础医学与临床医学日渐分离，而临床医生在临床、科研和教学之间往往不得不有所抉择。这在当代美国的医学体系中最为显著，医生可以选择专门从事临床工作、教学辅以临床工作、科研辅以临床工作三者之一。

源自于美国医学教育革命的"老协和"体系仍然旨在培养出医教研兼顾而又十分出色的医学人才。时代的进展在考验着协和的教育体系，而协和的医学教育也在审时度势中不断改进。1979 年第 3 次复校后的课程即增加了科研训练的内容，并且同时覆盖基础医学科研和临床医学科研，加强科研实践。这样，协和医学生毕业时不仅有着扎实的临床基本功，也有着初步的科研能力，理论上前程远大。然而，现实却是残酷的，目前的就业市场已经悄然改变：短学制医学教育 + 专科培训 + 多多益善的 Sci 论文才是各大医院青睐的对象；而"5 + 3"规培制度的大规模推广也正在为这一趋势推波助澜。在当前的评价体系下，如何提高协和毕业生的竞争力？又如何能培养出当代的刘士豪和史轶蘩？这将是协和医学教育所面临的严峻挑战。

Liu Shihao and Shi Yifan – The Two Generations of Masters in Endocrinology at Peking Union Medical College

Li Naishi

Li Naishi, M. D., Ph. D., graduated from Peking Union Medical College (8-year curriculum program) in 2000. In 2013, he was granted a Ph. D. from Department of Molecular Genetics of University of Groningen, Netherlands. Now, he is the vice chief physician at the Department of Endocrinology, Peking Union Medical College Hospital, and tutor for master degree candidates. He is serving as the vice chairman of Youth Committee of Beijing Medical Association Internal Medicine Branch, and executive member of Medical History Profession Branch of the Chinese Society of Science and Technology, member of the editor boards of "Chinese Health Management Journal" and "Chinese Medical Humanities".

Peking Union Medical College (PUMC) has made a great contribution to endocrinology both in China and internationally. As such, PUMC has paved the way for China's endocrinological research community and developed a prestigious international reputation. Despite growing competition, PUMC has managed to maintain it's place as a leader in endocrinology research within the Chinese academic community. PUMC is responsible for edifying many who have gone on to play an extraordinary role in the field of endocrinology in China, such, as; Liu Shihao (刘士豪, also as Liu Shih-hao), Zhu Xianyi (朱宪彝), Wang Shuxian (王叔咸), Zhou Shoukai (周寿恺), Shi Yifan (史轶繁), Zeng Zhengpei (曾正陪), Li Guangwei (李光伟), Xiang Hongding (向红丁), and Dai Weixin (戴为信), to name a few. This article briefly presents the intertwined path of two pioneers, Liu Shihao and Shi Yifan. These two masters of endocrinology will be described both in terms of their achievements at PUMC, and the manifesting influence on medical education in China in two era.

Liu Shihao (1900 ~ 1974)

Journey from Xiang-Ya School of Medicine to Peking Union Medical College: An overview of Liu Shihao's earlier educational experiences

Liu Shihao came from Wuchang in Hubei Province, born into a timber merchant family during a time when business was in decline. In 1913, Liu entered Boone Middle School (文华中学) in Wuchang, and completed the 6-year-course of study within 4 years, graduating two years earlier. In 1917, he passed exams and was admitted to the prestigious Hunan-Yale Premedical School. Two years later, Liu Shihao graduated from the premedical school, he did not follow the standard path of becoming a student of Hunan-Yale Medical School. [1] Instead, Liu took the entrance examination for PUMC and became a PUMC student. From 1919 to 1920, Liu transferred and continued on the third year of the premedical course at PUMC, and then began the preclinical education program at PUMC.

As a medical student Liu Shihao was exemplary, and at the end of his first year at PUMC he along with another classmate were top of their class after their exams. As a result, Liu shared the "Trustee scholarship". However, for the next four consecutive academic years, Liu Shihao ranked the first, and thus won the "Wenham Prize." Even as an undergraduate medical student, Liu had started to demonstrate his aptitude for scientific research.

In 1924, under the guidance of George Harrop - an expert in adrenal endocrinology, Liu observed of two girls suffering ricketsia who had been hospitalized after tetany seizures. Liu demonstrated improved treatment efficacy of cod liver oil using the metabolic balance method. In 1925, Liu published a report based on the research of the two cases in the *Chinese Medical Journal*, entitled "*The influence of cod liver oil on the Calcium and Phosphorus metabolism in tetany*". Therefore, Liu Shihao's clinical research started during his early years as an undergraduate at PUMC.

Journey from resident to professor – growing with the "old PUMC"

When Liu Shihao started work with the department of internal medicine at PUMC in 1925, PUMC was not fully established. . In 1926, Liu Shihao became the second chief resident doctor in the department of internal medicine, preceding Dr. Zhang Xiaoqian. In 1928, after promotion to the attending physician, Liu went to the Hospital of Rockefeller Institute for Medical Research in the US for a fellowship,[2] working under the famous biochemist D. D. van Slyke. Until his return to China in 1930, Liu systematically studied biochemistry and further developed the method of blood gas analysis under the guidance of D. D. van Slyke who was as established as Folin, another leading biochemist in related research. This experience greatly influenced Liu Shihao who would go on to lead the department of biochemistry at PUMC in the future.

During the early 1930s, and based on previous accomplishments, PUMC was gradually becoming more visible in international medical stage and this intensified when Liu Shihao returned to PUMC. At that time, Liu was mainly engaged in clinical practice and research in the field of metabolic endocrinology, and he eventually became research leader in this field at PUMC. After American professor, R. R. Hannon had left PUMC, Liu attained the more senior role and became leader in both endocrine and metabolic research. This placed Liu in charge of the metabolic laboratory and the wards for metabolic diseases. A position which he then held for a long time.

The team Liu Shihao led focused research efforts mainly on calcium and phosphorus metabolization. During this time, they accumulated a wealth of information around how the body distributes and utilizes calcium and phosphorus. Liu's team managed to garner this new knowledge using the metabolic balance method, attracted the attention from the international community and indeed the series of studies conducted by Liu and his team culminated in the classification of the disease, "renal osteodystrophy". This classification first appeared in an article co-authored by Liu Shihao and Zhu Xianyi and was published in *Science* in 1942. Later in 1943, the full text report was published in *Medicine*.

Liu Shihao and his team continued their research using the metabolic balance method to study calcium and phosphorus metabolization in patients suffering renal failure complicated by osteomalacia. Their unified goal was to identify unique characteristics of these patients, as well as to determine the effectiveness of dihydrotachysterol solution (DHT) which is a synthetic vitamin D analog. Classifying 'renal osteodystrophy' had led to a divergence in clinical understanding which resulted in more specified research and developments in diagnostic techniques as well as interventions.

In other areas of endocrinology research, Liu Shihao's team also made considerable progress. In 1936, Liu, Harold H. Loucks, Zhou Shoukai and others published findings on China's first case of insulinoma in *Journal of Clinical Investigation*. This team successfully removed a tumor and performed bioassays of insulin from the extracted tumor specimens. During the period 1938 – 1939, Liu went to London for another fellowship and conducted animal research on the pituitary gland using rats to investigate the pituitary/testicular axis and water metabolization across this juncture. This period is now recognized as the early stages animal modelling for human biological research, and Liu's research was considered cutting-edge study at that time.

In October 1941, Liu Shihao was promoted to Professor of Internal Medicine, the first PUMC graduate to be promoted to full professor. Unfortunately, later that year the Pearl Harbor incident occurred resulting in Japan's declaring war against the United States. The Japanese army swiftly landed on the eastern China and began to occupy all major facilities including PUMC. All the foreigners were placed under house arrest at PUMC and Chinese faculty and staffs were all driven out of the PUMC campus. This placed Liu Shihao in a precarious position. Liu opened a clinic in Wanliqiao Hutong (万历桥胡同), downtown Beijing to serve the Chinese people

Director of biochemistry department with multi-responsibilities and *"the connection between biochemistry and clinical medicine"*

In 1947, after World War II when PUMC resumed, Liu Shihao returned to PUMC and continued to serve as the professor of internal medicine. From 1948 to 1957, he simultaneously served as the Director of Beijing Tongren Hospital. However, at the beginning of 1951, PUMC was again taken over by the People's Liberation Army (PLA), and all PUMC staff including American citizens were expelled. William Adolph, who was the director of biochemistry department was sent home and Liu Shihao was appointed director which he was until 1958. Liu Shihao was director for both the Department of Biochemistry and professor of internal medicine, which demonstrates PUMC thought highly of Liu's establishment in both basic and clinical medicine. When he was the director of biochemistry department, Liu initiated formulating a variety of methods in endocrine hormone tests and functional detection in China. This also highlights Liu's drive for development not only in implementing radioimmunoassay of insulin, but also more generally reflecting his desire for advancement with his discipline.

When was working in the biochemistry department at PUMC, Liu organized four national biochemistry training classes, training biochemical talents from various medical institutions in China. Through these classes, Liu developed a theory and went on to publish an article which is now considered seminal work in 1957, entitled "*The Connection Between Biochemistry and Clinical Medicine*" by the People's Health Publishing House. This article aroused great interest in the field of internal medicine and it t was said that almost every physician in hospitals in Beijing held a copy. Professor Zhang Zhinan (张之南), (class of 1954 at PUMC), a famous hematologist also repeatedly mentioned this far-reaching book in his writing. In one essay entitled "*Clinical Teaching at Old PUMC*", Zhang wrote: "Professor Liu Shihao, an expert in metabolic diseases and biochemistry, related to his work and wrote a book entitled " *the Connection Between Biochemistry and Clinical Medicine* ", which is not only practical in the content, but also sets up an example of combining basic scientific research with clinical work. " Now, it seems the book was indeed very advanced and visionary, placing Liu Shihao as a pioneer in the concept of Translational medicine.

Liu Shihao wrote in the forward of *The Connection between biochemistry and clinical medicine*, "If this book can make biochemists engage in clinical work, and clinicians engage in biochemistry, so that the two work closely together and march toward medical science, then the purpose of this book as the humble trailblazer has been realized. " This seminal work encompasses 20 chapters with over 300, 000 words, and the intention was clearly to influence clinical practice and thinking. At the same time, in the field of biochemistry, this book is considered the first monograph of clinical chemistry. Liu Shihao himself highly regarded this book; however, being so methodical he continued to make note of revisions, in planning a second edition. Unfortunately, due to the Cultural Revolution, a second edition was never published, much to the detriment of the international medical community.

Establishing the Department of Endocrinology at PUMC

In 1958, the Ministry of Health intended to transform the original German hospital (presently known as the Beijing Hospital) into an endocrine research institute and to appoint Liu Shihao Head of the Department. As a result, Liu looked to consolidate a team from the Biochemistry Department and endocrine group within Department of Internal Medicine of PUMC in order to establish the new department of endocrinology. They planned to relocate to German Hospital in August that year and this was to be China's first department of endocrinology. However, after all the logistics of relocating had been completed they received a new notice that the original German Hospital was changed to the hospital specifically used for leaders. So, Liu Shihao's team had to move back to PUMC in October and was subsequently downgraded to a discipline group within the Department of Internal Medicine which lasted until the end of 1961, when the Department of Endocrinology was resumed. Since then, the endocrinology department of PUMC has flourished, organized into four areas of advanced fellowship in endocrinology, training many who have become the bedrock of the endocrinology community in China.

Establishing radioimmunoassay of insulin and the epidemiological study of diabetes mellitus at Shougang (首钢) - the Capital Steel Plant

In 1959, Yalow and Berson successfully established the radioimmunoassay of insulin and published findings in 1960. Liu Shihao was able to see the significance of this research and understood the importance of this method. With the radioimmunoassay of insulin, protein hormones could be quantitatively tested, which led to a revolution in clinical endocrinology. In 1962, when the postgraduate program began to be reimplemented, Liu Shihao began recruiting Chen Zhizhou (陈智周) as his postgraduate fellow whose primary research interest was the establishment of radioimmunoassay of insulin. At that time, all the bovine serum albumin (BSA) used in experiments had to be imported from outside China which was quite expensive, considering the economic level China was facing at that time. As a result, Liu Shihao suffered from a lot of criticism, however he insisted on carrying out the project in spite of the tremendous pressure. Finally in 1965, the project was deemed a success, and Chen Zhizhou defended his thesis and graduated. Chen's thesis defense committee included senior academicians; such as, Zhang Xiaoqian (张孝骞), Wang Shizhen (王世真), Xie Shaowen (谢少文) and others, who unanimously thought highly of the application of Chen's research findings.

During the same period, Liu Shihao also performed another attempt: investigating the prevalence of diabetes mellitus among the workers at Shougang. Since 1964, Shi Yifan (史轶蘩)、Pan Xiaoren (潘孝仁) and other clinicians such as Deng Jieying (邓洁英), Sun Meili (孙梅励) as well as other researchers engaged themselves in the investigation and collected a lot of information. Abundant fruitful results could have been achieved through their efforts in the cross-sectional investigation, establishing the cohort study of diabetes mellitus and combination with application of the precise test of insulin. However, with the onset of the Cultural Revolution, the information was never sorted and lost forever by 1969. It was such a tremendous regret, however, the investigation provided project members with sound scientific training. The survey at Jiuxianqiao (酒仙桥) led by professor Chi Zhisheng (池芝盛) in the early 1980, and the survey at Daqing (大庆) led by professor Pan Xiaoren, could be regarded as a result of the influence by Liu Shihao.

Introducing the stress theory and adopting the Chinese translation of the word "stress" - "Yingji"

The stress theory was first proposed in 1936 in a paper by Hans Selye published in *Nature*. In the 1950s, the Soviet scholars discussed this concept extensively, so that it stimulated debate within the academic community in China. In the summer of 1962, the Tianjin Physiological Society held a lecture on the stress theory of Selye. In the process of the discussion, Liu Shihao suggested that the Chinese translation of the word "stress" should be changed from "*Yingli*" (应力) into "*Yingji*" (应激), with which all the participants agreed. Since then, the translation of "Yingji" (stress) was widely accepted by the academic society. In 1962, Liu Shihao complied and published "A brief introduction to the stress theory of Selye" (《塞里应激学说概要》). In this book, Liu systematically introduced the stress theory which played a pivotal role in the promotion of this theory throughout the country.

In summary, the first half of Professor Liu Shihao's life went exceptionally smoothly. In addition to his extraordinary talent, the medical education within "old PUMC" also played an instrumental role in guiding Professor Liu's career. Although, he suffered a great deal through political turmoil at a later stage, academically he was highly respected, and he contributed to the development of endocrinology of China in many different ways.

Shi Yifan (1928 ~ 2013)

"The PUMCer" after the first resumption of PUMC in 1946

Shi Yifan, whose family originated from Liyang, Jiangsu Province, was descended from the famous "Family Shi of Liyang". When she went to primary school, the Sino-Japanese War broke out. Shi Yifan and her siblings trekked through different places and united with their parents in Qingdao where she entered the famous "Tsingtao Anglican Church Middle School for Girls" (青岛圣公女中). She excelled in her studies and was able to rank highest in her class every year. In 1946, she was accepted to the premedical program of Department of Biology, College of Science, Yanching University. Then in 1949, she was formally offered a place to study at PUMC. In the summer of 1950, along with her classmates Zhang Zhinan, Sun Ruilong and Liu Lisheng, she was awarded the Golden Key Award which was issued by the Phi Tau Phi Scholastic Honor Society (φτφ) of the College of Science, Yanching University. This is a highly prestigious award as only 10 people won the award. In 1954 when she graduated, Shi, Zhang Zhinan, and Sun Ruilong were give the title of 'Outstanding graduates'.

When Shi Yifan was at the College, the Sino-Japanese War had just started. At that time, Yanching University and PUMC were both occupied by the Japanese army which came immediately after the Pearl Harbor incident on December 8, 1941. Both the President of Yanching University – John Leighton Stuart and the President of PUMC – Henry S. Houghton were arrested by the Japanese army and imprisoned until the end of the war. The devastated Yanching University reopened in September 1945. PUMC, however, had been used as the "headquarters for peaceful coordination". PUMC did not fully resume until 1947; however, after 1947 civil war broke out. Up to the beginning of 1949, Peiping (Peking) was surrounded by the PLA (People's Liberation Army) and therefore the situation was not conducive to studying. Although, Yanching University was in the suburbs, and it was not under artillery fire, the college could continue delivering high quality education, the influence on the teachers and on the students was not minimum.

In the fall of 1949, when Shi Yifan entered into the preclinical program of PUMC, Peiping had already been liberated by PLA. The faculties of PUMC were already dominated by Chinese professors, most of whom were graduates of "old PUMC". Still, the college enjoyed a strong capacity in teaching and research, with both the curriculum and teaching being similar to that delivered in the past. In other words, PUMC managed to maintain the highest standards in education and clinical practice. Then, in January 1951 PUMC was nationalized, and PUMC became a negative example of cultural aggression by American Imperialists in China. All kinds of political movements occurred, causing tremendously negative impact on students.

In 1950, all the students on the premedical program in Yanching University were transferred to other departments and since 1951, no new students were to be enrolled, and the "elimination system" (fail then drop out) was abandoned. Although, the teaching system endured, many courses underwent an overhaul. For example, clinical rotation was originally done in all departments, but when Shi Yifan was in her final year it changed. Clinical practice was more like a clerkship at a specialized department. Thus Shi did rotations on wards within the internal medicine department for a year. This was something Shi would later regret, never having had the opportunity to take a clinical rotation within the departments of surgery, obstetrics and gynecology. In short, despite all kinds of interference, Shi Yifan went through the whole program of the eight years of medical education at PUMC, laying a good foundation for her subsequent growth.

Experiences prior to the Cultural Revolution

After graduation, Shi Yifan was assigned to work in the Department of Internal Medicine in PUMC Hospital. When she served as a medical resident, Shi Yifan was known for her healthcare excellence. She was not only dedicated to the medical profession but also engaged in teaching less experienced students. In her later years, she used to talk about her working style with her students: every night she would ponder the teaching content and teaching methods for the next day, and read the reference books to make the fullest preparation for an optimal teaching effect. Wu Ning, a female doctor two grades lower than Shi at that time (who later became a Professor of Cardiology – a famous professor at PUMC Hospital), recalled that when she and her classmates were interns at the hospital, Shi Yifan used to ask the interns in the ward how they could judge the effectiveness of the treatment for heart failure in a simple way. Shi was able to tell it simply by observing the changes with patients when she removed the two pillows that the patient normally reclined on lying on the bed. The experience benefited the medical students throughout their whole life.

In 1958, when China's first endocrinology department was established at PUMC, Professor Liu Shihao appointed Shi Yifan to be the acting attending physician and in charge of the ward. As the political movements at that time were overwhelmingly in number, career promotion became unpredictable, thus Shi Yifan did not become a confirmed attending physician until 1963. However, Shi Yifan was always the attending physician and someone Professor Liu Shihao regarded highly. Lin Lixiang, who attended advanced training classes of endocrinology, could still remember very clearly years later, that Professor Liu Shihao asked her to go to the ward for clinical training to be mentored by Shi Yifan. At that time only four students could be enrolled to the advanced training classes of endocrinology and therefore the students who completed this training were highly valued and have become academic leaders within this field all over China.

Since 1954 Shi Yifan engaged in the clinical study of meningitis in 1955, and was responsible for the summary work of clinical cases. After the establishment of the Department of Endocrinology, Shi Yifan's clinical research work focused on the clinical summary of a variety of endocrine diseases. In 1964, when the first national symposium of Endocrine and Kidney Disease was held in Guangzhou, Shi Yifan was unable to attend, but she contributed three papers, namely: "*The diagnosis and classification of Cushing's syndrome*" (Shi Yifan, Liu Shihao); "*The outcome of Cushing's Syndrome*" (Shi Yifan, Liu Shihao); "*The clinical manifestations and Cytological Examination of the* 12 *cases of primary ovarian dysgenesis*". According to the later record, every time Shi Yifan included these three academic publications she also included her curriculum vitae, which demonstrates her own belief in this research.

After Professor Liu Shihao established the endocrinology department, with his vision, he took the lead in establishing China's first radioimmunoassay of insulin at about the same time in 1964 when he carried out the screening project for diabetes mellitus in Shougang – Capital Steel Corporation (CSC). If there had been no interference from the "Cultural Revolution", the combination of these two tasks could have made China produce a number of research on diabetes mellitus of the advanced international academic standard. Shi Yifan participated in the investigation of Capital Steel Corporation (CSC) . She did have access to the in – depth radioimmunoassay research, and this important work was likely to have a far-reaching impact on her. Later, she always emphasized the importance of the establishment of hormone determination method, and put into practice herself.

In sum, before the Cultural Revolution, Shi Yifan did an excellent job in clinical, teaching and research. On one hand it was because of her talent and effort, and on the other hand it was contributable to the guidance of her famous teacher Liu Shihao and the academic atmosphere in the Department of Endocrinology at that time.

The clinical environment and research during the "Cultural Revolution"

The "Cultural Revolution" in 1966 was a disaster for the scientific community generally and this was no exception for the medical professions. As the example of cultural aggression to China by the American Imperialism, PUMC became a severely afflicted place when the tenured professors, such as; Zhang Xiaoqian, and Liu Shihao were all criticized as examples of capitalist thinkers. They were not allowed to teach, and they were also forced to be reviled, persecuted, and worked as janitors cleaning the public toilets.

However, after all, the hospital was a special institution with medical rigor stipulated as a prerequisite. Except for the castigated "old experts" who were not allowed to work, doctors who actively participated in the Cultural Revolution were unable to undertake this clinical work. Only a group of young doctors like Shi Yifan remained on wards, overloaded to meet patient needs. They were facing all kinds of challenging and complex diseases, which required intensive care and treatment. In the absence of superior physicians, Shi Yifan needed to make clinical decisions for treating patients all by herself. Sometimes, Shi Yifan would secretly go to find Professor Liu Shihao (who was cleaning the toilets) to ask for his advice and guidance which she would then implement.

After years of experience through many social and political changes Shi Yifan had become an effective clinical practitioner. In 1970, after the earthquake of Tonghai in Yunnan Province, PUMC sent a rescue team. Among all the rescue cases, one of the most successful cases was done by the surgical team led by Professor Zhu Yu who cured a patient with multiple fractures. Another patient with Type I diabetes was saved by Shi Yifan simply using fluid infusion, rather than insulin therapy which would normally be administered. Although, 10 years of the *Cultural Revolution* brought countless negative effects, Shi Yifan was able to garner advanced clinical skills as well as laying solid foundation for further clinical research.

In the late "Cultural Revolution", Shi Yifan found opportunities to conduct trials of using new treatment methods. One of the most prominent was in the preparation of the drug used for pheochromocytoma. This disease is caused by a tumor on the adrenal site that secretes catecholamines, intermittent or continually release catecholamines, leading to paroxysmal or persistent hypertension (or persistent hypertensive paroxysmal aggravation). The preferred therapy of the disease is surgery; however, before the preoperative alpha receptor antagonists were available, mortality from surgery was high. The earliest suspected pheochromocytoma cases was recorded at PUMC Hospital in 1939, when there were no means to confirm the diagnosis. It was not until 1950s that successful cases of removal pheochromocytoma began. According to surgeon, Wu Jieping who performed the operation, his experience was that surgery should be done very fast to remove the tumor ASAP, otherwise it would significantly increase the risk of death. In 1970s, Shi Yifan was the first in China using α receptor antagonist pheochromocytoma on patients for preoperative preparation. The procedure gradually became the gold standard and was promoted throughout the country. Pheochromocytoma is no longer a disease associated with high risk and this treatment has gradually become a routine, standard procedure.

After the *Cultural Revolution*, Shi Yifan in her fifties, became passionate about the revival the Department of Endocrinology PUMC. On the one hand, she made a systematic summary of a variety of endocrine diseases diagnosed and treated at PUMC Hospital. The most prominent included the finding that Chinese people with primary hyperparathyroidism were often accompanied by softening of the bones, and she proposed the idea of "early risk manifestation" toward the diagnosis and treatment of hyperthyroidism, playing an important role in guiding the clinical treatment. On the other hand, the endocrinology department divided into different groups to improve diagnostics and treatments. As the group leader of the newly established pituitary group, Shi Yifan paid special attention to the various pituitary hormone determination methods. She started from established radioimmunoassay. From then on, she has led a series of pituitary disease-related clinical and basic research, and eventually won the First Prize of National Science and Technology Progress Award.

At National Institutes of Health (NIH)

In January 1981, Shi Yifan flew to the NIH, and began a two-year fellowship. Her mentor, R. Sherins was a very well established doctor and scientist in the field of male reproductive endocrinology. Shi Yifan engaged in Professor Sherins' clinical work and basic research in male reproductive endocrinology and was also actively involved in various forms of discussion on various endocrine diseases. Shi eventually published two papers based on her work at NIH. One is "*Long-term stability of aqueous solutions of luteinizing hormone-releasing hormone assessed by an in vitro bioassay and liquid chromatograph"*, and the other is *"Increased plasma and pituitary prolactin concentrations in adult male rats with selective elevation of FSH levels may be explained by reduced testosterone and increased estradiol production.* " These two papers were highly praised by Professor Sherins and regarded as an important supplement to the understanding of the pathophysiology mechanism of male gonadal endocrine disease in that era.

Shi Yifan gradually became more aware that the causal factors of pituitary disease laid in evaluated hypothalamus activity and particularly between the pituitary/target gland axis function. The priority was the determination of various pituitary hormone for the hormones whose results were not accurately measured. Due to excessive fluctuations, functional tests became very important, the research of which accounted for huge part of Shi's research after she returned to China. Shi Yifan's original research at NIH mainly resided in animal experimentation although she became acutely aware of how animal testing would complement clinical research. . Later, Shi emphasized the combination of clinical research and basic research methods, and led by example, which shows an obvious influence of her experience at NIH.

Clinical and basic research on hormone-secreting pituitary adenoma

The study of hormone secreting pituitary adenoma began in 1979. Earlier the method for the determination of growth hormone was established, but how to evaluate whether the growth hormone of a patient was too much or too little had not been studied in detail. After Shi Yifan became the Head of the Pituitary Group, she set the research direction and organizational goals which were the establishment of radioimmunoassay for other various pituitary hormones and the establishment of hormone normal value vs. pathological value range. After Shi's returning from NIH, this direction was further strengthened. For those diseases that could not be clearly determined by a hormone test, the corresponding functional tests were established to assist in clinical diagnosis. For example, for children with growth hormone deficiency, simply by measuring serum growth hormone levels alone, doctors could not diagnose growth hormone deficiency, because normal children showed low levels of growth hormone at default state i. e. no difference from that of children with growth hormone deficiency. Shi Yifan recognized that it was necessary to establish a growth hormone excitement test, stimulated appropriately, the normal children's serum growth hormone levels could be activated, while the patient children were impossible; so as to distinguish the patient children from normal children, to avoid missed diagnosis and misdiagnosis.

When the research into "Hormone secretion of pituitary tumors" was nominated as the candidate for the national award, the establishment of six kinds of hormone determination and eight functional test methods served as an important evidence for improving the diagnostic level. Of course, the importance of the use of such technology as CT in assisting the location diagnosis, visual field examination and the value of pathological diagnosis is self-evident. In addition to diagnosis, Shi Yifan's team promoted the progress of treatment, surgical treatment, radiation therapy and drug therapy, all of which became an important option for pituitary tumor treatment. The meticulous observation on the side effect of somatostatin – its inhibitory effect on gallbladder contraction was discovered first in the international community. For further study of the mechanism, Shi Yifan designed animal experiments for further illustration. Therefore, the PUMC's endocrine research attracted attention once again from the international academic counterparts. The professor of endocrinology of the Southwest Medical Center in the US wrote a special report on the Department of Endocrinology PUMC Hospital in the American Journal of Clinical Endocrine and Metabolism.

The significance of pituitary tumor research led to the social benefits. In 1979, the diagnosis of pituitary tumors in China almost entirely relied on experiences, while in 1992, when Shi Yifan's team applied for the National Science and Technology Progress Award, almost all types of pituitary tumors could be dealt with appropriately in line with international level of treatment. A great contribution in pituitary tumor and other areas, Shi Yifan was elected as the academician of Chinese Academy of Engineering in 1996 and was awarded the Ho Leung Ho Lee (何梁何利) Science and Technology Progress Award the same year.

Adolescent development research, obesity research and others

After the successful completion of pituitary tumor research, Shi Yifan's interests turned to adolescent development and obesity. The first step was the establishment of normal values as was in the previous years. Shi, in her 70s still led her graduate students to Da Qing to conduct a survey of child and adolescent development, in an effort to establish a normal age range for the onset of adolescent development in Northern China. The idea was to understand thresholds for the onset of precocious puberty and to understand youth development delay and other adolescent diseases in China. Shi also engaged in the development of the current diagnostic criteria for obesity and overweight in China. She was trying to isolating active ingredients from the traditional herbal medicine. Led by Shi Yifan, the Endocrine Key Laboratory of Ministry of Health was established in 1988 in Peking Union Medical College Hospital, which was the first endocrine laboratory of ministerial level set up in the hospital.

Shi Yifan also made important contributions to the development of China's clinical pharmacology research. As early as 1983, soon after she became the director of Department of Endocrinology PUMC Hospital, the department was designated as the Ministry of Health's clinical pharmacology base. Since then, for a variety of new endocrine drugs, such as Bromocriptine, clinical trials were completed at here and in 1995, Shi Yifan founded the Clinical Pharmacology Center of PUMC Hospital and served as director. At the same time, she also engaged in drafting the Good Clinical Practice (GCP), making remarkable contribution to the standardization of clinical pharmacology in China.

Reflecting on Professor Shi Yifan's life, her learning stage was to a certain degree interfered, but she graduated with honors. After the establishment of the Department of Endocrinology at PUMC Hospital, Shi Yifan's spent most of her time in clinical work, especially during the "Cultural Revolution" period. This was the heavy and stressful clinical work but also enabling her to develop highly advanced clinical skills. After the Reform, the training experience at NIH improved Shi Yifan's scientific mindset and scientific research ability rapidly. Then after return to China, in her study on the pituitary tumor, she closely linked the basic research to clinical research, and ultimately won the national Scientific and Technological Progress Award, and was elected member of the Chinese Academy of Engineering.

Reflections on the Academic Growth and Educational System from the Cases of the Two Masters in Endocrinology

As the leading academic authorities in endocrinology of two generations in China, both Liu Shihao and Shi Yifan headed the endocrine field at PUMC. Their success is uncontested, which also demonstrates the success of PUMC's medical education. Although, there is nearly 30 years difference between the two, the two were alumni, with a teacher student relationship. Their academic development trajectory is surprisingly similar. The medical education system they went through is a combination of great changes and continuity. Whether the advanced medical education system then is still considered the most advanced nowadays, and whether it is still instrumental in cultivating the medical leader, is in fact, a subject worth serious consideration.

The "old PUMC" medical education system was the most advanced medical education system based on the Flexner report. It emphasizes on premedicinal education, bedside teaching, practice, and self-study. The graduates of the 20 year period from 1924 to 1943 can be said the products of the practice of the education system in China. Liu Shihao was a graduate of the second class in graduate session. Although the education system did not yet reach best practice state. For example, premedical education was undertaken at PUMC not as it was in Yenching University. PUMC's premedical education was entirely based on the idea of the new American education system. Hence, Professor Liu Shihao can be regarded as one of the best representatives of the education system.

The college and hospital placed high attention on his academic career after graduation. Liu Shihao obtained a number of good opportunities to continue education throughout his career. Plus, he was hard working and extraordinarily talented. When he was 41 years old, PUMC offered him a professorship. The eight years of medical education he obtained, including; premedical, basic and clinical medical education, then graduate studies. His first working experience was with residency training, and then he was promoted to chief resident because of his excellent work, after that he was an attending physician. Not long after, he had the opportunity to go abroad to study. He went to the advanced Rockefeller Institute for Medical Research in New York and followed the famous biochemist Van Slyke, laying the foundation for his research in biochemistry. He published a number of papers before that, but these were basically case reports and clinical summary.

After returning from his study in the United States, Liu Shihao's competency in basic medical research greatly improved, which served as the basis for qualifying the Deanship of Department of Biochemistry later in his career. After being appointed assistant Professor, Liu Shihao once again got the opportunity to study abroad. This time, he went to Middlesex Hospital in Britain, and learned the very advanced experimental animal research technology. Therefore, Liu Shihao's two overseas experiences can be said to be two leaps in his scientific research, so that his later academic level was greatly acknowledged in both the biochemistry and endocrine society. If it had not had for the impact of various "movements" after the founding of PRC, Professor Liu Shihao's achievements would have had a far wider reach.

Professor Shi Yifan's academic growth trajectory is more complicated than that of Professor Liu Shihao. Enrolled as a PUMC student, Shi went to pre-medical program at Yanching University after PUMC resumed after the Second World War. Though there was further interference caused by the civil war, the program still followed the previous education system. When she entered the preclinical program at PUMC, Peiping (Peking) was liberated. However, at the beginning, as an American institution, PUMC did not suffer too much from the impact until the breakout of the Korean War. In January 1951, PUMC was put under the military control and nationalized. Therefore, Shi Yifan's clinical stage of learning was done at PUMC after the PUMC was nationalized and no longer enrolled students, so that the information about Shi's study in this phase is lacking. One can only imagine the impact on the medical students from a variety of political campaigns.

Conversely, although the learning environment underwent dramatic changes, strong teaching traditions at PUMC did not change much, considering that the overall situation of the faculty did not change dramatically. As a result of the Korean War, a large number of doctors from surgery related departments were loaned to other institutions. The doctors who remained at PUMC Hospital could still continue and guarantee the teaching quality of small class size. The tradition of emphasizing bedside teaching and self-learning to a certain extent made sure that the quality of teaching more mainly depended upon the quality of the students rather than the teacher's teaching experience. Therefore, it is justifiable to conclude that the "old PUMC" education system continued to play a core role in the education of the students after the PUMC resumed in 1946, so that classes of 1945 – 1949 followed the "old PUMC" education concepts.

Different from Liu Shihao whose career path was smooth after graduation, Shi Yifan entered the Department of Internal Medicine and later worked at endocrinology after graduation. Shi basically engaged in clinical work, and had few opportunities to do systematic clinical research, let alone to go abroad to study. Liu Shihao was clearly very talented both in basic and clinical medicine, so that he could have opportunities to study and do research in the endocrinology on wards. However, for Shi, during the so called *10 year Cultural Revolution*, she could only devote her effort in clinical work, and developing extraordinary clinical skills under the extremely stressful clinical circumstances. Shi's research competence has also driven research thanks to her fellowship in NIH. Shi learned to complement clinical research with animal testing which led to her direct involvement in hormone determination analysis.

After Shi returned to China, she made the quantitative determination of pituitary-related hormones as her primary task. Shi made a series of studies on the role of hormone determination in clinical practice, ensuring the diagnosis and treatment of pituitary disease in China kept pace with international standards. Throughout the course of her research, Shi made some original discoveries, and eventually won the Science and Technology Progress Award. In addition, Shi Yifan had access to the most advanced clinical research at NIH, which also partially aroused her attention to clinical pharmacology. Later, she established the Clinical Pharmacology Center at PUMC Hospital and served as the first director.

In reality, the academic growth trajectory of Liu Shihao and Shi Yifan's has a lot in common. Access to various disciplines in general education in their premedical program and both were equipped with the highly attuned scientific thinking. During their basic medical learning stage, they received sound training in scientific experimentation and in their clinical learning stage, both developed strong competency in self learning through a quality bedside teaching model, laying the foundation for becoming scientists. After intensive residency training, they went to abroad to learn the most advanced scientific research ideas and scientific research methods. Then after returning to China, they combined what they had learned with their own research interests. Based on their high-quality clinical work, they made innovative academic contributions. In other words, the PUMC eight year education cultivated their scientific quality and basic clinical skills, and their clinical skill reached a higher level after the residency training. By going abroad, they studied and conducted research within the leading international research arena. They brought back the cutting edge scientific research methods to PUMC and combined them with the clinical work. Both made significant breakthroughs on the basis of sound preparation and in a consistent way. Although, Liu Shihao went to the United States as early as 29 years old, while Shi Yifan was already in her 52 years old when she went abroad, it is obvious that their overseas experience enhanced their scientific research capacity.

The second half of the twentieth century saw the robust development of life sciences. The rise of molecular biology led to the emergence of a series of new disciplines, so that the depth and breadth of basic medicine is quite different than the "old PUMC" era. Therefore, it is unlikely to produce such experts as Liu Shihao who excelled both in biochemistry and clinical medicine. The emerging statistics permeated almost every field of clinical medicine, so that the dependency of clinical research on statistics was unprecedentedly intense after the rise of evidence-based medicine. This results in the increase in separation of basic medicine from clinical medicine, while clinicians had to make choice between clinical, scientific research and teaching. This is most visible in contemporary medical system in the United States, where doctors can choose one from the three: clinical work, teaching and assisted in clinical work, scientific research assisted in clinical work.

The "PUMC" system, which originated from the American medical education revolution, aimed at nurturing excellent medical talents who excel in clinical work, teaching and research. The dynamics of the era is constantly testing the education system of PUMC, and PUMC's medical education is also in the continuity of improvement. In 1979, after PUMC reopened for the third time in its history, PUMC incorporated more content of scientific research training in the teaching model, covering basic medical research and clinical medicine research simultaneously, strengthening scientific research and practice. In this way, PUMC's medical students not only possess solid basic clinical skills, but also the basic scientific research capability after graduation. Theoretically, they have a brightfuture; however, the reality is cruel. The current job market has quietly changed. Hospitals favor those graduates with short-term medical training, specialized training and SCI papers. Meanwhile, the large scale promotion of "5 + 3" system is also fueling this trend. Under the current evaluation system, how to improve the competitiveness of PUMC graduates? How can we cultivate contemporary Liu Shihao and Shi Yifan? This will be a huge challenge to Peking Union Medical College.

"新协和" 的医学专业化 （1951－1966）[1]

胡　成

　　胡成，1998 年南京大学历史学博士，现任南京大学历史学教授，出版了《学者的本分：传统士人、近代变革和现代学术制度》（社会科学文献出版社，2017 年）、《医疗、卫生与世界之中国》（科学出版社，2013 年）、《近代转型与史学反思》（北京三联书店，2013 年）等学术专著，并还刊发了多篇学术专题论文。

　　1950 年夏，时任西南军区军政大学，也就是前二野军政大学教育长的张之强，经军委卫生部副部长傅连暲的介绍，因肺结核住进了北京协和医院的头等病房。那时协和西门口还挂着"私立北平协和医院"的牌子，尚未断绝与美国洛克菲勒基金会旗下的罗氏驻华医社（后更名，本文统称 CMB China Medical Board）的联系。1949 年解放军占领南京之后，张之强也曾住过该地的中央医院。那所医院创办于 1929 年，1930 年由南京国民政府划归卫生部（后改为卫生署）管辖，是国民政府规模最大、设备最完善的国立医院。不过，当张之强住进协和之后，留下深刻印象的是医生与医生、医生与护士之间的工作语言均用英文，大夫查房很严格、病史问得很详细；病房里很安静，听不到大声说话和走路的声音，从而让他感到"和南京中央医院有明显的不同"。

　　尽管如此，张之强在当时对协和却持有一种意识形态意义上的憎恨情结。他在五十多年之后，即 2006 年刊发的回忆录中写道："我过去在北京上学时，就听说协和是全国医疗水平最高的医院，但因为它是美帝在中国办的医院，情感上总有些不舒服。"[2]这是指他曾于 1936 年在北平师范大学教育系就学，知道有这么一家美国人办的医院。1938 年他加入中共后不久奔赴延安。然而，1950 年在协和住院的他，还不知道这家医院将在 1951 年初由政府接管，自己将被任命为政委、党委第一书记。直到 1965 年调任卫生部，他都是负责协和全面工作的第一把手。

概括说来，医学专业化的意义在于治疗不只是医生与病患的个人之事，且还包括职业共同体的基本利益、内在化了的核心伦理，以及取得成就之后的荣誉和奖励。[3]就欧美发达国家的医学专业化发展来看，这是通过职业共同体的竞争、角力，以及民族国家的立法而逐渐形成。例如 1815～1848 年间，法国关于医学专业化改革的九项创议；1840～1858 年期间，英国议会通过十八项有关医学专业化的法令；以及 1847 年美国医学协会（American Medical Association）的成立。与之不同，中国的医学专业化是由欧美的医疗传教士、通商口岸的外籍医生，日本殖民当局，以及数以百计的中国留日学生，根据各自境况而碎片化地引入——不同地区、不同医学机构的发展相当不平衡。洛克菲勒基金会于 1914 年成立罗氏驻华医社，并投入巨资于 1917 年创办北京协和医学院。在整个中国，乃至在整个东亚，北京协和医学院都被公认为拥有最高医学专业化水准。[4]然而，1950 年之后面临的严峻问题是：如果将"协和"与"美帝"绑定，再以新政权将医疗卫生的重点放到农村，力图极速改善普通民众缺医少药的落后境况，那么"旧协和"矢志与西方发达国家同步的医学专业化，在新政权的管控之下将会有怎样的一些发展？

清除"美帝"影响与热火朝天的思想改造运动

建国之后，以往协和的医学专业化标准首先受到政治冲击，这是在 1950 年 11 月 8 日。中央政府卫生部、教育部和军委卫生部为解决志愿军伤病员的医疗问题，与时任协和医学院院长李宗恩、医院院长李克鸿商谈，想向协和借用二百五十张病床成立一所新的医院。李宗恩对政府此举很不情愿，最初婉拒的理由是驻协和的罗氏驻华医社代表娄克斯（Harold H Loucks，1894－1982）于当年 6 月 28 日返回美国，校方没有办法单独决定此事。后来在强大的政治压力之下，两人不得已做出妥协，同意如数借出病床，并于 11 月 20 日参加了政府主持成立关于协和未来发展的咨询委员会。12 月 22 日，该委员会讨论决定新成立的医院将与协和医院合作，共同收治志愿军伤病员。具体分工是前者负责伤病员的组织工作，后者负责医疗合作，行政管理和财政各自独立，并由双方派出有关人员组成行政、医疗、经济三个小组，分别进行工作。[5]

就李宗恩在抗战及后来北平解放没有流亡海外的表现来看，应该是不缺"爱国主义"情怀的。此时他之所以没有识时务者为俊杰，慷慨借出这二百五十张病床，就是想维持协和的医学专业化标准，而非对中国参入朝鲜战事的抵触。在一年后思想改造运动的检查中，他坦承自己此时有三点顾虑：首先，协和总共只有三百五十张病床，借出二百五十张病床后，剩下的一百张病床，就没有办法维持正常教学秩序；其次，既然协和还被政府视为医学教学机构，就应当保证医疗教学设备齐全而可向其他医院求借；再次，让协和与新成立的医院合作，一定会"乱七八糟，协和标准很难维持"。[6]可对于新政权来说，这正是那些受过去协和医学专业化之影响，从而不能积极适应新社会需要的消极表现。张之强说，他们向协和借用二百五十张病床，有人就不大愿意，经过多次做工作，才勉强接受。实际上，这类摩擦就已经出现过。如 1949 年 9 月第一届全国政治协商会议在北京召开时，政府向协和商借学生宿舍，以供与会政协委员住宿，可是"就有人坚决不同意而只得作罢"。[7]

再让政府感到忧心忡忡的，尽管于 1951 年 1 月 20 日接管了协和，党组织随即发动了大规模政治宣传运动，声称一个"新协和"的开始；但仍然有不少人身陷昔日的医学专业化标准之中而执迷不悟。1950 年 3 月 22 日、4 月 19 日的《人民日报》分别刊发了"读者来信"以及协和医学院的检讨，称协和医学院有许多人不看党的报纸，漠不关心于政府大力号召民众支持的抗美援朝、增产节约和"三反"运动。这篇文章列出的数据是，三百多人中（包括教授、大夫、护士、助理员），约有二分之一基本上不读报。以拥有各种资料最多而自傲的协和图书馆甚至连一份《人民日报》都不订。原因在于一些教授、大夫们只晓得整天忙于专业学术研究、跑病房，对于外事不闻不问。个别教授认为参加学习小组，是一件令人生厌的麻烦事。更让这几位读者感到愤慨的是："上学期，当学生们要求分出一定时间学习政治的时候，教授们竟然不接受这一意见，（说）课程表上没有规定一分钟的政治学习时间。"[8]

作为应对，党委提出"改造旧协和，建设新协和"的口号，大张旗鼓地动员师生们投身到"彻底肃清美帝文化侵略影响"的运动之中。这最初只得到与所谓"旧协和"关系不太深的少数进步学生的响应。他（她）们撰文批判说："旧协和"毕业的三百二十名学生中，百分之七十三留在城市，百分之十四去了外国，没有一个人前往解放区。究其原因，进步学生们认为是"旧协和"提供的优渥条件之所致。这篇文章批判道：直到抗日战争爆发之前，该校每位同学每月的饭费高到六十银元。早餐有牛奶、鸡蛋、水果，下午四、五点有茶点。吃饭时每桌有四碟菜，一个汤、五六个人吃。如果一个人来，照样可以开一大桌。喜欢吃哪一个菜，吃完了可以再要，到够了为止。饭后还有冰淇淋，每张桌子上放了一个呼叫佣人的按铃。每四张桌子安排了一位专门负责添饭的"茶役"（table boy）。吃完的学生敲一下碟子，马上就有人过来负责添饭。这些西服笔挺的学生被培养出来，远远脱离了广大中国人民的生活水平，造成严重的享乐思想。这篇文字最后说："结果就是使人安于这个舶来的'现实'，不愿想什么中国革命的问题。"[9]

党委接下来进一步揭露"披着绅士、学者外衣的帝国主义分子"，批判火力集中如娄克斯这些曾在协和任职的美国教授及外籍管理人士身上。宣传动员最初同样难以奏效，如娄克斯长期担任外科主任，在协和兢兢业业地工作了二十年，有较高学术声望和良好人缘。在1950年6月他回国之前，校方组织了欢送会。他在答谢致辞中说自己在中国几十年，最让他在回国之时难以忘怀的，是学生对先生的景仰和友谊，并称："这是中国学生的特质。"娄克斯讲这番话时的态度和蔼，语调平缓，充满了感情，在场很多学生被"深深感动，眼泪就在眼眶上"。由于学生会就此活动仅仅写了一封简单的祝贺信，很多同学还感到不满，认为对娄克斯太冷淡了。学生会主席为此做了抗辩，称娄克斯是帝国主义分子。但是大部分同学并不随声附和，反而说协和与帝国主义的文化侵略没有什么关系。甚至到了1951年2月，学校开展进一步肃清美帝国主义影响的学习运动之时，还有学生不认为娄克斯是帝国主义分子，相信自己"所抱的态度是科学的、客观的"。[10]

更严厉的批判还在后面。1951 年 11 月 30 日，中央下发《关于在学校中进行思想改造和组织清理的指示》，要求更为彻底清理"三美"（"亲美"、"崇美"、"恐美"）主义，娄克斯遂不容置疑地被定性为狡猾的帝国主义分子。1952 年 5 月《新协和》刊发的一篇批判文章写道：此人平日装成"绅士"、"学者"，从不当面骂人，使得很多外科大夫对他常有好感，不会想到就是他在掌握协和的实权。美国的文化侵略政策，就是通过他来执行。这篇文章揭发他一贯行使小恩小惠，如送实习大夫每人一条领带，住院总医师结婚时，送二十元美钞等，并时常请外科大夫们分批到家里吃饭，大肆宣扬美国生活方式和美国的民主等。解放后他假装同情新政权，说回到美国后发表了同情新中国的言论，被美国人指责为"同情共产主义者"，以博得中国人民对他的信任。当然，这篇文章少不了批判娄克斯推崇的"旧协和"的医学专业标准。如他总叫大夫们把经验和心得写成论文，送到美国杂志上发表。1949 年冬，当他得知政府将抽调协和学生参与防疫时，愤怒地表示这样做会妨碍协和的教学计划。[11]

这场运动采用"人人洗澡，个个过关"的方式，设置了所谓"大盆"（全院大会）、"中盆"（全系）或"小盆"（科室小组）的自我思想检查，与娄克斯关系密切之人自然要被推出来表态。1935 年进入协和、1940 年毕业、长时间作为娄克斯属下的外科大夫曾宪九（1914－1985），撰文检查自己对娄克斯的"学术关心"缺乏警惕。他交待了娄克斯返回美国之后寄来的三封信。起因是他写了两篇文章，请娄克斯批评指正。娄克斯的第一封信说正在修改他的论文，第二封信提了些修改意见。第三封信，是娄克斯知道无法回到中国后所写的，表示自己会将这两篇论文送出发表，并提到此后他虽然不能再写信了，但仍希望与曾宪九等外科同仁保持学术上的联系，以"能继续过去协和外科的诚实与好奇的传统"。娄克斯的信中还写道："因为国际间的猜疑，使远东为阴魂阴云所笼罩，不过他相信终会有一天人类可以和平共处，追求真理与学术。"他自己"无论在何时何地，外科同仁将永远与他的心同在"。就此，曾宪九的大会深刻思想检查是："当时看了这封信后，很受感动，觉得娄克斯对外科同仁是何等关心、何等亲切、也觉得他是反对战争的。因为他不能回协和，感觉惋惜。"[12]

　　与娄克斯关系不那么密切的医生们，也要检查自己深受"旧协和"推行的医学专业化之影响。1951年5月12日晚上，妇产科、小儿科、公共卫生科、眼科举行了联合控诉大会。一位妇产科的年轻医生反省道，当自己收到世界卫生组织请求调查中国新生儿的身高、体重的信函后，毫不犹豫地接受了任务，甚至不惜加班加点。该检查说所有参加者都感到很光荣，以为国际友人很重视我们的工作而要感谢他们；相反，对于"政府要我们抽一部分时间为解放军干部治疗，我们就以为共产党'侵略'到我们头上来，拼命推却。推不掉，才很不愿意的接受了。对于美帝，我们就赶任务，对于为我们流血的人，我们敷衍，推诿抗拒。"同一期刊物还刊登了另一位担任志愿军病房护士长的自我检查，更是触及"旧协和"医学专业化的实质——那就是不愿意协和被政府接管，认为将来的出路被断送了。这份检查说，当自己被调到志愿军病房（五楼二层）时，最初的想法是美国人对协和很好，为什么与他们打仗，惹起大祸来可受不了。她再看到来到协和的志愿军伤员大都是休养的，对自己的医疗技术没有什么提高，接到调令后就颇有抵触。她随即到医务部请求调至别的病房，遭到否决后，"回去大哭了一场，自认'倒霉'。"[13]

　　1952年9月27日，《人民日报》刊发了协和资深教授林巧稚的《打开"协和"窗户看祖国》，标志着此次思想改造运动获得了巨大成功。张之强对这篇文章的评论是，"在协和高级知识分子中也有代表性"。[14]的确，林巧稚集中火力批判了所谓的"协和标准"。文章的开头，她追溯当年因为羡慕"协和"的"国际标准"，不顾一切困难地离开家乡，考进"协和"之后非常得意。她说：三十年前一位女学生从厦门到北京"协和"，不是一件小事。在协和读书期间，她念的全不是中国书，写的不是中国字。1929年毕业后留校工作。当然，林巧稚在文章最后也要表示感谢，说这次思想改造运动唤醒了她……[15]

　　历次政治运动都是这样过来的，有进步的；就有不进步、落后乃至反动的。时任院长李宗恩，被认为恪守"协和标准"而冥顽不灵，过关需要经过全院大会的"大盆洗澡"。一些思想改造的积极分子，批评李宗恩强调"尽力在维护'协和标准'和制度，并无政治的用意"，是企图蒙混过关。李宗恩辩解说他不是不与政府合作，而是想拿出主人翁的态度，对国家负责。他宣称以一个有医学教育经验的专家身份，认为"协和标准"高，对国家是有帮助的。然而，积极分子们则提出诸多质问，如在召开政治协商会议前后，李宗恩常与美国人通信，将会议的内容向美帝份子汇报，"为了维护协和一个小机构的标准，必须这样立刻时时向美帝分子汇报政协的情形吗？"[16] 好在，这次运动除了有确凿证据的现行反革命分子之外，即使思想问题严重的，也只是做自我批评和大会检查而没有太多政治处罚。不过，李宗恩此后虽然还担任院长，但已经被严重边缘化。到了1957年的"反右"运动，他被作为全国闻名的大右派而被重点批判。《人民日报》发文说：从8月到10月，经过"两个月的说理斗争，十几次大小辩论会，协和医学院专家教授驳倒了李宗恩"。当时举出的罪证之一，是李宗恩的书面意见书写有："协和业务质量方面是降低了……协和这几年的损失必须要有一定的时间，以恢复元气。"这篇批判文章指称由此可以看出他的别有用心——叫嚣协和的医学专业水准"今不如昔"，"是有组织、有计划、有纲领的为美帝国主义文化侵略服务的半殖民地奴化医学教育制度。"[17]

要把"新协和"办得比"旧协和"更好

　　不论从哪方面来看，李宗恩不是位图谋不轨的政治反对派，而是太执着于"旧协和"的医学化专业标准而不知退让。就如当年在协和主持这场运动的张之强，多年后为其不幸被打成右派，几年后客死他乡而表示了内疚和自责。除此之外，张之强还从实际主持这场运动的切身体会，道出其时中共之所以发动一系列政治整肃的深层原因。他用了毛泽东所说"知识分子工农化、工农分子知识化"的那句话，认为"这是有所指的"。[18] 早在1951年春天，张之强当得知自己将被任命为军事代表接管协和之时，心里十分惶然。他的焦虑是深知协和作为一所国际知名的医学校，肩上的担子太重。因为高层领导在决定将协和收归国有后，就认定这是关乎国家声誉的一件大事，"如果办得不好，美帝国主义和其他的反华势力，就会趁机进行反华叫嚣。"[19]

说到把"新协和"办得比"旧协和"更好的口号，还要把目光回溯到 1951 年 1 月 20 日该校被宣布正式收归国有，全体师生员工约一千人参加庆祝大会。与会的卫生部领导宣读了政务院关于处理接受美国津贴的文化教育、救济机关及宗教团体的法令，宣布全体职工一律原职，按照大约是其时北大、清华等学校薪酬两倍的原薪留用，旧有教学制度将予以维持。与会的教育部、军委卫生部领导信心满满地宣称：在摆脱美国帝国主义的侵略影响后，中国人民有能力、有信心把协和医学院办得更好。接着，协和的领导、工会、学生会代表纷纷表态，表示坚决拥护政府决定，说他们也相信"属于中国人民的协和医学院，前途是无限远大的。"[20]一个月后，刚创刊的《新协和》进而写道：他们将尽量收集全院各方面的意见和报道以充实内容，除大力肃清美帝文化侵略的影响之外，主要目标还有"改正我们服务的态度，使教学和医疗的工作面向工农兵大众，这样才是'新协和'的使命！"[21]

1952 年 1 月，协和被划归军队管辖，首要任务被确定为满足国防卫生建设需要——基础研究服从于临床治疗，临床治疗服从于实际需要。接着，为创办解放军 301 医院，总后从协和临床和基础部抽调包括十七名教授，二十名主治医师等一大批专业骨干，致使其教学和科研力量受到了很大削弱。[22]在 1952 年至 1956 年期间，协和医院诊治的病患多是军人干部，其住院人次、门诊人次、急诊人次几乎占到二分之一。1953 年春协和就停止招收医学生，开始成为医疗卫生干部的进修学院。[23]为了满足各地医疗卫生的需要，协和举办了来自全国各地、不同岗位，医学基础知识参差不齐的各种训练班。如为落实 1950 年 8 月全国第一届卫生工作会议关于预防为主的决议，培训当时迫切需要的公共卫生护士，该院公共卫生护士班的人数一下子比过去增加了 4～5 倍。资料记载说："由于教学人员不足，公共卫生护士也担当了实习教学工作。"[24]1957 年 8 月，为反击李宗恩《人民日报》提供的数据也只是说："旧协和"的 22 年中，仅培养了 310 名毕业生；建国以后的"新协和"通过进修和短期训练班等形式，培养了 937 名医务干部，245 名医学生毕业，以及接收了来自全国各地 120 个医疗单位的进修生。[25]

1956 年，协和被重新划归卫生部领导，1958 年卷入了超英赶美的"大跃进"。那时响彻云霄的口号是医疗治疗和科学研究的"多快好省"。作为该院先进而被大力表彰的妇产科，过去作简单的全部子宫切除术平均需要两小时半，此时部分子宫切除术缩短为一小时半。速度更快的是，施行一个部分子宫切除术，仅一小时十五分钟就结束了。结扎输卵管手术，以前一般在产后六至二十小时内进行，此时改进到产后二至三小时内进行。皮肤切口由丝线缝合改为肠线皮下缝合，病人不必等待五天后拆线，出院日可以提早三天，已试行 3 例而效果良好。[26]更鼓舞人心的是，有些积极分子提出"五年内征服肿瘤"。抗生素系的先进分子们筛选有效药物，工作速度提高 215 倍，他们"决定在半年内找到抗癌抗生素"。[27]这也让张之强非常振奋，在一次总结会上说协和已经发生了翻天覆地的大变化，一天等于二十年，并强调"协和维持了 30 年的美国标准一夜之间就被冲垮了。"[28]

此时领导人之所以大力强调对"旧协和"的"破旧立新"，原因在于高标准的专业化影响太根深蒂固。那些顽固恪守当年"旧协和"医学专业标准之人，总对群众性的"大跃进"风言风语，冷嘲热讽。当时一篇文章批判道：这些人说"旧协和"冷冷清清，研究成果却是国际水平，"言外之意，今天轰轰烈烈，却是一事无成"。[29]作为针锋相对，这篇文章说"新协和"发扬了当年革命军队办医院的光荣传统——即被"旧协和"蔑视的所谓"游击习气"和"农村作风"。如"旧协和"主张按照世界一流水准办学，认为科学研究必须掌握国际进度，深入追踪英文世界发表过的国际文献，研究的成果须得到外国人的承认。然而，是年五月初，院党委组织了四周的相关务虚会议，发动全院对科学研究中的"旧协和"／"新协和"进行讨论。在 5 月 29 日的全院辩论大会上，党委领导谈到科学研究中的"国际水平"问题时，斩钉截铁地说："我们所强调的'国际水平'，是为人民生产解决实际问题的国际水平，所谓填补英美文献中空白点的'国际水平'……实际上是立场问题，必须予以彻底批判。"[30]后来刊发的另一篇文章的口气更是豪迈，声称："我们不要顾虑外国人承认不承认。我们六亿人民承认了，外国不承认，也不要紧。"[31]

再与那个时代的意识形态格格不入的，是"旧协和"在医疗过程中"等级森严"。一篇文章批判道：旧协和有这样一种传统：层次繁多，等级严明，任何人不得越雷池一步。上级大夫的话是金口玉言，即使是错误的，下级医生也不能提出反对意见。结果造成医师职级越高，越脱离病人的实际。那些幸运升到讲座教授之人，高高在上，埋头于"高深理论"和个人兴趣。然而，资历浅的大夫却只有和病人打交道的资格，对研究工作无权过问。这篇文章说："高级医师有时下来查房，总以外国文献套病人实际。甚至摆出权威架子，无端训斥下级医师，弄得下级医师噤若寒蝉。"[32]此时走在最前面的是脑系科破除"权威"和"等级制"的全面大跃进。该系科自10月初以来，所有高级医师都被下放到门诊和病房，在面向实际和为病人服务的基础上开展研究工作。为了让医师们集中力量治疗，护士们担负起医师们的部分常规治疗工作，如打针、输血、输液、穿刺等。同样，医师们利用一切机会做护理。每遇开饭时间，给病人喂饭的不仅有护士，也有医师。此外，他们坚决地推进了技术民主，以党组织为核心，在治疗过程中不只是专家说了算，青年们在集体讨论中也可以提出新的疗法和建设性意见，有些老教授"过去惯于用'姜是老的辣'这句话去训斥青年，现在再也听不到这句话了"。[33]

另一项温馨动人的改进，是"新协和"大力倡扬"全心全意为人民服务，医院如同家庭，使病人感到亲切、温暖"的新型医患关系。[34]在他们看来，"旧协和"如同衙门，使人感到冷酷森严，广大人民可望而不可即。就如当时许多医院实行了三班门诊制，有的医院还实行了二十四小时门诊和星期日门诊，基本上消灭了排队挂号。目的是方便工人职员们利用下班时间就诊，不致耽误工作和生产。天津医学院附属医院、上海第一医学院的六个附属医院，还开办了每天只收住院费一角二分，病人自带伙食、衣物的简易病床、大大减轻了病人的负担。然而，协和很多医生却不愿给劳动人民看病，认为他们笨、脏、说话啰嗦。此时一位熟练工人的月工资不超过四十元，可在协和看一次门诊，挂号、药费平均是一元八角，住一天医院平均费用是七元一角九分。很多群众反映，在协和治好了病，多带着眼泪出院——病治好了，也倾家荡产了。当然，最让人民群众不满意的，是挂号后十天半月才能看上病。[35] 作为一项最重要的医疗惠民的举措，协和于当年 6 月 3 日晚上正式开始二十四小时的门诊，科主任、教授亲临门诊。简易病床也连夜准备就绪，计划第二天开始收容病人。新闻报道说："当夜来到北京的癌症患者，用不着等到第二天，就可以立即到肿瘤医院就诊。湖南到北京来的一位患者，本来听说到'协和'看病如何困难，没想到 4 月 1 日到'协和'就看上了病，真是喜出望外。"[36]

"党的领导加旧协和" 与八年制医学院的重建

尽管在那些年里"旧协和"被政治敏感化，并上升到意识形态的高度，但要求恢复其医学专业水准的呼声，一直不绝于耳，挥之不去。张之强在回忆录中写道："协和划归中央卫生部领导以后，他们的专家教授们大多都希望恢复协和医学院的老传统，以担负起培养高级医学教育、临床医疗和科学研究人才的任务。协和人的意愿和要求是强烈的，但迫于当时的政治气候，又都不愿、也不敢直接提出来，只是在言谈说话之间，总流露出认为协和的专家教授'比较有经验'的看法。"[37] 不过，1956 年 1 月，中央召开了关于知识分子问题的会议，纠正了此前只强调知识分子的思想改造，提出其绝大部分已经是工人阶级的一部分。毛泽东在会议的最后一天做了讲话，号召全党努力学习科学知识，同党外知识分子团结一致，为迅速赶上世界科学先进水平而奋斗。接下来在"向科学进军"的口号感召之下，直到 1957 年 7 月 "反右"之前，政治空气一下子宽松了许多。知识分子们和学者，开始敢于畅所欲言，建言献策，没有太多后顾之忧。

作为新中国成立以来首次公开为"旧协和"医学专业化发声的，是时任协和解剖系主任的张鋆教授（1890 - 1977）于 1957 年 7 月刊发在《人民日报》上的一篇文章。在文中他呼吁不应抛弃"旧协和"的高水准，并直言说："我认为协和医学院过去在培养高级医学人才方面还是有一定经验的，在基础科学、临床实习和实验室工作的训练上是十分重视的，因此协和的毕业生在医学岗位上是起到一定的作用的。在学术研究上，过去有的方面也曾达到世界水平。"[38]与此同时，协和另一位重量级人物，即时任内科主任的张孝骞教授也上书党的高层，建议恢复"旧协和"采用的八年制医学教学体系。他认为医学是一门应用科学，需要极为坚实的理论基础，因此医学人才的培养是一桩艰巨繁复的工作。在高等教育中，医学应当是年限最长、课目最多、自然科学训练较为全面的一科。张孝骞坦率地批评道，由于国家的迫切需要，建国以来的医学教育不得不照顾数量，缩短年限而降低了质量。此时的医学院学制是学习苏联的五年制，医预科课程极不充实。"由于学生人数过多，师资、设备、病床都感缺乏，教学也很不够理想。"[39]

相对于只在教学方面有重要影响的张鋆而言，张孝骞由于还担任中南海的保健医生，上书比较容易抵达高层而更可能产生实际效用。如最初在筹建中国医学科学院的过程中，虽有老协和之人提出恢复医学院的意见，但以张之强为首的党委没有给予考虑。因为这是一个政治上比较敏感的话题，且涉及到中国医学科学院方方面面的复杂人事关系。如来自原中央卫生实验研究院的有些领导就表示不满，不服气协和的独大影响力。他们在党委会上提出反对意见，说："协和虽是原来的庙，但早已不是原来的神了！"[40]不过，事情出现转机的是在1959年春，时任中宣部部长、国务院副总理同时也是主管高等教育工作的陆定一因病入住协和。一天，他约张之强到自己的病房谈话。陆定一告诉张之强，说协和有教授向他反映，希望恢复协和医学院，想听听张之强的意见。作为有丰富政治经验的张之强，自然揣摩到作为高层领导的陆定一说这番话的倾向性。他写道："当时陆定一个人似已同意恢复协和，当然他还要向有关部门和领导商量、研究。他说我可以先在医科院党委内部吹风，听听大家的意见。"[41]

1959年9月，重建的八年制医学院如期开学。即使在此时，"旧协和"还是一个时时需要注意撇清干系的话题。9月5日，在东单三条胡同礼堂召开的中国医科大学成立大会和开学典礼上，只有曾是协和 1924 年的毕业生、时任中国医学科学院院长的黄家驷，当着二十九名插班生和五十名新生，以及北京市、卫生部领导的面，讲话中没有贬斥"旧协和"，而是称赞"我们许多老教授过去在八年制的协和医学院积累丰富的教学经验"。[42] 作为大会压轴发言的，是卫生部李德全部长的讲话。当话题转到"旧协和"时，谈及有人怀疑"旧协和"会死灰复燃，她斩钉截铁地说："决不可能回到旧协和资本主义道路上去，这一点是无可怀疑的。"接着，她在讲话中提到，这所八年制医学院所以被命名为"中国医科大学"，是有着特定的革命意义。在筹备成立之初，中国医学科学院最初拟定的名称是"人民医学院"，后来定为"中国医科大学"。这是抗战时期党在延安创办的，直到 1956 年以前，此名还由后来改名为沈阳医学院沿用。李德全部长说，采用这个具有光荣革命传统的名称，就是希望新创办的这所八年制的医学院，艰苦朴素，接近群众，教育工作结合生产劳动，结合群众卫生工作——继承和发扬这些老解放区的医学教育传统。[43]

标准不立，方向不明，相应的制度自然也就难以确立。这所新创办的八年制医学院的医疗和教学秩序最初颇为混乱。先就医疗而言，1960年，林钧才（1920～2015）由南京调任协和医院院长兼党委书记。到任之后，他看到的是该院医疗基础工作制度破而未立。这具体表现在秩序混乱，医院任务庞杂，战线过长，力量分散，人员不稳定，工作重量不重质。此外，医疗质量下降，事故增多；医、教、研关系失调，高级知识分子情绪消沉，谨小慎微，青年知识分子怕走"白专"道路。林钧才写道："人们把当时的协和医院的形象概括为'忙、乱、脏'"。[44] 面对这种情况，主管教学的黄家驷心急如焚，提出应当按照当年"旧协和"的医学标准，尽快组建起一支专职教师队伍。1961 年 11 月，章央芬（1914～2011）由上海第二医学院的副院长，调任该校担任教务长、党委常委，主管教学工作。按照张鋆教授的说法，协和自 1951 年 1 月被政府接管，划归军队领导之后，"来了很多部队的同志，他们和我们的生活习惯不大相同，谈心也很少，虽然没有什么大问题，但关系是不大融洽的。"[45] 再可以作为旁证的，是张之强在回忆录中也讲述 1957 年召开"向科学进军"的动员大会上，他号召党政干部要做好后勤保障工作，为科学工作者服务，一些来自部队的干部表示不理解。他们说："老子打北京时，你们还在为美帝国主义侵略服务呢。"[46]与这些人不同的是，章央芬虽然1938年参加新四军，但成长于江南城市、毕业于上海医学院（六年制）。一个可资参照的具体事例，是章央芬的丈夫，当时也是新四军野战医院医生的吴之理的回忆：即使在最为艰苦的战争年代，章央芬每天给自己的孩子洗澡，且不许陌生人抱。群众有反映，说她太娇气了。时任新四军第三师师长的黄克诚得知后，在一次群众大会上说："章大夫是大学毕业的医生，能到敌后抗战，就是爱国进步的表现，她爱清洁，怕给孩子传染上疾病，是讲科学。你们不能对人这样说三道四。"[47]

好在，此时"大跃进"的风头已过，一些较为务实的高层领导人开始以审慎、冷静的态度，不再那么讳言"旧协和"医学专业化的正面意义。1959年5月6日，中国医学科学院在吉祥剧院召开党员大会，陆定一到会讲话。他说："中宣部和卫生部一致认为协和医学院多年来培养了一批有真才实学的人才，有一套医学教育的经验。只要有党的领导，可按旧协和医学院的办法办。"[48]就现在披露的资料来看，当时不只是陆定一、中宣部和卫生部，甚至更高位阶的中央领导人也发表过类似言论。上面提及被调往协和医院担任领导的林钧才，1960年12月前往卫生部报到时，副部长向他传达了周恩来总理的指示："协和医院在亚洲乃至全世界是很有名望的，我们一定要把她办好，办不好影响不好。"[49]张之强的回忆录也写道：1960年，周恩来曾询问恢复老协和的情况和困难，说协和是世界有名的学校，恢复协和不能单纯从业务技术方面来看，她对医学界和国际上都是有影响的。更早些还传来了邓小平的指示，也是说协和要办好，要发展，协和的传统要保持，并派人专门前往协和进行调研。此外，彭真在一次讲话中更明确地指出："中苏友谊医院按苏联的（模式）办，协和按老协和的办。比如，不仅规章制度、传统作风，就连大夫、护士、职工的服装样式都要按老协和的样式，有什么不好。"[50]

1961年底至1962年初，"党的领导加旧协和"的办学方针被陆定一正式提出，并在这其时名为"中国医科大学"的"新协和"深入人心。教务长章央芬走马上任伊始，立刻就感到继承当年协和医学专业化传统的强大气场。章央芬写道：常委分工主管医大，兼医大校长的黄家驷，以及教学处处长张茝芬，都是"旧协和"毕业的高材生，对于吸取其经验办好医大坚定不移。例如在医大教学大楼内部建筑设计，教室、实验室、实验台、学生宿舍、食堂都是黄家驷按照旧协和标准、按照每年级120名学生设计的。他选定的教研室主任都是旧协和毕业生或在旧协和工作多年的老教授，都能很自觉地实行旧协和教学工作的好经验。"只要有一点偏差，黄校长、张处长就要提出意见：'这点没协和严，那点没协和细'，我很欣赏他们这种精神。"[51]这其中最石破天惊的一步，是1962年2月在黄家驷、章央芬的多次建议下，经卫生部批准，以中国医学科学院党委的名义召集旧协和毕业的专家教授开座谈会。经过七天的反复研究探讨，会议形成的历史性成果，由"旧协和"1942年毕业生、时任教务处长的张茝芬执笔，再经黄家驷修改，党委讨论后以名为《老协和医学院教学工作经验初步总结》的定稿。[52]

　　这份被付诸实施的文件，蓝本是协和当然效仿美国约翰·霍普金斯医学院的"小班、个体化、手把手"，即"导师制"的培养训练模式。1961年9月，作为建国之后首批"导师制"培养下的20名六年级的学生，来到协和医院临床学习。此时采用的是"旧协和"的医学临床教学巡诊和示教的方式，由导师带领学生围绕具体病人进行检查讨论，教授随时提问，启发思考，并引导学生讨论疾病的发生、发展、诊断、治疗和预防、预后等问题。以曾被誉为旧协和"三宝"之一的书写病历为例，有位学生刚开始写得很简单。导师看完她写的病历之后，递过几份协和医院过去的病历，叫她仔细地翻阅。这位学生看到协和的旧病历不仅记载了病人从出生、长大、结婚到有了孩子所患过的疾病，而且记载了每次疾病的发生、发展和治疗的情况。这位导师的教诲是："一个好的临床大夫，诊断的诀窍之一就是全面地向病人询问病情，仔细地进行体格检查，认真地书写病历。"[53]另外，还有一个可被数据计量的变化，是协和的研究人员借阅书刊数量逐月增加。一篇文章称1961年9月份，协和医学院图书馆平均每天借出图书130多本、10月份160多本；上架书刊（主要是阅后放在架外的书），8月份平均每天460多本，9月份平均每天610多本，10月份平均每天890多本。原因在于当时党委承诺保证研究人员每周有五个工作日，能够用到医疗、教学、研究工作上，希望由此为医务人员创造一个良好的，能够全神专注的发挥其专长，不受干扰的环境。这也致使他们"一有空就钻图书馆，经常了解国内外医药学发展的最新动向和成就"。[54]

结语

1966 年 6 月，"文化大革命"爆发，"党的领导加旧协和"被标签为"企图复辟旧协和的教育制度，培养的是资产阶级的接班人"[55]而遭到无情声讨和严厉批判。不过，自 1978 年"改革开放"之后，该校先以"首都医院医科大学"命名，继以"中国医学科学院"，又以"中国首都医科大学"，再以"中国协和医科大学"命名，并终于在 2007 年 5 月 18 日正式复名为"北京协和医学院"。相对于二十世纪以来美国人、欧美教会在华创办的所有大学，如在北京的"燕京"，在南京的"金陵"，在苏州的"东吴"和在上海的"圣约翰"等，"协和"是唯一被得到正名和在某种意义得到了"平反"的高等教育和科学研究机构，这就表明"协和"及其曾大力推进的医学专业化在当下中国已不再是一个高度政治敏感化的字眼。那么，在今天中国走向世界，世界接纳中国，全球学术交流日益密切，并不断精益求精而追求卓越的大背景之下，我们当如何评价 1949年之后"新协和"的医学专业化呢?

如果抛开非此即彼、非黑即白的紧身衣，而是从疾病、医疗与经济、社会、政治和文化之关联的视角来观察，似可以认为现代中国医学专业化发展本身就充满着深刻矛盾和尖锐冲突。熟悉"旧协和"历史的人都知道，[56]该校自创办以来就一直受到传教士和中国政府的批评——即其课程设置周期太长，全部用英文教学，以及培养的学生过于物质主义而只在都市工作。尽管该校在 1930 年代已努力参与北平公共卫生实验，以及河北定县的乡村卫生重建工作，但那只是部分介入而非其医学专业化发展之重心，也没有在资金和人员方面全力以赴地投入。毕竟，当时的中国疾病丛生、传染病肆虐，医疗卫生资源十分缺乏，民众的患病率和死亡率极高。就像面对无数饥肠辘辘、饥不可堪的难民，救济者首先应当提供最易填饱肚子的几片面包或一碗浓浓的热汤，而非满桌珍馐美馔的皇家大餐。"旧协和"采用霍普金斯的模式，在这个贫穷的国家推进最发达国家花费最昂贵的医学专业化之发展，确有其奢侈、华丽或过于超前的一面。

1956 年提出"向科学进军"的口号，中国以举国之力推进公共卫生事务，采取强大的群众动员模式控制鼠疫、霍乱、伤寒、血吸虫等烈性传染病的蔓延和传播。这些举措一定程度上改善了普通民众的医疗卫生条件，人民的预期寿命有了较大幅度地提高。再随着 1953～1957 年第一个五年计划的推进，工业化、城市化又得到了进一步的发展，国家开始需要尽可能地提升医疗专业化水准，在城市创办一批治疗条件更好、设备更加完善的医疗机构，以控制对全民健康有更多危害的心血管系统疾病和不断增高的肿瘤发病率。所以，此时"旧协和"虽还与"美帝文化侵略"紧密捆绑在一起，但其办学理念和各项制度、举措，则是国家在提升医学专业化水准而不能不继承的一项优质学术传统资源。

这里不必重复上面谈及较多的历史细节，最值得浓墨重彩的还是在那个年代极"左"的政治高压之下，一批曾由"旧协和"培养出来的精英，也是其时中国医学专业化发展的领军人物，冒着被解职、被迫劳动改造和被关押监禁的风险，始终坚持和恪守着医学专业化的最高准则。如 1962 年 4 月，个性温和、慎重的黄家驷院长主持召开关于"老协和医学院教学工作经验初步总结"会议，用当时意识形态最能接受的语言充分肯定了"老协和"的医学专业化对于中国高端医学发展的正面意义。[57]还有教授林巧稚，私下里不时赞颂"'旧协和'的好传统、好经验"。[58]再到最激进批判"旧协和"阴魂不散的"文化大革命"之时，曾作为娄克斯下属同事的协和外科医生曾宪九，虽被戴上有严重"崇美思想"的高帽，却无所畏惧地直言道："我确实认为美国的科学发达，医学技术高超。科学是没有国界的。"[60]1957 年访问中国的《柳叶刀》（The Lancet）的主编福克斯（T. F. Fox）也有类似记述。他说尽管中共大力号召向苏联学习，但中国医学界对欧美更相似。全国十五份医学期刊，或用中文、或用英文，却没有一份是用俄文出版的。福克斯总结出来的原因是《很多资深研究者为海外留学回国之人，在精神上与我们的事业紧密联系在一起。"[61]由此，我们从学者共和国（republic of literati）的世界主义之立场出发，更能理解洛克菲勒二世（John D. Rockefeuer, Jr）于 1951 年 4月写的一封信——他虽为协和被政府接管而深感遗憾，却认为："有谁敢说，这不是上帝的旨意，以这样的方式，达成其创建者最初的目的。尽管这种方式与我们心中所想的完全不同。让我们希望，祈祷并相信：最终一切都能达到最好的（Let us hope, pray and believe that all may be ultimately for the best）。"[62]

参考书目

1. 本文使用了藏于美国洛克菲勒档案馆的《新协和》等档案。

2. 张之强《我的一生》，自印本，出版不详，2006 年，第 200 页。

3. Stephen J. Kunitz，"Professionalism and Social Control in the Progressive Era：The Case of the Flexner Report," *Social Problems*, Vol. 22, No. 1, Oct., 1974, pp. 16 – 27; Toby Gelfand, From Guild to Profession：The Surgeons of France in the 18th Century, *The Humanities and Medicine*, 32 no. 1, Spring 1974, pp. 121 – 34; Jeanne L. Brand, *Doctors and the State：The British Medical Profession and Government Action in Public Health*, *1870 – 1912*, Baltimore, 1965; William G. Rothstein, *American Physicians in the 19th Century：From Sects to Science* Baltimore, 1972.

4. Mary E. Ferguson, *China Medical Board and Peking Union Medical College：A Chronicle of Fruitful Collaboration*, *1914 – 1951*, China Medical Board of New York, Inc.; 1st edition, 1970, p. 192.

5. 中国协和医科大学：《中国协和医科大学校史 1917 – 1987》，北京科学技术出版社，1987 年，第 45 页。

6. 《李宗恩的检查》，《新协和》1952 年 6 月 13 日，思想建议特刊第 14 期，第 1 版。

7. 张之强：《我的一生》，第 209 页。

8. 读者来信：《医务工作者不应该忽视读报》，《人民日报》1952 年 3 月 22 日，第 2 版；中国协和医学院：《协和医学院关于忽视读报工作的检讨》，《人民日报》1952 年 4 月 19 日，第 2 版。

9. 学生会：《美帝文化侵略在协和》，《新协和》创刊号，1951 年 2 月 20 日出版，第 2 - 21 页，China Medical Board，Inc. Box：128，Folder，937，Rockefeller Archive Center，RAC.，Sleepy Hollow，New York，United States.

10. 祝寿嵩：《我的先生》，《新协和》创刊号，1951 年 2 月 20 日出版，第 21 - 22 页，China Medical Board，Inc. Box：128，Folder，937，Rockefeller Archive Center，RAC.，Sleepy Hollow，New York，United States.

11. 范度：《娄克斯——披着绅士学者外衣的帝国主义分子》，中国协和医学院节约检查委员会宣传组编：《新协和》，1952 年 5 月 9 日，《思想建设特刊》第 1 期，第 2 版。

12. 曾宪九：《我认识了娄克斯‘学术活动’的真正目的》，《思想建设特刊》第 13 期，《新协和》第 2 版，中国协和医学院节约检查委员会宣传组编，1952 年 5 月 14 日，第 2 页。

13. 《志愿军病房护士长杨英华控诉，美帝文化侵略使我敌我不分，不爱志愿军》，中国协和医学院节约检查委员会宣传组编：《新协和》1952 年 5 月 24 日，第 18 期，《思想建议特刊》第 13 期。

14. 张之强：《我的回忆》，第 210 页。

15. 林巧稚：《打开"协和"窗户看祖国》，《人民日报》1952 年 9 年 27 日，第 3 版。

16. 林巧稚：《李宗恩，你的问题和我们的不一样》，《思想建设特刊》第 35 期，《新协和》，1952 年 7 月 31 日，第 52 期，第 2 版。

17. 新华社：《从美帝文化侵略堡垒变成人民医疗机构，协和医学院解放后在医疗、教学、研究和建设等方面已经起了根本变化》，《人民日报》1957 年 8 月 20 日，第 4 版；新华社：《两个月的说理斗争，十几次大小辩论会，协和医学院专家教授驳倒李宗恩》，《人民日报》1957 年 10 月 6 日，第 3 版。

18. 张之强：《我的一生》，第 111 页。

19. 张之强：《我的一生》，第 200 - 201 页

20. 新华社《中央人民政府卫生部正式接收北京协和医学院，该院师生员工千人集会欢欣庆祝》《人民日报》1951 年 1 月 21 日，第 1 版；《中国人民的新协和万岁》，《新协和》创刊号，1951 年 2 月 20 日，第 1 页，China Medical Board，Inc. Box：128，Folder，937，Rockefeller Archive Center，RAC.，Sleepy Hollow，New York，United States.

21. 《'新协和'的使命》，《新协和》1951 年 2 月 20 日，创刊号，China Medical Board，Inc. Box：128，Folder，937，China Medical Board，Inc. Box：128，Folder，937，Rockefeller Archive Center，RAC.，Sleepy Hollow，New York，United States.

22. 张之强：《我的一生》，第 219 页。

23. 中国协和医科大学编：《中国协和医科大学校史 1917–1987》第 48 页。

24. 中国协和医科大学编：《中国协和医科大学校史 1917–1987》，北京科学技术出版社，1987 年，第 45 页。

25. 新华社《从美帝文化侵略堡垒变成人民医疗机构，协和医学院解放后在医疗、教学、研究和建设等方面已经起了根本变化》，《人民日报》1957 年 8 月 20 日，第 4 版。

26. 《妇产科加强配合改进操作，缩短手术时间和术后住院日》，《中国医学科学院院报》1958 年 6 月 7 日，第 4 版。

27. 《抗生素系筛选速度提高 215 倍，决定在半年内找到抗癌抗生素》，《中国医学科学院院报》1958 年 7 月 16 日，第 1 版。

28. 《在首次献宝献礼大会上廿个单位报捷并宣布跃进新指标》，《中国医学科学院院报》第 5 号，1958 年 6 月 19 日，第 1 版。

29. 苏芋：《斥"冷冷清清"的爱好者》，《中国医学科学院院报》1959 年 12 月 10 日，第 3 版。

30. 《揭穿科学研究中的资产阶级本质，明确科学必须为生产大跃进服务》，《中国医学科学院院报》1958 年 6 月 4 日，第 2 版。

31. 《学习协和脑系科的革命创举》，《中国医学科学院院报》1958 年 12 月 29 日，第 1 版。

32. 《为游击习气恢复名誉以后——协和脑系科大破资产阶级传统经过》，《中国医学科学院院报》1958 年 12 月 29 日，第 1 版。

33. 郭少军、熊世琦：《大破"权威"和"等级制"协和医院脑系科的全面大跃进》，《人民日报》1958 年 11 月 10 日，第 6 版。

34. 《徐运北副部长在我院全体人员上的报告摘要，卫生工作必须大力改革，坚决贯彻党的总路线》，《中国医学科学院院报》1958 年 6 月 7 日，第 1 版。

35. 《徐运北副部长在我院全体人员上的报告摘要，卫生工作必须大力改革，坚决贯彻党的总路线》，1958 年 6 月 7 日，第 1 版。

36. 《中国医学科学院在总路线的光辉照耀下，砍掉迷信美英的奴隶思想，面向病人，面向实际，敢作敢为》，《人民日报》1958 年 6 月 8 日，第 2 版；《破迷信、插红旗、订规划、搞革新，中国医学科学院壮志凌云、干劲冲天》，《健康报》1958 年 6 月 25 日，第 4 版。

37. 张之强：《我的一生》第 222 页。

38. 张鋆：《帮助党办好医学教育》，《人民日报》1957 年 6 月 4 日，第 7 版。

39. 张孝骞：《恢复医学生教育》，第 69—71 页。

40. 张之强：《我的一生》第 222 页。

41. 张之强：《我的一生》第 224 页。

42. 《黄家驷院长在中国医科大学成立及一九五九年开学典礼大会上的讲话》，《中国医学科学院院报》1959 年 9 月 10 日，第 2 版。

43. 《卫生部李德全部长的指示》，《中国医学科学院院报》1959 年 9 月 10 日，第 3 版。

44. 林钧才：《协和医院成功之路：在北京协和医院八年的回顾》《解放军医院管理杂志》1996 年第 3 期，第 87－89 页。

45. 张鋆：《帮助党办好医学教育》，《人民日报》1957 年 6 月 4 日，第 7 版。

46. 张之强：《我的一生》第 214 页。

47. 吴之理：《一名军医的自述》，华夏出版社，2004 年，第 92 页。

48. 中国协和医科大学编：《中国协和医科大学校史 1917－1987》第 61 页。

49. 林钧才：《协和医院成功之路：在北京协和医院八年的回顾》，《解放军医院管理杂志》1996 年第 3 期，第 87 页。

50. 张之强：《我的一生》第 314 页。

51. 章央芬：《自豪的回忆》华夏出版社，2004 年，第 170 页。

52. 中国协和医科大学编：《中国协和医科大学校史 1917－1987》第 63 页；章央芬：《自豪的回忆》第 168 页。

53. 朱彬：《当大夫之前——中国医科大学六年级教学见闻》，《人民日报》1962 年 6 月 3 日，第 2 版。

54. 熊世琦：《医药工作者的密友——记全国医学中心图书馆》，《人民日报》1961 年 12 月 6 日，第 4 版。

55. 《我院广大革命工人、革命同学、革命干部，热烈响应院党委向资产阶级代表人物，向一切牛鬼蛇神，向一切资产阶级和封建的意识形态猛烈开火》，《中国医学科学院院报》，1966 年 6 月 10 日，第 1 版。

56. John Z. Bowers, *Western medicine in a Chinese palace*：*Peking Union Medical College*，*1917 - 1951*，（The Josiah Macy，Jr. Foundation 1972）；Mary B. Bullock，*an American Transplant*：*The Rockefeller Foundation and Peking Union Medical College*，（University of California Press，1980）；Bridie Andrews and Mary Brown Bullock ed.，*Medical Transitions in Twentieth-Century China*，（Indiana University Press，2014）．

57. 中国协和医科大学编：《中国协和医科大学校史 1917－1987》第 73 页。

58. 章央芬：《自豪的回忆》第 177 页。

59. 中国医科大学红小兵：《从洛克菲勒到中国赫鲁晓夫》，《人民日报》1968 年 2 月 24 日，第 4 版。

60. 钟守先：《忆我的恩师曾宪九教授》，http：//www.pumch.cn/Item/11768.aspx。

61. T. F. Fox, " the New China, Some Medical Impressions", *The Lancet*, Nov. 23, 1957, p. 1057.

62. *China Medical Board and Peking Union Medical College A chronicle of Fruitful Collaboration* (*1914 – 1951*), pp. 227；《美国中华医学基金会和北京协和医学院》，闫海英、蒋育红译，中国协和医科大学出版社，2014 年，第 210 页。

The New PUMC and Its Professionalism（1951 – 1966）

Hu Cheng

Hu Cheng, Ph. D, graduated from History Department of Nanjing University in 1998, now professor of history at Nanjing University. He published a number of books include: "The Original Role of Scholars: traditional scholars, modern change and modern academia" (Social Science Literature Publishing House, 2017), "Medicine, Health And China In The World" (Science Press, 2013), "Modern transformation and Historical reflection" (Beijing Sanlian bookstore, 2013) and others, as well as a number academic papers.

In the summer of 1950, Zhang Zhiqiang（张之强）was admitted to the first-class ward in PUMC Hospital with tuberculosis. At that time, there was a plaque *"the Private Peking Union Medical College"*（私立北京协和医学院）hung on the West Gate, and PUMC had not cut off its ties with the China Medical Board（once affiliated to the Rockefeller Foundation）in the United States. While in the hospital, Zhang Zhiqiang found that PUMC had a higher standard of medical professionalism and better medical conditions than the Central Hospital（中央医院）in Nanking（南京）that he was once hospitalized in during the summer of 1949 when the CCP occupied Nanking. Established by the Nationalist Government in 1929, the Central Hospital was the largest and best equipped public hospital then. However, Zhang was impressed by the PUMC Hospital, where doctors and nurses talked in English, the rigorousness demonstrated in ward rounds and the detailed inquiry about patient's history. Also, he noticed that the wards were very quiet and there were no loud noises and sound of walking. Zhang felt that "It is remarkably different than the Central Hospital"

However, with many ideological grievances in mind, he said, "When I studied in Peking, I heard that the PUMC was a hospital having highest standard of medical services nationwide. But the fact that it was established by American imperialism (美帝) always made me uncomfortable sentimentally. "[1] He had studied in the Department of Education at Peiping Normal University (北平师范大学) in 1936 and went to Yan'an (延安) in 1938 after joining the CCP. Zhang Zhiqiang did not expect that the PUMC hospital would be taken over by the government and that he would be appointed the NO. 1 Party Secretary of the CCP organization of the College. This early remark quoted above was full of mixed emotions and feelings which prophesied a stormy path that PUMC had yet to face.

The medical professionalism of PUMC had its origins in the mid-19th century and early early 20th century when the dynamic development of Professionalism in different specialties such as law, engineering, journalism, or medicine was driven by the continuous development of urbanization and industrialization in Europe and America. [2] As regard to medicine, the medical Professionalism in the advanced countries in Europe and America was more than between the doctors and patients; it also evolved with the competition and struggle of the professional communities and the legislation of the nation state. For example, from 1815 to 1848, France had announced nine initiatives on the reform of medical Professionalism; from 1840 to 1858, the British Parliament had passed eighteen acts about medical Professionalism; and in 1847, the American Medical Association was founded. In contrast, the development of medical Professionalism was introduced into China in a fragmented form under various circumstances by Western medical missionaries, foreign doctors from treaty ports, the Japanese colonial authorities, and hundreds of Chinese students studying in Japan. Therefore, the development among different regions and medical institutions was considerably uneven. On the whole, the PUMC, founded by the Rockefeller Foundation in 1917, was regarded as the representative of the highest standard of medical professionalism in China and possibly in the East Asia. [3] Problems arose after 1950: could PUMC maintain the "old PUMC's" legacy of a high standard of medical professionalism against the backdrop of China's "anti-Americanism" movement and the national health agenda shifted to rural areas and addressing medical shortages?

Rooting Out the Influences of the "the Greatest Bulwark for Cultural Aggression of American Imperialism" and the heated Ideology Reform Movement

The discordance between the "old PUMC" and the CCP surfaced on November 8, 1950. At that time, the PLA had entered North Korea to fight the United Nations troops and the massive propaganda campaign to "Resist U. S. Invasion and Aid Korea" (抗美援朝) was launched nationwide. On that day, the representatives from the Ministry of Health, Ministry of Education and Ministry of PLA Health Administration of the Central Government approached the Director of PUMC, Li Zongen (李宗恩) and the superintended of the PUMC Hospital, Li Kehong (李克鸿) and requested to borrow 250 beds from the hospital in order to set up a new hospital for the sick and wounded of the PLA from the Korea War. However, Li Zongen was very reluctant to this request and declined it with the excuse that the two couldn't make the decision since Dr. Harold H Loucks (1894 – 1982), the representative of China Medical Board in PUMC, had returned to U. S. on June 28th. Later under pressure, they were forced to compromise and agreed to lend the exact number of beds. Then, they attended the meeting of forming the advisory committee on the future development of PUMC held by the government on November 20th. On December 22nd, the committee made a decision that a newly-founded military hospital would cooperate with PUMC to treat the sick and wounded of the PLA from the Korean War together. They made arrangements that the newly established hospital was in charge of organizing the wounded and sick soldiers whereas the

PUMC was in charge of medical care, administration. PUMC Hospital was financially independent, and both parties appointed representatives to form three specific groups in charge of administration, medical care, and finance respectively. [4]

Judging from Li Zongen's act of not exiling overseas during the Second Sino-Japanese War and after Peking was taken over by the CCP in 1949, he did not lack a "patriotic" sentiment. His reluctance was not to oppose China's involvement in the Korean War, but rather to insist on the standard of medical professionalism in PUMC. For Li, why not be aware of the timing and lending out the two hundred and fifty beds generously at the moment? Over a year later in The First Intellectuals Ideological Reform Movement（第一次知识分子思想改造运动，1951 – 1952）, he confessed his three concerns over the matter：firstly, if two hundred and fifty beds were borrowed, the beds in PUMC would be reduced from total three hundred and fifty to one hundred, which couldn't maintain the normal teaching arrangement；secondly, so long as PUMC was regarded as a medical teaching institution by the CCP, it should be fully equipped with medical facilities for teaching while the Government could borrow the beds from other hospitals；thirdly, cooperation with the new hospital must cause "a mess, and it's hard to maintain PUMC's standard". [5] However, despite all these considerations, the CCP saw this reluctance to lend sickbeds as the political disobedience of the "old PUMC" and reluctance to adapt to the new society. Zhang Zhiqiang therefore said, "Some people in PUMC were very reluctant to lend out those two hundred and fifty beds; after much persuasion, they grudgingly agree to." In fact, there had already been frictions between the CCP and the "old PUMC" back in September, 1949, when the first Chinese People's Political Consultative Conference（政治协商会议）was held in Beijing. The CCP approached PUMC and negotiated to borrow the dormitories as the accommodations for political consultative members；however, "there was someone's strong disagreement". [6]

What worried the CCP more was the fact that although they had taken over PUMC since January 20th, 1951, and started a huge propaganda campaign claiming the beginning of a "new PUMC", there were still many people who indulged obsessively in the medical professional standards of the "old PUMC". On March 22nd and April 19th, 1950, *the People's Daily* (《人民日报》) published respectively two articles – the "Readers' Letters" and the "Self Criticism of PUMC", alleging that many people in PUMC didn't read the Party's newspaper and were indifferent to the government's call for resisting the U. S. invasion and aiding Korea, Increasing Production and Lowering waste, and the "Three Anti Movement" ("三反运动", 1951 – 1952). The article cited the statistic that about half of the three hundred people or more (including professors, doctors, nurses and assistants) hardly read any newspapers. The PUMC library which boasted its largest collection of resources didn't even subscribe to the *People's Daily*. The reason was that some professors and doctors were too busy with academic research or ward-rounds to care about what happened outside. Several professors even thought that joining political study groups was annoying and troublesome. What made the authors of the readers' letters even more angry was that, "last semester, when students asked to allocate some time to study politics, the professors refused their requests and said there was not a single minute designated to study politics in the class schedule."[7]

In reply to these criticism, the Party Committee of PUMC came up with the slogan "transforming the Old PUMC, building the New PUMC" (改造旧协和，建设新协和) and mobilized the faculty and students with a great fanfare to join the campaign of "thoroughly eliminating the influences of the cultural aggression of the American imperialism". The first cohort to respond was the progressive young students who had no close tie to the "old PUMC". They wrote articles criticizing that among the three hundred and twenty graduates from the "Old PUMC", none of them went to the Liberated Area occupied by the CCP while 73 percent stayed in the cities of the Kuomintang (KMT) and 14 percent went abroad. From the progressive students' perspective, the fundamental reason of the phenomenon was the superior living and working conditions of "Old PUMC" offered to them. The article pointed out that before the outbreak of the Sino-Japanese War, the meal cost of each student of PUMC amounted to sixty silver dollars a month. There were milk, eggs, fruits for breakfast, and refreshment at four or five o'clock in the afternoon. During the meal, each table was seated five or six people with four courses and a soup. Even if there was only one person at the table, the courses were still the same. Students could ask for more if they finished their favorite dishes till they had enough of it. After the meal, they could have some ice-cream. There was a bell on each table that could ring for the servant and a so-called "table boy" for every four tables, who was responsible for filling students' bowls. Once a student finished a course and tapped the plate, the table boy would come to refill. The graduates trained from the college wore suits and had lived far better than the living standards of the majority of the Chinese people, and indulged deeply in hedonism. The article concluded in the end, "As a consequence, these people were content with this "reality" introduced from overseas, and preferred not to think about any issue of the Chinese revolution. "[8]

Besides, the CCP PUMC Committee further exposed those "imperialists in the guise of gentlemen and scholars". Their criticism centered on Dr. Harold H. Loucks, who was the last representative of the CMB in China. The initial propaganda was not working well, because Loucks had served as the head of the Department Surgical of for years and was very dedicated to PUMC for twenty years, winning him relatively high academic reputation and popularity. For example, just before he went back to the US in June 1950, the College held a farewell party for him. In his acknowledgment speech, he said that most unforgettable during his stay in China for decades was the students' admiration and friendship, which "was the Chinese students' special endowment". His speech showed so much affection with an amiable and gentle tone that many students present "were deeply touched and had tears in their eyes". Many students were even critical of the Student Union for only writing a simple letter of congratulation and being too indifferent to Loucks. In defense of these behaviors, the president of the Student Union called Loucks an imperialist. However, most students didn't agree with him, instead saying that PUMC had nothing to do with the cultural aggression of imperialism. Even when the College mounted the study campaign to further the elimination of the influences of American cultural imperialism in February 1951, there were still students who didn't think of Loucks as an imperialist and believed that " attitudes they held were scientific and objective". [9]

The more severe criticism was yet to come. On November 30th, 1951, CCP Central Committee issued *Instructions on the Ideology Reform and the Rectification of the Organization in Schools*, ordering to eliminate the "Three Americanism" (三美主义), including worship-America (崇美), pro-America (亲美), or fear-America (恐美) more thoroughly; Loucks was thus characterized as a crafty imperialist without any doubts. In May 1952, a critical paper published in *New PUMC* (《新协和》) mentioned that this man pretended to be a "gentleman" and "scholar" in daily life, never speaking ill of others to their faces. His disguise made many surgeons show a favorable view of him without expecting him to be the one that held the real power of PUMC. The American policy of cultural aggression was implemented through him. The paper revealed his typical likelihood of giving petty presents and favors to people. For example, he gave ties as presents to the interns and twenty dollars to the newly married chief resident as wedding gifts. He also often invited groups of surgeons to have meals in his home and propagated American lifestyles and democracy. After 1949, in order to win over Chinese trust, he pretended to sympathize with the CCP, saying that he was accused of being a "communism sympathizer" by Americans because of his statements favoring new China after he was back to America. Certainly, the paper couldn't do without criticizing the medical professional standards of the "old PUMC" which Loucks highly recommended. For instance, he always asked the doctors to write articles on their experiences and ideas, submitting them to be published in American journals. In the winter of 1949, when he knew that the CCP would borrow some students of PUMC to help with the epidemic prevention, he said with great anger that this would disrupt the teaching plans of PUMC. [10]

This campaign ran in the way of so-called "everyone has to wash him or herself inside out and passes the test one by one" ("人人洗澡，个个过关") which means to self examine one's ideology. The college carried the self-examination in three levels , each analogous to three sizes of bathtubs – "large" (大盆 refers to self examinations at the institutional level), "medium" (中盆 refers to departments level), or "small" (小盆 refers to groups level) . Everyone who was close to Loucks was naturally pushed to take a stand. Surgeon Zeng Xianjiu (曾宪九 Tseng Hsien-chiu , 1914 – 1985) entered PUMC in 1935 and graduated in 1940, who had long been Loucks' subordinate, wrote to reflect on his unwariness to Loucks' "scholarly concerns" . He admitted that Loucks wrote three letters to him from America. The letters were about two articles Zeng wrote and asked Loucks for suggestions. After Loucks was back to America, he mentioned in the first letter that he was making revision to the papers, while he offered some suggestions on revision in the second letter. Knowing that he couldn't come back to China anymore, Loucks wrote the third letter, telling Zeng that he would help him publish the two articles and although he couldn't write to him anymore, he still would like to keep in touch academically with Zeng and other colleagues in the Surgical Department, hoping to "continue the traditions of integrity and curiosity of the Surgical Dpartment of PUMC" . Loucks also said in this letter, "the Far East is clouded by the international distrust, but I believe people will live in peace one day and seek after truth and science together. " He said, "no matter when and where, my heart is always with the Surgical Department. " Thus, Tseng said in his incisive self-criticism, "I was deeply moved by this letter, thinking that Loucks was so caring and kind to our surgical colleagues that he must be against the wars. I felt a shame that he couldn't come back to PUMC. " [11]

Those who were not so close to Loucks also needed to examine themselves and talked about how they were profoundly affected by the medical professionalism of Old PUMC. On the night of May 12th, 1951, the Departments of Gynecology and Obstetrics, pediatrics, public health and ophthalmology held a joint meeting of accusation. A young doctor in the Department of Gynecology and Obstetrics reflected that after receiving a letter from the World Health Organization requesting to do a survey on the height and the weight of Chinese newborns, she took this assignment without any hesitation, even being willing to work for extra hours. The self-criticism mentioned that all participants in this assignment were proud of themselves and thanked foreign friends for valuing the work; on the contrary, "when our government asked us to take some time to treat cadres of the PLA troops from the Korean War, we exerted all efforts to refuse, supposing that CCP made an invasion upon us. If failed to refuse, we accepted it with great reluctance. For American imperialism, we work overtime to meet the deadline; however, for the Chinese soldiers in this War who shed their blood for us, we only made a perfunctory effort or shifted our responsibilities. " Another self-confession, which was written by a head nurse from this PLA's ward and was published in the same issue of the journal, touched on the essence of the medical professionalism in the "old PUMC" which was the unwillingness to accept the government's takeover of PUMC considering the takeover as the ruin of their future. In this self-criticism, the Head nurse said when she was transferred to this ward, she didn't quite understand at first why they fought a war against Americans who had been very kind to PUMC, and worried about the potential disaster of the war with the US. What's more, she was very resistant to the order of being transferred to this ward after finding that these wounded soldiers in PUMC came here to recuperate. This kind of work there couldn't help her to improve her medical techniques. She then went to the Medical Department and asked to be transferred to other wards. After being rejected, she "burst out crying at home and accepted her 'bad luck'" .[12]

The paper *"Open the Window of "PUMC" to See Our Motherland,"* written by PUMC senior professor Lin Qiaozhi (林巧稚, Lim Kha-t'i) published in *the People's Daily* on September 27th, 1952, marked the great success in the campaign of ideology reform. The Party secretary Zhang Zhiqiang's comment on this paper was "being able to represent the higher intellectual Staff of PUMC". [13] Indeed, in this article, Lin concentrated her criticism on the so-called "PUMC standard". At the beginning of this article, she looked back upon the years she left home regardless of all difficulties because of her admiration for the "international standard" of "PUMC". She was very proud of herself when she was admitted to PUMC. She said, it was a big deal for a female student to go to PUMC in Beijing from Xiamen (厦门) thirty years ago. While studying in PUMC, she never read Chinese books or wrote in Chinese. In 1929, upon graduation, she stayed at PUMC teaching. The "PUMC" system, plus the thoughts of seeking for fame and promotion, naturally drove her to a path arranged by the American imperialists, worshiping the America's academics and admiring its "democracy", and judging China by American standards in all respects. Certainly, Lin expressed her gratitude at the end of the article, saying that this campaign of ideology reform woke her up, "making me determined to abandon the 'PUMC standards' that I clung to for years, opening up the window that had closed for over thirty years, looking out and 'singing our beloved motherland, rising toward rejuvenation...'" [14]

Similar to every political movement, in which there are the progressives, there will simultaneously be the non-progressives, the laggards or even the reactionary. Li Zongen, the Director of PUMC at that time, was considered to be stubborn and insensitively adhering strictly to the "PUMC standard" (协和标准) and needed "a bath in the large bathtub" – institutional conference to pass the test. Some activists in the ideology reform criticized Li for his emphasis on "just trying to maintain the 'PUMC standard' and the programs without any political intention", saying that he just said so to muddle through. However, Li argued that he was not unwilling to collaborate with the government; he was actually having a sense of ownership and being responsible for the country. He claimed that as an expert on medical educator with experiences, he thought the high "PUMC standard" was beneficial to the country. However, the progressives poured in lots of questions. For example, before and after the first Chinese People's Political Consultative Conference, Li Zongen often corresponded with Americans and reported the content of the conference to the American imperialists. They asked him, "is it necessary to constantly report to the American imperialists about the Conference just for the maintenance of the standard of such a small institution like PUMC?" [15] Fortunately, in this movement, except for those proven active reactionaries, even those who had serious ideological problems just had to made a confession in the meetings and this was done without any political punishment. However, from then on, even though Li Zongen still served as the director, he was severely marginalized. In the "Anti-Rightist" (反右) movement in 1957, he was regarded as a notorious Far Rightist (大右派) and was the key target of castigation. *The People's Daily* issued an article, saying that from August to October, after "a dozen debate meetings big or small for two months, experts and professors in PUMC confuted Li Zongen". One evidence of his guilt was his written comment, "the performance of PUMC has declined...The damage to PUMC in the past few years must take time to fix in order to resume its dynamics." The castigating article said this was a proof of his ulterior motives – claiming that the current standard of medical professionalism was "inferior to the previous time," aiming to preserve a semi-colonial and enslaving medical education system in an organized, systematic and programmed way, which served the cultural aggression of the American imperialists. [16]

Making the "New PUMC" Better Than the "Old PUMC"

Making the "new PUMC" better than the "old PUMC" were the key words in the political propaganda of that era, which were shouted out loudest. On January 20th, 1951, PUMC was formally declared nationalized and over a thousand students, faculty members, and staffs attended the celebration. The leaders of the Ministry of Health who were present at the meeting announced government regulations and orders related to the takeover of American sponsored cultural and educational institutions, the relief agencies, and religious organizations; declaring that all faculty and staffs would retain their positions of the college with their original salaries, which was twice as much as the salaries in Peking University（北京大学）or Tsinghua University（清华大学）at that time, and the old teaching program would be maintained. Leaders of the Ministry of Education, and of the Administration of Health of the PLA present claimed with great confidence that Chinese people had the ability and confidence to make a better PUMC after rooting out of the influences of American imperialist's aggression. Then, representatives of PUMC leaders, labor union, and student union expressed that they firmly supported the decision of the CCP, saying that they believed "PUMC which belongs to the Chinese people has an extremely promising future. "[17] A month later, the newly founded journal, *New PUMC*（《新协和》）published an editorial and said they would try best to enrich the content by collecting opinions and reports from the whole institution and in all respects. In addition to thoroughly eliminating the influences of the cultural aggression of the American imperialists, other goals included "correcting our attitudes toward services by turning the education and medical work towards workers, peasants, and soldiers, which was the right mission of the 'new PUMC'!"[18]

Rather than being a political opponent intending to sabotage the CCP, Li Zongen was just too obsessed with the standards of medical professionalism of the "old PUMC" and refused to make concessions. Years later Zhang Zhiqiang, who led this movement in PUMC in those days, felt compunction and was full of remorse for what happened after Li was labeled as a Far Rightist and died in a remote area not long thereafter. Years later, when Zhang reflected upon the ulterior reason why CCP carried out the political purging reform, he referred to Chairman Mao's saying that " intellectuals casted to be workers and peasants, while workers and peasants intellectualized " and said this saying had its connotation. [19]

In view of this, one of the important reasons that Li was purged politically was that he couldn't keep pace with the era and thought the "new PUMC" after the Liberation was not as good as the "old PUMC" when it was run by the Americans, which was the weakest part of the new regime and last thing to be attacked upon. In addition, as early as in the spring of 1951, Zhang felt very worried and panic of knowing that he was appointed as the military representative to take over PUMC. His anxiety arose from the responsibilities or heavy burdens of knowing that PUMC was an internationally recognized medical school. The top leaders of the CCP had already said that this takeover was an important event concerning the national reputation, "If it is not done right, the American imperialists and other anti-China forces would seize the chance to cry out loud the anti-China sentiment". [20]

However, the "new PUMC" had problem in its professionalism at the beginning of its nationalized stage. In January 1952, PUMC was under the leadership of the PLA, with its top priority of meeting the needs of national defense health development – that was to say, basic research was subordinated to clinical treatments, while clinical treatments were subordinated to real life needs. Then, a large number of backbone professionals, including seventeen professors and twenty attending physicians, were transferred from the clinical and basic medical departments of PUMC to establish The General Hospital of the PLA; the transfer weakened the education and scientific research of PUMC. [21] From 1952 to 1956, almost half of the inpatients, outpatients visits, and emergency room visits of PUMC were military cadres. [22] In the spring of 1953, PUMC stopped enrolling new students and started to become the training college of medical care cadres. In order to meet the medical needs all over the country, PUMC held various training courses for people with different levels of basic medical knowledge and who came from different posts across the country. For example, in order to implement the resolution of putting major effort in prevention proposed in the First National Health Conference in August 1950, the number of trainees in public health nurses training program increased 4 – 5 times in face of the urgent needs for public health nurses. According to data resources, "Because of the lack of teachers, even public health nurses acted as instructors for practice."[23] In August 1957, in order to refute Li Zongen's claim that the "new PUMC" after the Liberation "was not as good as the 'old PUMC' when it was run by the Americans", *the People's Daily* briefly cited the data that during the twenty-two years of the "old PUMC", they only had produced 310 graduates; whereas the "new PUMC" after the Liberation had trained 937 medical cadres and 245 medical graduates by advanced training and short-term training courses, accepting graduate trainees from 120 medical departments all over the nation.[24]

PUMC was put under the leadership of the Minister of Health again in 1956 and was involved in the "Great Leap Forward"（大跃进）that aimed at outpacing the UK and catching up the US. At the time, the slogan of providing medical treatment and conducting scientific research in a "more, faster, better, and economical"（多快好省）manner pitched high to the sky. Surgeons in the Department of Gynecology and Obstetrics which was the role model department and was lauded a lot at PUMC used to do a simple total hysterectomy in two hours and a half on average, now shortened the time of doing a subtotal hysterectomy to one hour and a half. The faster surgeons could even do a subtotal hysterectomy in one hour and fifteen minutes. The tubal ligation, which used to be performed between six hours to twenty hours after delivery, now was improved and was given between two to three hours after delivery. The surgeons changed the method of closing the incision from silk suture to cat gut suture, which made it possible for patients to leave hospital three days earlier instead of waiting five days to take out the stitches. They had tried the method in three cases and had good outcome.[25] What was more inspiring was that some activists proposed to "conquer cancer in five years". Activists in the department of antibiotics made their work of screening effective drugs two hundred and fifteen times faster, and "decided to find anticancer antibiotic in half a year" .[26] Their words made Zhang Zhiqiang so excited that he said in a summing-up meeting that in PUMC an earth shaking change had taken place and one day today passed for twenty years in the past; he emphasized that " the American standards that kept 30 years in PUMC was washed away overnight" .[27]

At that time, the reason why the leaders made great effort emphasizing the eradication of the old PUMC and establishment of the new one was that the professional influences of the "old PUMC" was deep-rooted at PUMC. Those "obstinate" people who strictly clung to the standards of medical professionalism of the "old PUMC" always spoke ill of and made sarcastic remarks against the nationwide "Great Leap Forward" . An article then castigated: those people said that the "old PUMC" was quiet but the academic achievements it made were of international level, just wanted to "imply that today's PUMC was louder and more visible but achieved nothing" .[28] To fight against this statement, the paper said the "new PUMC" carried forward the glorious traditions which was that the revolutionary army established the hospital years ago – the tradition that was derogated by the "old PUMC" as "guerrilla habits" ("游击习气") and "rural styles" ("农村作风") . For example, the "old PUMC" advocated running the school with world standards, believed that scientific research must know the international progress, investigate and follow up the international papers in the English language world, and that the research findings must be recognized by foreigners. However, in early May of the same year, the Party committee of the College held a four-week strategy-discussing meeting, mobilizing all PUMC people to discuss the "old PUMC" / "new PUMC" in scientific research. In the College's debate conference held on May 29th, when the Party leader talked about the "international level" in scientific studies, they said firmly "the 'international level' that we emphasized here referred to the one that would solve practical problems for people's production; whereas the

one that filled the blanks in the British and American literature...was actually
the issue of political side that people take and must be thoroughly castigated. "[29]
The tone of the words in another article published later was even audacious,
saying, "we should not care about foreigners' recognition. It does not matter as
long as the six hundred million people acknowledge it. "[30]

Another thing that couldn't fit into the ideology of that age was the strict
hierarchy in medical care in "old PUMC". An article raised criticism that with
multiple academic layers and distinct boundaries, people in PUMC upheld the
tradition of never crossing the hierarchical line. Orders from senior doctors were
so undisputable that junior doctors couldn't raise any objections even if they
found the orders were wrong. The tradition resulted in a phenomenon that the
higher the rank of the doctors is, the more they cut themselves off from the
patients. Those who were fortunate to be promoted to full Professors were aloof
high above from the masses and reality, indulging themselves in "abstruse
theories" and personal interests. However, inexperienced junior doctors only
could meet with the patients and were not qualified to do research. The article
said, "Sometimes, when senior doctors made the rounds of the wards, they
simply used the foreign literature mechanically to the actual case of the
patients. They even put on airs of an authority and scolded junior doctors for no
reason, making junior doctors "as mute as fish. "[31] At that moment, the
example was Division of Neurology with its overall great leap forward in breaking
away with the "authority" and "hierarchy". Since the beginning of October,
all senior doctors in this division were transferred down to out-patient department
and wards, doing research based on reality and services for patients. In order to
make doctors concentrate on the treatment, nurses undertook some of doctors'
conventional treatment such as injection, blood transfusion, infusion, or
puncture. Likewise, doctors used every chance to do nursing work. In the
mealtime, it was not only nurses but also doctors who fed patients. Moreover,
the Party firmly pushed forward technical democracy. In the medical procedures,
the specialists were not the only ones to make decisions; the youths could offer

new treatment methods and constructive suggestions in the group discussions as well. Some senior professors "got used to saying 'the older, the wiser' to scold the youths in the past, but now people no longer hear words like this."[32]

Another warm and touching improvement was the new doctor-patient relationship that the "new PUMC" advocated, which was "serving the people heart and soul, making the hospital more like home, and making patients feel familiar and warm."[33] In people's eyes, the "old PUMC" was cold, grim and majestic like an authority court (Yamen 衙门), inaccessible to the majority of the people. At that time, many hospitals instituted a three-shift outpatient system; some even had 24 hours outpatient service and outpatient service on Sundays, and almost eliminated the lining up of registration at hospitals. The aim of instituting the system was to help workers and clergies to see the doctors in their after-hours, without delaying their work and productions. The affiliated hospital of Tianjin Medical College and the six affiliated hospitals of Shanghai First Medical College also had simple sickbeds practice that only charged 0.12 yuan, in which needed patients bring their own food and clothes, greatly alleviating patients' economic burden. In contrast, many doctors in PUMC didn't want to treat the working classes, thinking that they were stupid, dirty, and could not articulate themselves succinctly. The wage for a skilled worker was no more than 40 yuan a month at that time; however, for an outpatient visit at PUMC, they spent 1.8 yuan for registration and drugs on average; and hospitalization for one day charged for an average of 7.19 yuan. Many people said they were cured, but with tears in the eyes when they left PUMC – healthy but broke. Certainly, what dissatisfied the people most was they had to wait about half a month after registering.[34] This would be an important medical measure to benefit the people, so PUMC formally opened the twenty-four-hour clinic at the night of June 3rd that year; chiefs of the departments and professors showed up there. Simple sickbeds also were ready overnight to take in patients the next day. The news reports said, "cancer patients who came to Beijing at the night didn't have to wait until the next day to see the doctors in cancer hospital. A patient came from Hunan（湖南）to Beijing was overjoyed when he saw the PUMC doctor on April 1st – the day he arrived in Beijing, which was unexpected for him because he heard of the difficulties of seeing doctors at PUMC. ”[35]

“The Party's Leadership Plus the Old PUMC” – the 8-year Curriculum Medical School Resumed

Although the "old PUMC" became a sensitive subject in politics and even lifted to ideological matters, the voice of resuming its medical professionalism lingered on. Zhang Zhiqiang wrote in his memoirs, "After PUMC was put under the leadership of the Central Ministry of Health, most of its specialties and professors hoped to resume the old traditions of PUMC so as to bear the responsibilities of training professionals in high level medical education, clinical medicine, and scientific research. Despite the strong desire and willing from PUMC people, no one wanted to or dared to speak it out loud under the pressure of the political climate at that time. They only revealed the signs of their thoughts in their daily conversations, mentioning that specialties and professors in PUMC 'were more experienced'. ”[36] However, in January 1956, the CCP held a conference on the issue of the intellectuals, correcting the deviation of solely emphasizing the ideology reform of the intellectuals, pointing out that most intellectuals had already been part of the working class. Mao Zedong gave a speech in the last day of the conference, calling on the whole Party to study science and unite the non-Party member intellectuals and to strive to catch up with the advanced world levels. Then inspired by the slogan of "Advancing Toward Science"（向科学进军）, the political tension was eased until "the Anti-Rightist" movement began in July 1957. In this period, intellectuals and scholars started to have the courage to speak their minds freely and make suggestions without many political worries.

An article published in *the People's Daily* in July 1957 by professor Zhang

Jun（张鋆 1890 – 1977），the chief of the Department of Anatomy of PUMC, was the first one who spoke out publicly for the "old PUMC" since 1950. In the article, he cried out that the traditions of medical professionalism of the "old PUMC" should not be abandoned, and said straightforwardly in the article, "I think the old PUMC had some experience in cultivating top medical professionals and attached great importance to the training in basic science, clinical practicum, and working in labs. Thus, the graduates from PUMC had played a role in their medical work. In academic research, they also reached the world level in some aspects". [37] At the same time, another established PUMC professor Zhang Xiaoqian（张孝骞, Chang Hsiao-ch'ien 1897 – 1987），the chief of the Department of Internal Medicine, also submitted a written statement to the top leaders of the Party, suggesting to resume the eight-year medical education program. In his opinion, medical science, as an applied science, needed extremely solid theoretical basis. Therefore, the training of medical talents was difficult and complex. In higher education, medical science should be the one with the longest length of schooling and involving the greatest number of subjects – comprehensive training of natural sciences. He made a frank criticism, saying that because of the urgent needs of our country, the medical education after the foundation of new China had no choice but focused on increasing the number of the students; thus shortening years of study in sacrificing of the quality. The length of the school year at the time in the medical school followed the Soviet Union's five-year model, with extremely limited premed courses. "Because of the excessive number of students, the teachers, equipment, and sickbeds were all insufficient and the teaching was not good." [38]

Compared with Zhang Jun, who only had great influence in teaching, it was much easier for Zhang Xiaoqian to submit his statement to the top leaders and he was able to produce real effects since he was responsible for the medical care of the top leaders of the CCP. In the previous preparation tasks for the setting up of Chinese Academy of Medical Science（CAMS, 中国医学科学院），some who had worked at old PUMC for a long time proposed to resume the old medical school; but the proposal was not considered by the CCP under the leadership of Zhang Zhiqiang. The reason was because this was a sensitive subject in politics and involved complex interpersonal connections in all respects of the Academy. Some leaders in the original Central Health Laboratory Research Institute (中央卫生实验研究院) were discontent with the dominance of PUMC's influences. They opposed at the meeting of the Party committee, saying that "PUMC is in the same palace but the people there are no longer the same. "[39] However, things turned around in the spring of 1959, when Lu Dingyi (陆定一, 1906 - 1996), the minister of the Central Propaganda Department (中共中央宣传部) and vice-premier of the State Council (国务院副总理) who was responsible for higher education, was sick and admitted to PUMC Hospital. One day, he called Zhang Zhiqiang to his ward. He told Zhang that some PUMC professors came to him and expressed their desire to resume the PUMC and asked his opinion. With abundant political experiences, Zhang figured out the implied preference in leader Lu Dingyi's words. He wrote in his book, "at that time, Lu Dingyi seemed to have already agreed to resume the PUMC personally, and was going to discuss it with leaders in relevant departments. He said that I could reveal some details inside the Party Committee of the CAMS and listen to what people say about it. "[40]

In September 1959, the resumed eight-year medical school started the new semester as scheduled. But even at that moment, the "old PUMC" was still a subject people ought to stay away from. On September 5th, in the opening ceremony of China Medical University held in the auditorium of Chinese Academy of Medical Science at Dong Dan San Tiao, only Huang Jiasi (黄家驷, Huang Chia-ssu 1906 - 1984), a graduate of Class 1924 and then President of this College in 1958, did not derogate the "old PUMC" in his speech made in front of audience, including 29 transferred students, 50 new students, and the leaders of Beijing Municipal government and Ministry of Health. Instead, he praised that, "many of our old professors had accumulated rich teaching experiences in the eight-year-program of PUMC. "[41] The speaker giving closing remark at the ceremony was Li Dequan（李德全, 1896—1972）, the Minister of Ministry of Health. When talking about the suspicions of the resurgence of the "old PUMC", she categorically said, "No doubt, we will never go back to the old PUMC's capitalist road". Then she mentioned in the speech that the name "China Medical University"（中国医科大学） – eight-year medical school had certain revolutionary meaning. At the beginning of the preparatory stage, Chinese Academy of Medical Science originally decided a tentative name- "People's Medical School"（人民医学院） and changed to "China Medical University" later. This name was created by the CCP in Yan'an during the period of Sino-Japanese War, and continued to be used by the later Shenyang Medical School before 1956. Minister Li said: By using this name with glorious revolutionary tradition, we hope this newly founded eight-year medical school can carry forward those traditions of medical education in the old liberated areas（Yan'an）, which was hardworking and plain-living, being close to the masses, combining education with productive labor and health care of the masses. [42]

Without standards and clear directions, the system could not be established. Initially, the medical and teaching arrangements this newly founded eight-year medical college was in utter chaos. In medical care, Lin Juncai（林钧才, 1920 – 2015）was transferred from Nanjing to PUMC as the president and the Party secretary of the hospital in 1960. Upon assuming the posts, he saw that the basic medical care in PUMC Hospital was disrupted and had not resumed yet. More specifically, with excessive, complicated and long-term tasks, the hospital was in a state of chaos and staffs worked inefficiently with frequent changes of positions. The hospital sacrificed quality for quantity. In addition, the quality of medical care was degraded and malpractice increased; the relationship among clinical practices, teaching, and research was imbalanced; senior intellectuals were low-spirited and overcautious, while young intellectuals were afraid of taking the road of "being a capitalistic expert". Lin wrote "the general image of the PUMC Hospital at that time was 'busy, disordered, and dirty'". [43,44]

Facing the problems, Huang Jiasi, who was responsible for education, was very anxious. He proposed to build a team of full-time faculty in accordance with the medical standards of the "old PUMC". In November 1961, Zhang Yangfen (章央芬, 1914 – 2011), the then vice-president of Shanghai Second Medical College, was transferred to serve as the dean and member of the standing committee of the Party of PUMC, taking charge of education. According to professor Zhang Jun, since PUMC was taken over by the CCP and put under the jurisdiction of the Army in January 1951, "many comrades from the army whose living habits were very different from us came here; we didn't have many heart-to-heart talks, and although there was no conflict, we still didn't get along very well." [45] Another evidence of the situation was from Zhang Zhiqiang's memoir. It was said in the mobilization conference of "advancing toward science" in 1957, when he asked the cadres of the CCP to do a better job in the logistical work and serve the scientific workers, many cadres from troops showed dissatisfaction. They said, "When I was in the army and attacked Beijing city, all you scientific workers still served for the aggression of the American imperialists." [46] Unlike them, although Zhang Yangfen joined the New Fourth Army (新四军) in 1938, she grew up in the city of the south and graduated from Shanghai Medical College (上海医学院 six-year-program). A more specific case that could be used as a reference was from the memory of her husband – a doctor in the field hospital of the same army: Even in the hardships of wartime, she still bathed her children every day and did not allow strangers to hug her children. Some people said she was too finicky. However, after the commander of this army heard about the remarks, he said, "Doctor Zhang was a college graduate who came to the enemy's rear area to fight. That's the manifestation of patriotism. She respects science and cares for hygiene, she doesn't want her children to be infected with diseases. You shouldn't be judgmental about her." [47]

Luckily, the "Great Leap Forward" was over. Being more prudent and sober, some pragmatic top leaders of the CCP no longer avoided mentioning the positive side of the medical professionalism of the "old PUMC". On May 6, 1959, Lu Dingyi made a speech in the Party convention held by Chinese Academy of Medical Science. He said, "all leaders from the Propaganda Department of the Central Committee and Ministry of Health agreed that PUMC had developed a cohort of competent and well-trained talents with a set of medical education experience over years. As long as it is under the leadership of CCP, we could run the institution in the way of old PUMC."[48] Judging from the published materials available, Lu Dingyi, and the Propaganda Department and Ministry of Health made such speeches; so did higher level leaders. The above mentioned Lin Juncai, who was transferred to PUMC to lead the hospital, also received the instruction from premier Zhou Enlai (周恩来) through the vice minister of the Ministry of Health when he reported to duty there in December, 1960. The instruction said, "PUMC was famous across Asia and the world; we must do a good job running the school, if not, the influence will be unfavorable".[49] In Zhang Zhiqiang's memoir, he also wrote: In 1960, Zhou Enlai used to ask about the situation and difficulties of resuming the old PUMC. He said that PUMC was a prestigious university with influences in medical field of the whole world. The resuming of PUMC couldn't just simply focus on the professional and technical aspects. There was also instruction from Deng Xiaoping (邓小平) much beforehand, saying we must run PUMC well, develop it, and maintain its traditions. He also sent special investigators to PUMC for surveys. Moreover, Peng Zhen (彭真) made it more clear in a speech, "China-Soviet Friendship Hospital runs in a soviet way; PUMC runs in an old PUMC way. For example, the rules and regulations follow the old PUMC way, so do the clothing styles of doctors, nurses, and staffs. Is there anything inappropriate?"[50]

From the end of 1961 to the beginning of 1962, the policy of "the leadership of the Party plus the old PUMC" ("党的领导加旧协和") raised by Lu Dingyi had taken deep root in this eight-year curriculum medical college. In her first day in PUMC, Dean Zhang Yangfen immediately felt the strong prevailing atmosphere of carrying forward the traditions of medical professionalism of old PUMC. She wrote: Huang Jiasi, designated by the standing committee of the Party PUMC in charge of the College and concurrently as President of the PUMC, and Zhang Chaifen (张茝芳), the director of the teaching department, were all top students graduated from the "old PUMC" and stood firm on running the school based on experiences of "old PUMC". As an example, the interior design of the teaching building, including classrooms, laboratories, test beds, dormitories, and dining rooms, was done following the standards of the old PUMC and now on the basis of 120 per grade. All professors he appointed as chiefs of the teaching and research departments were graduates from the old PUMC or long-standing professors who had worked at the old PUMC for many years. They could all apply their good teaching experiences gained in the old PUMC consciously. " Whenever slight deviation, if any, occurred, President Huang and Director Zhang would give their opinions and said, 'this is not as strict as the old PUMC; that is not as detailed as the old PUMC's standards.' I admired their spirits. "[51] Of course, the most remarkably astonishing step was the workshop held in February 1962, upon the advice of Huang Jiasi and Zhang Yangfen, with the permission of the Ministry of Health. It gathered specialties and professors who graduated from the old PUMC, in the name of the Party committee of Chinese Academy of Medical Science. After seven days of repeated discussions, the historical achievement of the workshop was made – the creation of the final draft of *the Preliminary Summary of the Teaching Experience of Old PUMC*. It was written by Zhang Chaifen , revised by Huang Jiasi, and resolved after the discussion within the Party committee.[52]

This summary was put into effect. Since its establishment in 1921, PUMC followed the Johns Hopkins model and established its education tradition of "small class, individualization, and mentorship" . All students able to be enrolled in PUMC were trained under the "mentorship system". In September 1961, twenty students in six grades, who were the first cohort to study under the "mentorship system" after the founding of new China, went to PUMC hospital for clinical rotation. Using the method of clinic round visits and demonstration inherited from the Old PUMC, professors guided the students in the examination of the individual patients and discussed with students about the patients. Professors would ask questions at any time, enlighten students to think and guide the discussions of the occurrence, development, diagnosis, treatment, prevention, and prognosis of certain disease. Take the writing of the medical record as an example, it was regarded as one of the old PUMC's "three treasures" （三宝）. One of the students wrote a very simple medical record at first. Her mentor gave her some medical records written in the past after seeing her writing and asked her to read it carefully. This student found that this old medical record of PUMC not only recorded all the diseases the patient had from his birth to adulthood, from his marriage to the birth of his child, but also recorded the details of the occurrence, development, and treatment of those diseases. This professor inculcated the student, "one of the diagnostic secrets of a good clinician is asking in details about a patient's condition, carefully performing a physical examination, and writing the medical record seriously."[53] In addition, another visible change was that the number of books borrowed by researchers in PUMC library increased month by month. A report said, the library of PUMC lent out over 130 books on average per day in September 1961, and over 160 in October; books and magazines available on the shelves (returned ones) were around 460, 610, and 890 on average per day in August, September, and October respectively. This change was due to the fact that the PUMC party committee promised to guarantee five working day a week to be spent on medical care, teaching, and scientific studies, hoping to create a good environment for them to focus on their specialties without any interruption. Consequently, they "went to library as soon as they were free, equipped themselves with the latest development and achievement of medicine at home and abroad".[54]

Conclusion

In June 1966, the "Great Proletarian Cultural Revolution" ("无产阶级文化大革命") broke out; the principle of "the leadership of the party plus the old PUMC", for the purpose of "adjustment, consolidation, enrichment, and improvement" ("调整、巩固、充实、提高") after the "Great Leap Forward", was then labeled as the revisionist's path for education and castigated. Needless to list the abundant castigating papers here, the prevailing clamor was to denounce the bourgeois "specialists", "scholars", "masters" and "capitalist roaders in power in the CCP", as well as those who attempted to resume the education program of the old PUMC and train successors of capitalists". [55] Without doubt, that frenzy and insane age was only a snap of the fingers in the one-hundred-years history of PUMC. Subsequently, after the "Economic Reform" in 1978, the College changed its Chinese name from the "Medical University of Capital Hospital" (首都医院医科大学) to "Chinese Academy of Medical Science" (中国医学科学院), then "Chinese Capital Medical University" (中国首都医科大学), later changed to "China Union Medical University" (中国协和医科大学). Finally it was changed back to "Peking Union Medical College" (北京协和医学院) on May 18th, 2007, which naturally demonstrated that "PUMC" was no longer a highly sensitive topic in politics. Compared with universities that were also set up by Americans in old China, such as "Yenching" (燕京) "Nanking" (金陵), "Soochow" (东吴), and "St. John's" (圣约翰), PUMC was the only one that was resumed its original name which somehow redressed the earlier injustice. From this, it can be seen that PUMC was more closely related to the history, the present, and the future of China compared with other universities established by the Americans. However, for the development of medical professionalism, and even to some of current studies of "anti-Americanism", what's the historical significance of the "old PUMC" which faded in and out, then lingered in the great changes of the passage of time?

If we disregard the ideological vest of either white or black, only looking at PUMC through the disease, medicine, society, politics, culture, and economic point of view, we can see that the Chinese society has been full of conspicuous conflict and controversy. All of those who have familiarized themselves with the history of PUMC know that since the beginning of the PUMC, the Western missionary societies in China and the Chinese government always criticized PUMC for its long-term program, small number of students enrolled, English instruction, so that its students dwelled and indulged in urban materialism rather than serving for the majority poor rural populations. [56] Even though the College was involved in Peking's public health experimental program in 1930s and the rural reconstruction work in Dingxian County, this part of its work had never been the focus of the medical professional development, nor did the college dedicate all possible funding or human resources in it. After all, China was an epidemic ridden, infectious disease ravaged, medical and health resources deprived country, with extremely high morbidity and mortality rate. It was analogous to starving refugees who would eat anything available and the relief agency would give them bread and a bowl of hot soup easily to feed them rather than serving them a royal feast. On the one hand, "Old PUMC" adopted the Johns Hopkins model and set a rich standard in a poor country, but it did have the extravagant, flashy side that was ahead of its time.

In 1956, some pragmatic Chinese top leaders proposed the slogan "advancing toward science". China was already under a model of highly centralized power, so that it would use the capacity of the whole country to promote public health and adopted the mass mobilization model to control the spread of plague, cholera, schistosomiasis and other virulent epidemic of infectious diseases. It greatly improved the medial care of the people, so that the life expectancy of the Chinese people greatly improved. From 1953 to 1957, with the implementation of the first five year plan, industrialization and urbanization greatly pushed forward, the country made great efforts to upgrade its medical care and establish a number of better equipped medical facilities in the cities. A lot of measures were taken to lower the prevalence of cardiovascular diseases and cancers. Therefore, even though PUMC was still bound with Cultural Aggression of the American Imperialism, the professionalism of the College in every aspect was the heritage needed most by the country.

There is no need to reiterate more historical details, but what is worth mentioning most was that under the extreme "left" pressure, a cohort of the elite educated from the Old PUMC, also the leading figures of the professionals in Chinese medical world, were under the risk of being sent to reformation through labor or put into jail, nonetheless adhered to the highest standard of medical professionalism. For example, in April 1962, Huang Jiasi, who was mild tempered and cautious organized the meeting on the Preliminary Summary on the Teaching Experiences of the "Old PUMC" and he used the languages that most acceptable in the ideological environment at that time speaking positively about the significance of the professionalism of the "Old PUMC" toward the development of China's advanced medicine. [57] Lin Qiaozhi who published the most visible paper about "anti-Americanism" in *the People's Daily* in all previous political movements, praised passionately in private "the great heritage and good experiences of the 'old PUMC". [58] Surgeon Zeng Xianjiu, who was Loucks' junior colleague, and under political siege for the "pro-Americanism" during the cultural revolution when PUMC was castigated most, [59] still bravely stated outright: "I really think that America is scientifically advanced and medical technically superior. Science has no national boundary." [60] The chief editor T. F. Fox, who visited China in 1957, also documented a similar account. He said although the CCP called for learning from the Soviet Union, the Chinese medical society felt more akin to Europe and America. The fifteen medical journals in the whole nation were all published in Chinese or English; none of them was published in Russian. Fox concluded that it was because many senior and established researchers were Chinese with overseas experience and therefore "though many of the seniors have worked abroad, and are mentally in contact with what the rest of us are doing, very few of the younger ones have done so."[61] So, from the point of view of the cosmopolitanism of republic of literati, we can have a better understanding of the letter written by John, D. Rockefeller Jr. on April 4th, 1951. Even though he was very sorry for the takeover of PUMC by the CCP, he still thought that, "but who are we to say that this may not be the Lord's way of achieving the intent of the founders, although it be a way so wholly different from that has been in our mind. Let us hope, pray and believe that all may be ultimately for the best"[62]

Bibliography

1. Zhang Zhiqiang, *My Life* (《我的一生》), Self-printed, no record of press, 2006, p. 200.

2. Stephen J. Kunitz, "Professionalism and Social Control in the Progressive Era: The Case of the Flexner Report," *Social Problems*, Vol. 22, No. 1, Oct., 1974, pp. 16 – 27; Toby Gelfand, "From Guild to Profession: The Surgeons of France in the 18th Century," *The Humanities and Medicine*, 32 no. 1, Spring 1974, pp. 121 – 34; Jeanne L. Brand, *Doctors and the State: The British Medical Profession and Government Action in Public Health*, *1870 – 1912*, Baltimore, 1965; William G. Rothstein, *American Physicians in the 19th Century: From Sects to Science* Baltimore, 1972.

3. Mary E. Ferguson, *China Medical Board and Peking Union Medical College: A Chronicle of Fruitful Collaboration*, *1914 – 1951*, China Medical Board of New York, Inc.; 1st edition, 1970, p. 192.

4. *The History of Peking Union Medical College* (1917 – 1987) (《中国协和医科大学校史（1917 – 1987）》, compiled by Peking Union Medical College, Beijing Science and Technology Press, 1987, p. 45.

5. "Lee Chung-en's Confession" (《李宗恩的检查》), New PUMC (《新协和》), June 13, 1952, Special publication on Ideological Construction (思想建设特刊), Vol. 14, p. 1.

6. Zhang Zhiqiang, *My Life*, p. 209.

7. Readers' letters, "Medical Workers Should Not Neglect Reading Newspapers", (《医

务工作者不应该忽视读报》），*People's Daily*（《人民日报》）Mar. 22，1952，p. 2；PUMC，"Self-criticism of Neglecting Reading Newspapers,"（《协和医学院关于忽视读报工作的检讨》），*People's Daily* ，April 19，1952，p. 4.

8. Student Union，"American Imperialism 's Cultural Aggression in PUMC"（《美帝文化侵略在协和》），*New PUMC*，The first issue，Feb. 20，1951，pp. 2 – 21，China Medical Board，Inc. Box：128，Folder，937，Rockefeller Archive Center，RAC.，Sleepy Hollow，New York，United States.

9. Zhu Shousong（祝寿嵩），"My Teacher"（《我的先生》），*New PUMC*，The first issue，Feb. 20，1951，pp. 2 – 21.

10. Fan Du（范度），"Loucks-Imperialist in Gentry-Scholar's Coat,"（《娄克斯——披着绅士学者外衣的帝国主义分子》），*New PUMC*，May 9，1952，Special publication on ideological building，Vol. 1，p. 2.

11. Zeng Xianjiu（曾宪九）， "I Realized the Real Purpose of Loucks' s Academic Activities,"（《我认识了娄克斯'学术活动'的真正目的》），*New PUMC*，May 14，1952，Special publication on ideological building，Vol . 13，p. 2.

12. " The Accusation of the Head Nurse Yang Yinghua of the Ward of PLA，Cultural Aggression Makes Me Unable to Distinguish Between Friends and Enemy，Don't Love the PLA Soldiers ,"（《志愿军病房护士长杨英华控诉，美帝文化侵略使我敌我不分，不爱志愿军》），*New PUMC*，May 24，1952，Special publication on ideological Construction，Vol. 18，p. 2.

13. Zhang Zhiqiang，*My Life*，p. 210.

14. *People's Daily*，Sept. 27，1952，p. 3.

15. Lim Kha-t'I，"Lee Chung-en-Your Problem is not the Same as Ours,"（《李宗恩，你的问题和我们的不一样》），*New PUMC*，July 31，1952，Special publication on ideological building，Vol. 52，p. 2.

16. Xinhua News Agency（新华社）， "From Bastion of the Cultural Aggression of American Imperialism to the People's Medical Institution，After the Liberation，PUMC has Undergone Through Dramatic Changes in Medical Care，Teaching，Research and Construction"（《从美帝文化侵略堡垒变成人民医疗机构，协和医学院解放后在医疗、教学、研究和建设等方面已经起了根本变化》）*People's Daily*，Aug. 20，1957，p. 4；Xinhua News Agency："Two Months' Reasoning and Fighting，Dozens of Debate Meeting，Big or Small，PUMC Experts Knock Down C. U. Lee"（《两个月的说理斗争，十几次大小辩论会，协和医学院专家教授驳倒李宗恩》），*People's Daily*，Oct. 6，1957，p. 3.

17. Xinhua News Agency， " The Ministry of Health of Central Government Formally

Took Over PUMC, and a Celebration Involving a Thousand People of the Teachers and Students of this College Was Held," (《中央人民政府卫生部正式接收北京和医学院，该院师生员工千人集会欢欣庆祝》) *People's Daily*, Jan. 21, 1951, p. 1; "Long live the Chinese People's New PUMC," (《中国人民的新协和万岁》), *New PUMC*, The first issue, Feb. 20, 1951, pl.

18. "The Mission of New PUMC," (《"新协和"的使命》), *New PUMC*, The first issue, Feb. 20, 1951, pl.

19. Zhang Zhiqiang, *My Life*, p. 111.

20. Zhang Zhiqiang, *My Life*, pp. 200 – 201.

21. Zhang Zhiqiang, *My Life*, p. 219.

22. *The History of Peking Union Medical College* (1917 – 1987), p. 48.

23. *The History of Peking Union Medical College* (1917 – 1987), p. 45.

24. Xinhua News Agency, "From the Bastion of the Cultural Aggression of American Imperialism to the People's Medical Institutions, PUMC's Fundamental Change in Medicine, Teaching, Research and Construction after Liberation ", *People's Daily*, Aug. 20, 1957, p. 4

25. "Obstetrics and Gynecology Department Strengthen Cooperation and Improve Procedure, Shorten the Operation time and Postoperative Hospital Stay," (《妇产科加强配合改进操作，缩短手术时间和术后住院日》), *CAMS* (Chinese Academy of Medical Sciences) *Newspaper*, June 7, 1958, p. 4.

26. "The Screening speed of the Antibiotics Department Increased by 215 times, Decided to Find Antibiotics Against Cancer within Six Months" (《抗生素系筛选速度提高215倍，决定在半年内找到抗癌抗生素》), *CAMS Newspaper*, July 16, 1958, p. 1.

27. "20 Departments Report Their Success and Announce the New Indicators of Great Leap Forward at the First Conference for Treasure Presentation," (《在首次献宝献礼大会上廿个单位报捷并宣布跃进新指标》), *CAMS Newspaper*, June 19, 1958, p. 1.

28. Shu Yu (苏芋), "Refute the Enthusiasts for 'Very Quiet' of the" (《斥"冷冷清清"的爱好者》), *CAMS Newspaper*, December 10, 1959, p. 3.

29. "To Expose the Bourgeois Nature of Scientific Research, Clarify that Science Must Serve the Production of Great Leap Forward," (《揭穿科学研究中的资产阶级本质，明确科学必须为生产大跃进服务》), *CAMS Newspaper*, June 4, 1958, p. 2.

30. "Learn from Revolution Pioneering in the Neurology Division of PUMC." (《学习协和脑系科的革命创举》), *CAMS Newspaper*, Dec. 29, 1958, p. 1.

31. "The Guerrilla Style Resumed its Good Reputation-the Account of the Brain

Department of PUMC Breaking Up the Bourgeois Tradition," （《为游击习气恢复名誉以后——协和脑系科大破资产阶级传统经过》）, *CAMS Newspaper*, Dec. 29, 1958, p. 1.

32. Guo Shaojun, Xiong Shiqi （郭少军、熊世琦）, " Break the System of Authority and Hierarchy, the Overall Great Leap Forward of the Neurology Division of PUMC," （《大破"权威"和"等级制", 协和医院脑系科的全面大跃进》 *People's Daily*, Nov. 10, 1958, p. 6.

33. Report Abstract of Vice Minister Xu Yunbei's made to CAMS, Health Work should be reformed thoroughly, sticks to the General Guideline of the Party （徐运北副部长在我院全体人员上的报告摘要, 卫生工作必须大力改革, 坚决贯彻党的总路线）, CAMS Newspaper, June 7th, 1958, p. 1

34. Report Abstract of Vice Minister Xu Yunbei's speech made to CAMS, Health Work should be reformed thoroughly, sticks to the General Guideline of the Party, CAMS Newspaper, June 7th, 1958, p. 1

35. CAMS Under the Sunshine of the General Guidelines, Break the Superstition of the Slavery Thoughts of the British and American, Facing Patients, facing Reality, Brave in Action, People's Daily, June 8th, 1958, p. 2., Break Superstition, Poke the Red Flag, Make Planning, Do Renovation, CAMS Aiming High, Ambitious is Action, Health Daily, June 25, 1968, p. 4

36. Zhang Zhiqiang, *My Life*, p. 222.

37. "Help Party to Have a better run of Medical Education" （《帮助党办好医学教育》）, *People's Daily*, June 4, 1957, p. 7.

38. "Resuming Medical Education," （《恢复医学生教育》）, *The History of Peking Union Medical College* （1917 – 1987）, p. 69 – 71.

39. Zhang Zhiqiang, *My Life*, p. 222.

40. Zhang Zhiqiang, *My Life*, p. 224.

41. "The Address of Huang Chia-ssu at the Convention of the Founding of the China Medical University and Opening Ceremony of 1959," （《黄家驷院长在中国医科大学成立及一九五九年开学典礼大会上的讲话》） *CAMS Newspaper*, Sep. 10, 1959, p. 2.

42. " The Address of Minister of Ministry of Health, Li Dequan," （《卫生部李德全部长的指示》）, *CAMS Newspap*er, Sep. 10, 1959, p. 3.

43. " PUMC Hospital's Road to Success,, a Review of Eight Years in this Hospital," （《协和医院成功之路: 在北京协和医院八年的回顾》）, *Journal of Hospitals Management of PLA*, （《解放军医院管理杂志》） Mar. 1996, p. 87 – 89.

44. *The History of Peking Union Medical College* （1917 – 1987）, p. 59.

45. "Help Party to Make a Better Run of Medical Education", *People's Daily*, June 4, 1957, p. 7.

46. Zhang Zhiqiang, *My Life*, p. 214.

47. Wu Zhili（吴之理）, *A Military Doctor's Self Statement*（《一名军医的自述》）, Huaxia Publishing House, 2004, p. 92.

48. *The History of Peking Union Medical College*（1917 – 1987）, p. 61.

49. Lin Juncai, "The Road to Success of Beijing Union Hospital, a Review of Eight Years in this Hospital," *Hospitals Management of PLA*, Mar. 1996, p. 87.

50. Zhang Zhiqiang, *My Life*, p. 314.

51. Zhang Yangfen, *Memory of Pride*（《自豪的回忆》）, Huanxia Publishing House, 2004, p. 170.

52. *The History of Peking Union Medical College*（1917 – 1987）, p. 63; Zhang Yangfen, *Memory of Pride*, p. 168.

53. Zhu Bing（朱彬）, "Before Becoming a Doctor – the Account of the Teaching at the Sixth Grade with the China Medical University"（《当大夫之前——中国医科大学六年级教学见闻》）, *People's Daily*, June 3, 1962, p. 2.

54. Xiong Shiqi, "The Close Friends of Medical Workers – An Account on the Library of the National Medical Center"（《医药工作者的密友——记全国医学中心图书馆》）, *People's Daily*, Dec. 6, 1961, p. 4.

55. "Revolutionary Workers, Revolutionary Students, Revolutionary Cadres of CAMS, Enthusiastic Response to the Call of the Party Committee, Fierce Attack on Bourgeois Representatives, All Evil Demons and Monsters, as Well as All Bourgeois and Feudal Ideology,"（《我院广大革命工人、革命同学、革命干部，热烈响应院党委号召，向资产阶级代表人物，向一切牛鬼蛇神，向一切资产阶级和封建的意识形态猛烈开火》）, *CAMS Newspaper*, June 20, 1966, p. 1.

56. John Z. Bowers, *Western medicine in a Chinese palace*：*Peking Union Medical College, 1917 – 1951*, （The Josiah Macy, Jr. Foundation 1972）; Mary B. Bullock, *an American Transplant*：*The Rockefeller Foundation and Peking Union Medical College*, （University of California Press, 1980）; Bridie Andrews and Mary Brown Bullock ed. , *Medical Transitions in Twentieth-Century China*, （Indiana University Press, 2014）

57. PUMC Press, The History of PUMC 1917 – 1987, p. 73

58. Zhang Yangfen, *Memory of Pride*, p. 168.

59. The Red Children Guard of China Medical University: From Rockefeller to Khrushchev, People's Daily, Feb. 24, 1968, p. 4

60. Zhong Shouxian (Head of the Surgical Department), "*Yi wo di enshi Zeng Xianjiu jiao shou*" (*On the Memory of My Teacher Professor Zeng Xianjiu http*: //*www. pumch. cn*/ *Item*/11768. *aspx.*

61. T. F. Fox, "the New China, Some Medical Impressions", *The Lancet*, Nov. 23, 1957, p. 1057.

62. *China Medical Board and Peking Union Medical College A chronicle of Fruitful Collaboration* (*1914 - 1951*), China Medical Board of New York, Inc. , 1970, p. 227.

中国医学科学院的成立及其早期运作（1956－1966）

蒋育红

蒋育红，现任北京协和医学院人文与社会科学学院副教授，翻译多本北京协和医学院、美国中华医学基金会历史丛书，发表多篇有关协和历史的文章。2017－2018 中美富布莱特研究学者。

对于 1949 年至 1966 年期间的中国医疗史、疾病史和卫生史的研究，这些年来较多集中在消除诸如血吸虫等传染病或"赤脚医生"等中国医疗卫生特有问题；对于医疗研究取向、医学知识共同体或机构的研究并不多见。本文希望能够在微观层面，更多探讨成立于 1956 年 8 月 11 日，1957 年与"中国协和医学院"[1]（当时"协和"的名称）合并、被定格为中国医学科学研究最高机构的"中国医学科学院"（简称"医科院"）的最初历史。除了利用彼时一些相关中文报刊资料之外，本文还利用了洛克菲勒档案馆及北京协和医学院档案馆收藏的一些档案资料以及当事人近年来刊印的回忆录、中国协和医科大学校史等。通过对这些历史资料的深描，本文将较前人更多关注特定人物及机构设置。

"苏联模式""中央性""计划性"

1956 年 2 月，党和政府成立了由总理周恩来领衔，副总理陈毅、李富春、聂荣臻参加的国家科学规划委员会。在接下来的几个月里，委员会调集来自全国各地的六百多位科学家和技术专家，反复讨论修改后编制出《1956 年至 1967 年科学技术发展远景规划》，落实到医学卫生的科学研究方面，规划中涉及到有：研究新的抗生素等药物和医学器材；总结和发扬中医理论和实践经验；加强劳动卫生、劳动保护的综合措施，以及防治主要职业病和职业中毒的研究等。其中最重要的，是期望在这一期间清除和预防对民众健康危害最大的几种主要寄生虫病和传染病——血吸虫病、疟疾、黑热病、丝虫病、钩虫病、脑炎、鼠疫、天花和性病等。此外，这份规划还强调中国科学研究必须按照党的指示："用最大力量来加强中国科学院，使它成为领导全国提高科学水平、培养新生力量的火车头。"[2]

在当时的政治背景下，设置全国最高科学研究机构，政府直接掌控各项科学研究活动，是追随和仿效了苏联模式。早在1950年代建国之初，由于国家采取了与苏联结盟的"一边倒"的政策。除了政府机构和军队系统，文化教育、科学研究等方面也掀起了学习苏联的高潮，并上升到"政治正确"的高度。1954年任北京医学院副院长，后任中国医学科学院副院长的薛公绰回忆道：刘少奇对他说过，要加强学习苏联领导，与苏联专家搞好关系，如果搞不好关系，"有理三扁担，无理扁担三"。[3] 具体措施如当时被认为科学研究水准最高的中国协和医学院，效仿苏联模式而建立起教研室，制定教学大纲和教学方案。为了尽快掌握俄语，1953年全院举办了七期，每期20天，共有622名教师及进修生参加的俄语突击学习速成班。另外，还有12个系科展开了苏联医学杂志的翻译工作。[4]

1956年党中央召开了关于知识分子问题会议，不久又发出"向科学进军"的号召，积极大力推进科学的发展。而1956年之前，唯一有着"中央"名分，被视为中国最高医学科学研究机构的，是设在北京的中央卫生研究院。该机构的前身是南京国民政府的中央卫生实验院，南京解放之后被人民政府接收。[5] 1950年卫生部召开的第一届全国卫生会议，做出加强医学科学研究工作的决定。呈请中央文委批准，将该机构总部从南京迁至北京，与其在北京分院合并，并于当年十月正式命名为中央卫生研究院。其原有的寄生虫学研究单位仍留南京，此外还有设在海南岛的一个疟疾研究站。1954年，该院建成八个研究单位，除南京、海南岛的两个分支机构之外，其余六个都在北京——即营养学系、微生物学系、卫生工程学系、药物学系、病理室与中国医药研究所。其时，全院共有专业科学人员 207 人，其中副研究员以上的高级研究人员 30 人。"此外还有院外有关高等学校及研究机关参加本院研究工作的专家共 13 人。"[7] 1956 年 2 月 23 日至 25 日，该院举行了首次学术专题研讨会，提交论文 50 篇，参加者有在京的医学人士和苏联专家 300 多人。[8] 作为领导的表态，是同一天的《健康报》刊发以《向科学进军》为题的社论，说这是中央卫生研究院响应党中央"向科学进军"的号召，为迅速赶上世界先进科学水平而总结部分研究工作的成就。[9]

　　1956 年 8 月，中央政府认识到中国医学科学发展要尽快赶上国际先进水平。为加强医学科学研究力量，将中央卫生研究院更名为中国医学科学院，[10] 这明显是仿效苏联的国家医学科学研究体制。苏联医学科学院创办于 1944 年，前身是苏联人民保健委员会组建的国家人民保健研究院和国家实验医学研究所。1932 年 10 月 15 日，苏联人民委员会决定将国家实验医学研究所改组为全苏实验医学研究所。苏联医学科学院以此为基础，将分散于各地的一些医学研究所整合而成。作为其时世界最大的高端医学科学研究机构，该院直属政府领导，是各加盟共和国、各省医学研究院效仿的典范。鉴于战后苏联各种医学专家和科学家奇缺，该院培养了大批高级人才及着手于提高医生们的业务能力，不仅保证了自身的需要，且在短短期间为国家输送了众多医疗卫生领导干部。1945 年至 1946 年，该院设立了 25 个研究所，有 60 名专任院士。[11] 1953 年，该院第八次学术会议召开之时，已有 99 位院士和 132 位通讯院士，全职科研人员已达 6000 余人。[12] 再为了追随其时医学科学发展的最新潮流，1956 年该院建立了心血管外科研究所，筹划设立首个针对单一疾病的科学委员会——研究恶性肿瘤的协调委员会（1959 年成立）。[13]

　　这一国家医学科学研究体制的特点，最引人注目之处是其"中央性"（centralization）和"计划性"（planning）。[14] 如苏联医学科学院，自 1947 年首次制订了首个全苏医学科学研究的五年计划之后，该机构不仅承担着很多科研项目，且还要规划、指导和业务监督全国各地科研任务的推进。同样，当中国医学科学院从中央卫生研究院更名而来，也面临着如何最有效地汇聚全国医学科学研究精英，计划和掌控最重要的医学科学研究项目。一份代表政府高层卫生官员的《健康报》社论说：必须解决当前工业化、农业集体化，在医学科学方面提出了一系列的新问题，中共的领导就是能够提供这样一种优越的制度保证。作为比较，这篇社论指出在国民党反动政府统治时期，各种研究机构都是残缺不全，设备简陋，人力分散。虽然不可否认，那种状况下仍有不少科学家是有浓厚的科学研究兴趣的，但是在这样的社会里是得不到政府的支持的，只能够各自为政，按照自己兴趣去做一些科学研究工作。这显然是按一种手工业式的方法进行的，其结果自然是缺乏计划性和整体性。"这种研究工作是和整个社会的要求，人民的需要是脱节的，所以成绩也就不会大。"[15]

与中国医学科学院同时期建立起来的医学科学研究机构的还有军事医学科学院、中医研究院。尽管如此，医科院并不具备能够统筹和领导全国医学科学研究的影响力。更名后的当年 10 月，该院一次性接收了130 多名来自各地医药学院和综合大学的毕业生以及 90 多名中专毕业生。当时的新闻报道说："一年中有这么多人涌入一个医学科学的研究机构，在我国医学科学史上是空前的。"[16]再就其时苏联医学科学院的院长的学术影响力来看，几乎都是全国学术声望极高的医学专家。其首任院长尼可莱（Nikolai Burdenko）博士，是苏联神经外科学的创始人，担任过红军的军医部长及苏联保健部医学科学委员会主席。[17] 1956 年前后，担任院长的是苏联心血管外科的奠基人之一的巴库列夫博士。[18]相比之下，中国医学科学院实力和领导力几乎没有达到当时在中国医学界的学科带头人或有影响力的人和研究领域。[19]

为了强化这种"中央性"和"计划性"，党和国家的高层领导人试图通过与其他高端研究机构协调，打造出一个学术影响更大，更有领导力的中国医学科学院。1957 年 3 月 20 日，时任中国科学院院长的郭沫若，在一份报告中强调科学研究的协调工作之重要性。他认为在医学研究方面，此时最突出的问题是军队和地方，中医和西医研究工作的协调。他坦率地指出："中国医学科学院现在已有十五个所（系），虽然作了不少工作，但领导骨干和设备都不足。"[20]一个月之后，即 4 月 16 日，时任国务院副总理、有着元帅军衔且也是主管中国高端科学研究（如核武器和人造卫星）的聂荣臻发表谈话，认为当下医学研究工作摊子铺得太大，力量分散，互不协作，浪费了大量人力物力，并阻碍了研究工作的开展。他认为应当按照"集中力量"的原则而尽快进行机构调整。[21]至于具体落实，最初是中央领导考虑先通过中国医学科学院与北京协和医学院的协调合作，等磨合成熟后将两个机构合并。不过到了 7 月底，聂荣臻迫不及待地将两个机构的"合作"改为"合并"。8 月 3 日，卫生部宣布了合并筹备委员会的组成名单，期望通过加强党的领导而加速这一进程。10 月 18 日，中共北京市委批准成立了推进两个机构合并事宜的临时党委。11 月 25 日，卫生部下发确认这一合并事宜正式文件。[22]中国协和医学院将不再招生，新命名的"中国医学科学院"开始作为中国医学科学研究的最高殿堂而被规划和建设。

苏联影响、"延安传统"与"老协和"

中国医学科学院虽然仿效苏联模式设立，但苏联那套以"学术官僚"为轴心的集体研究模式却无法顺利照搬。中国接触到苏联医学科学研究模式，还是缘自于 1951 年后向苏联大批派遣医学留学生。而 1956–1957 年先后有包括抗生素所所长在内的 12 名高级苏联科学家被派到医科院，医科院也对等派出了 8 人前往苏联进修，当 1956 年中国医学科学院成立之时，留苏学生中相当一批已经完成学业，陆续回国担任教职或参与科学研究工作。1956 年 6 月，中国科学院召集来参加讨论编制十二年科学规划医学组的专家，二十二位中已至少有四位是留苏的人。不过，这些留苏学者多是些三十岁出头、学历副博士、职称副研究员的年轻新秀，面对那些五十岁、六十岁，曾在欧美进修访学，或取得博士学位，1940 年代就已经是副教授、教授的资深学者，犹如学生见老师——在医学研究决策方面不会有太多话语权和决定权。

关键更在于，其时中国学者并不认为苏联医学科学研究的水准是世界领先，不值得全力仿效。1961 年春，英国生化学家、诺贝尔奖得主钱恩（E. B Chain，1906 – 1979）博士应中国科学院与中华医学会的邀请访华，曾在北京、上海与中国科学界和医学界人士频繁接触，广泛交流了双方对苏联医学的观感。钱恩指出，近四十多年来，苏联在诸如麻醉剂、镇痛药、硫胺类药剂、抗生素、维生素或激素等药物化学的任何一个领域，从未发明一种重要的新药。钱恩甚至认为："时下最令人感兴趣的更现代的有机化学领域，诸如高分子聚合物—蛋白质、核酸与合成塑料、树脂的研究，全都是西方发展起来的。在这些领域里，俄国人的贡献要么完全空白，要么非常平庸。"[23]中国学者当然颇有同感。在协和被划归军队管理时，协和血液专家邓家栋随国防部考察团访问苏联，得到的印象是水平不如预想的那么高。邓家栋写道："交谈中，我们觉得他们的临床专家对国外的信息不够了解，可能与他们缺乏和外界交流的机会有关。"[24]时任协和最高领导的党委书记，政治委员张之强（1915 – 2015）后来也回忆道，苏联的医学水平，完全不比协和高，但在当时强大的政治压力下，照搬了苏联的一套。张之强说："这引起协和教授们的强烈不满，但又不敢直言反对；我也认为改变协和医学院的性质不妥，所以曾向总后勤部领导提出异议，希望总后领导能重新考虑，结果受到了批评。"[25]

作为成功推翻南京国民政府统治的中国共产党，在武装夺取政权的过程中发展出一套自己的科学研究模式。尤其是党中央到了延安之后，很短时间里就在医疗卫生方面创办了中央医院、边区医院、白求恩国际和平医院、八路军野战医院、军委直属医院和当时颇有声誉的亚洲学生疗养院等五十多家医疗卫生单位。这些机构不仅为边区党政机关、部队服务，而且为当地群众服务，大大改善了人民群众的医疗卫生水平。除此之外，1939 年 5 月，中共在延安成立了自然科学研究院，1940 年 1 月将之改名为延安自然科学院。当时，延安受到国民党军队的重重包围，经济发展低下，文化水平落后。该研究机构虽是最高学术研究单位，却没有能力进行高深科学研究，只是为了加强对敌斗争而做些非常实用的仿制工作。不过，大多数当时在延安工作的自然科学工作者，自 1949 年之后就在科研领导工作中独当一面。再至 1949 年 11 月，在原国民政府的中央研究院、北平研究院和延安自然科学院的基础上，组建了中国科学院。一位研究者说："延安时期中国共产党播下的科学种子终于结出了丰硕的果实，中国共产党的科学事业也进入到了一个新的发展阶段。"[26]

　　在某种意义上来说，1957 年的中国医学科学院是按照这种"延安传统"建构的。虽则，自建国之后高层领导人一直强调学习苏联，但在"党的一元化领导"方面则一丝不苟地坚持中国特色。苏联实行党的属地管理制度，就像医学科学院这样的中央机构，院长是经院士选举产生。党的领导直属莫斯科，行政级别不能和院长平起平坐。再加上他们的院士制度也是要求凡事必须经过投票表决。与之不同，那时中国医学科学院是在延安就曾实行的党委领导制。1958 年 6 月《健康报》刊发卫生部医学教育司司长季钟朴（1913～2002）的讲话，称："苏联是校长负责制，学校党组织只起保证作用，而以教授为主组成学术会议，讨论全院重大问题，权力很大。苏联情况和我国不同，他们已经消灭了资产阶级，教授是又红又专，学校中党的领导十分巩固。"[27]时任上海第二军医大学校长的吴之理（1915～2008）回忆道，苏联专家建议在学校设立教授委员会，他和教授们是乐意的，"但党委会上有不同意见，称今后党的领导将会形同虚设。"[28]

　　这也意味着虽然是按照苏联医科院模式建立起来的中国医学科学院，但其决策体系和管理结构并没有完全照搬苏联的模式，而形成了自己的特有模式。毕竟，中国现代医学科学研究源自于北京协和医学院，以"科学济人道"当作其使命，秉承了美国约翰·霍普金斯大学（The Johns Hopkins University）医学院对医学科学的推崇及教育模式。该医学院拥有在当时中国乃至整个远东地区都可视为最先进、最完备科学研究的仪器、设备、实验室和图书馆以及生活、学习和研究的优越条件。该医学院在 20 世纪 20 年代至 40 年代的鼎盛时期，被视为是亚洲医学研究水准最高的学府之一。1948 年南京国民政府进行中央研究院院士选举，荣登医学类院士榜首的 7 人之中，有 6 人来自协和系统（在协和受过教育或在协和任职），占到总数的 85%。1955 年 6 月，中国科学院学部成立，被选为医学类学部委员会之人中已加入一些政治考量，被选上者不乏参加革命较早、政治立场坚定以及一些担任领导职务之人。尽管如此，在 16 名医学类的学部委员之中，协和系统有 9 人，占到总数的 56%。这表明即使在建国之后，协和的学术研究的影响力还是受人瞩目。

1956 年 9 月 1 日，中央决定将协和医学院从军队系统划归卫生部下属。[29]由此带来了人事问题，即该任命谁为此新成立科学研究机构的院长呢？这让负责向卫生部提出人选的张之强书记心里有点犯愁。他当时的想法，在这个并入诸多单位的新机构里，协和的影响太强，非协和之人不太服气，使之人事关系复杂，思想不稳定。张之强考虑到，如果院长能从"外边调入进来，工作起来就能会比较超脱一些"，遂提名由时任上海医学院副院长的黄家驷（1906~1984）担任。[30]相对于"老协和"的其他人来说，黄家驷思想进步，政治可靠。早在 1950 年冬朝鲜战争爆发之后，他就主动报名参加上海市志愿医疗手术队，担任总队长兼第二大队大队长。1952 年，时至中年的他早已过了学外语的最佳年龄，为了响应党提出的"学习苏联"之号召，从零开始挤时间强化俄语学习。1954 年，他还辛辛苦苦地翻译和出版了一部苏联学者撰写的《胸部外科学》。1955 年，黄家驷被聘为首批学部委员，并于 1956 年主持制订关于全国十二年科学技术发展规划。当然，黄家驷个性"谨慎从事，免招麻烦"。[31]在那个年代里，身居医学高位的他几乎从来没有指名道姓地批判过某人。1961 年，他主持学术会议，邀请学者介绍那些因政治不正确而一度被全盘否定的专业学说，"并纠正了片面学习苏联和将学术见解与政治观点混为一谈的错误倾向。"[32]

"一个机构、两块牌子"的运作方式

作为曾是 1933 年届毕业生，黄家驷的任命标志着该校在中国高端医学研究殿堂上的重新浮起。毕竟，建国之后不久，中美两国政府反目交恶，协和被贴上"美帝文化侵略中国的最大堡垒"的标签而被高度边缘化。协和先是被命令停止招生，接着划拨军方管制，接收各地进修生，负责培训那些参加革命早、文化水平低的老干部。此外，为了加强军队医学建设，该院临床和基础部专家学者被上级领导机关大批抽调至如解放军 301 医院等新的医疗机构。此时协和的科学研究虽未间断，但由于领导体制、教学任务不断变化，医疗任务繁重，研究题目多为解决临床诊断上的需要和教学上的问题，绝大多数属于一般医学的范畴。统计资料显示："1955 年各科汇总的 361 项研究题目来看，其中结合部队的研究题目占 7.5%，中医中药研究占 4.1%，高级神经活动的研究及理论研究占 14.6%，临床诊断及治疗的研究占 52.2%，其他占 21.6%。"[33] 当 1958 年黄家驷就职中国医学科学院的院长之后，认真调研各院所研究课题和工作情况，致力于重新激活协和以往的高端医学科学研究传统。他提出："尖端问题也必须进行研究。这是关系到目前任务和明天任务的问题。"[34]

　　为了实现国家科学战略规划，加强医科院实力，中国医学科学院在机构上开始了大规模的扩张。仅 1958 年的 1 月到 6 月，卫生部决定划归医科院的研究机构就有：北京皮肤病性病研究所和北京流行病研究所（南京皮肤病研究所的前身）；北京医院和北京第二医院；经聂荣臻副总理批准，军队所属的北京市胸科医院并入北京第二医院后，定名为"阜成门外医院"（中国心血管病研究中心／阜外医院的前身）；整形外科医院；位于天津的输血与血液学研究所（原解放军十三军医学校）；劳动保护科学研究所与卫生部的劳动卫生研究所合并、划归医科院。8 月 16 日，卫生部又批准将中国医学科学院原有 10 个系，改建为 5 个研究所（其中实验医学研究所在本书马超的文章中有详细记录，这里不再赘述）。[35] 直至 1962 年 10 月，中国医学科学院已经形成了高端医学研究的"国家队"，下辖有综合医院和专科医院、涵盖药物研究、抗生素研究、基础医学研究、公共卫生相关研究、血液病、寄生虫病、医学信息、生物工程等专业研究所，覆盖重要医学研究领域。[36]

　　将大批原来的教学人员调配到专业研究所，目的是为了加强科研的力量。除了 1958 年建立的医学仪器器械研究所（天津）、放射医学研究所（天津）由医科院自主成立的，其他各所都是卫生部直接下达政令，连人带设备及场地合并过来的。这体现了那个时代"集中力量办大事"的政府行为。也正是在这种"举国之力"体制之下，1958 年至 1966 年间的医科院的应用性科学研究，对解决中国医疗卫生问题与高端研究做出了相当大的贡献。具体说来，1958 年 11 月，地处昆明的医学生物学研究所，改建为中国医学科学院医学生物学研究所而集中力量研发脊髓灰质炎疫苗。1961 年 1 月 10 日，周恩来总理到该所视察，详细了解疫苗生产及科研情况，并观看了实验生产工作过程。1963 年该所成功地研制出"小儿麻痹糖丸"剂型，并进行了大规模地推广使用。该所接着又研制出了世界上第一个脊髓灰质炎减毒活疫苗糖丸新剂型，造福整个中国的儿童健康。再有，医科院在这一时段中，还成功地开展了中国的麻风病流行研究，以及完成了国内第一次人体心脏二尖瓣闭锁不全修补术和成功攻克绒毛膜癌的治疗难题（见本书刘德培文章）。同时，医科院还建立了我国第一个细胞遗传学研究组，并开创我国人体细胞遗传学和肿瘤细胞遗传学研究。

　　此时医科院的另一项重要发展，是期望推进医学科学研究与专业教学的相得益彰。最初，医科院领导体制和机构设置中，没有教学管理部门，大部分人员从事科学研究而基本不涉及教学。对于要不要办医学院，医科院内部意见分歧，不同意办医学院的领导也大有人在。早在 1957 年，时任协和内科主任张孝骞，建议恢复协和医学院的长学制的医学教育而上书有关领导部门。他在信中表示自 1953 年协和停止招生之后后备人才匮乏而感到担忧。针对很多人对于恢复医学院的担心，如教学工作是否会妨碍研究力量，张孝骞强调："教学诚然是个负担……但教学相长，这对于研究不仅没有矛盾，而且是相得益彰。中国科学院的科学家都乐于在高等学校义务任教，就是这个缘故。"[37]

　　除了张孝骞之外，黄家驷也是那些向中央高层领导提出这类意见的人之一。因为他从来就认为临床学科的研究，不能只留在临床观察和病例分析的水平上，必须开展客观性工作和研究理论问题，这样才能提出一些开创性的工作。他还明确表态：在八年制医科大学办学的同时，应当"致力于教学与研究工作相互促进，通过建校充实科研体系。而医学生、研究生的成长则加强了医学科学院的科研力量。"[38]正是在这批人的敦促下，1959 年 5 月 5 日召开的医科院第二次常务委员会议，通过了"关于筹办中国医科大学的初步方案"，黄家驷任筹备委员会主任。接着，在陆定一等中央领导的支持下，卫生部党组、北京市委以及中国医学科学院党委共同商讨，一致同意由中国医学科学院筹备，以原协和医学院为基础，恢复八年制的医学院。该校被命名为"中国医科大学"，校长由院长黄家驷兼任，并最终于 6 月 20、8 月 8 日先后得到卫生部党组、国务院的批复。1959 年 9 月 5 日，中国医科大学在东单三条礼堂召开了成立大会和开学典礼，从而开启了将临床医学教学与高端研究结合起来的一个新里程。

　　由于实行的是一个领导班子（党委）、一套组织结构、两块牌子、两个任务，在实际运作中最初有一个较为艰难的磨合过程。当年，新成立的医大通过全国高考统一招生、高分录取六十名新生，入学后先在北京大学生物系读医预科三年。再从包括北大、复旦、南开等五所综合性大学生物系调收来校读四年医学基础课的三十名肄业生，党委只是将他/她们安排给实验医学研究所，而没有常设专职机构负责。由于教师是兼职，主业在科研而非教学，教学实验室是借用研究所，教学设备还是旧协和零星留下来的，或是借用研究用的仪器，讲义教材往往是在课堂上和课后下发，致使开学不到两个月，学生们意见纷纷，反映根本不像一所大学而要求回到原来的学校。[39]

　　实际上，那时的医科院党委会对于如何办好医大，从来没有过统一意见。大部分党委领导更关注科研而非教学。每周三、六两次的党委常委会，讨论之事几乎全部是 13 个科研所遇到的问题。教学很难排到常委会的议事日程之上，有时好不容易排上一次，还会因为大多数党委常委不了解医大情况而难于发表意见。好在，曾任上海第二医学院教学副院长的章央芬于 1961 年被任命为医大主管教学的教务长，并担任了党委常委。由此，领导班子中除黄家驷院长之外，又多了一位对医大事务上心之人。正是通过黄家驷、章央芬的不懈努力，说服各位领导同意先组建了医大的人事科。尽管每次讨论此类问题时，在常委会上都不容易得到全数赞成，但黄家驷、章央芬等人耐心说服其他领导，同意逐步设立了独立的校长办公室、教材科、印刷厂、照相室、学生图书馆、食堂管理科等一整套专职医大的行政后勤机构。1963 年春，医大教学大楼建成，全部学生和教研室迁入，教学秩序和质量随即有了大幅提升。[40]卫生部于

1964 年组织的全国重点医学院校的教学质量测试，医大参试学生成绩名列前茅。1965 年，医大召开教改经验总结交流大会，得到了卫生部和兄弟院校的好评。更能体现医大作为当时全国顶级医学院的是规划其学生学业结束时，应在教授的领导和指导之下，单独或主要负责进行一个医学科学研究题目。鉴于那时主要与苏联等东欧社会主义国家结盟，这份规划承诺优秀学生中除可送到社会主义国家进修之外，破天荒地还提出"个别的也可送至资本主义国家进修。"[41]

结语

此时中国医学科学院与中国医科大学作为并列机构，虽然对外是两块牌子，两个印章，但日常科研和教学运作则是一个党委和一个行政。[42] 就能够发扬光大的"经验"来看，医学院与医科院共享一个机构，使科研力量得到了加强，的确十分有利于研究生的培养。医科院作为卫生部直接领导的"国家队"，又强化了协和在中国医学教育和科学研究中的领头军优势，大大推进了中国医疗卫生事业的改善。的确，正是医学科学院的成立，才在中国形成了比较高端的医学专业共同体。如顾方舟等留苏归国的科学家与出身于"老协和"的专家共同努力下，在高端医学研究方面取得了突破性的进展。这些都为 20 世纪 80 年代初乃至现今的医科院架构及医学科学研究的发展奠定了基础。

当然，有"利"就有"弊"。如果就应当吸取的"教训"来说，我们似乎可以看到行政力量的控制过于强大，在科学研究和教学过程中难免会加入一些"脑袋发热"的长官意志。1939 年参加革命，曾在八路军120 师卫生部工作，担任过中国医学科学院副院长的董炳琨就认为：这几十年的经验证明医科院"一套班子、两块牌子"的办法，难以使医本科教育完全到位。在他看来，"这种松散的联邦式的管理体制无法集中力量专心致志地搞教学工作，至于发挥协和优势和体现协和特色就更加困难……"。[43]毋庸置疑，同时期中国推进的原子弹爆炸、人造卫星、胰岛素合成、杂交水稻乃至 2015 年获得诺贝尔奖的青蒿素等项目，都是在最短时间动用举国之力，组织集体攻关的"大会战"以解决这些事关国防建设或国计民生的实际应用问题。然而，此时及随后一些最具原创性的医学科学研究，如 DNA 双螺旋结构、遗传密码、致癌基因、发育的基因调控、细胞凋亡、学习和记忆的机制等，几乎全都是发端于仅满足个人的好奇和偶然发现——通俗地说就是"只管耕耘，不问收获"的基础研究。相对而言，当时创办医科院的思路及其强调集体协作的制度设计，可能也造成了一定的人力、物力的浪费，且很大程度地还忽略了培育和发挥研究者们的开创性和探索精神。正如上引 1961 年 4 月至 6 月间访问中国的英国诺贝尔奖获得者钱恩所指出的，在其访问的中国科学研究机构中，感到震惊的是研究人员在智力和学识上的极高水平与其研究工作原创性的极低水平之间所形成的巨大反差。在他看来，那些即使在西方也可以看作出类拔萃之人，"从事的题目多半是低水平的应用性研究"。[44]由此说来，关于中国医学科学院的成立和早期运作的历史研究，就还是一个值得人们深入探讨的课题。

参考书目

1. 北京协和医学院于 1952 年改称中国协和医学院；1959 年 6 月 30 日 教育部（1959）入学宋字 431 号文批复同意更名为中国医科大学，学制八年。

2.《一九五六——一九六七年科学技术发展远景规划（修正草案）》，参见"中华人民共和国科学技术部网站" http：//www. most. gov. cn/ztzl/gjzcqgy/zcqgylshg/200508/t20050831_ 24440. htm。

3. 彭瑞聪：《回忆薛公绰同志在北医》，载徐守仁主编：《薛公绰纪念集》，北京科学技术出版社，2008 年，第 77 页。

4. 中国协和医科大学编：《中国协和医科大学校史（1917 - 1987）》，北京科学技术出版社，1987 年，第 49 页。

5. 沈其震：《感谢苏联援助，学习苏联先进经验，实现医学科学研究工作的更大跃进》，《中国医学科学院院报》，1958 年 11 月 5 日，第 1 版。

6. 还有中央防疫处。1945 年后，国民政府卫生署决定将中央防疫处迁回北平，改名中央防疫实验处。原防疫处旧址已被日军破坏，必须重建。国民政府不给建设经费，汤飞凡从联合国善后救济总署拨到几批面粉和一些剩余物质，又从美国医药援华会那里捐到一批仪器设备，新址于 1947 年增建了抗生素车间和研究室（后发展成为中国医学科学院抗生素研究所）。1949 年防疫处改名为中华人民共和国卫生部生物制品研究所，汤飞凡继续担任所长。

7. 沈其震：《中央卫生研究院成立四年来的工作概况》，《科学通报》1954 年 10 月号，第 33 页。

8. 《中央卫生研究院举行第一次学术论文报告会》，《健康报》1956 年 3 月 2 日，第 1 版。

9. 《向科学进军》，《健康报》1956 年 3 月 2 日，第 1 版。

10. 《卫生部决定加强医学科学研究力量，原中央卫生研究院更名为中国医学科学院》，《健康报》1956 年 8 月 5 日，第 1 版。

11. Henry E. Sigerit，《苏联的医学和保健》，宫乃泉译，华东医务生活社，1950 年，第 282－286 页。

12. 《苏联医学科学院第八次会议》，《科学通报》1954 年 1 月号，第 67 页。

13. 施忠道：《苏联医学科学院建院四十年》，《国外医学（社会医学分册）》1987 年第 3 期，第 128－185 页。

14. George C. Guins, "The Academy of Sciences of the U. S. S. R. ," *The Russian Review*, Vol. 12, No. 4（Oct. , 1953），pp. 269－278.

15. 《迅速开展科学的研究工作》，《健康报》1956 年 3 月 30 日，第 1 版。

16. 朱锡萤：《医学科学战线上的生力军》《健康报》1956 年 10 月 9 日，第 1 版。

17. Henry E. Sigerit，《苏联的医学和保健》，第 286 页。

18. 施忠道：《苏联医学科学院建院四十年》，《国外医学（社会医学分册）》1987 年第 3 期，第 128－185 页。

19. 时任中国医学科学院长的沈其震（1906－1993），就读于同济大学医学院、中山大学医学院。1927 年他留学日本，获东京帝国大学医学院医学博士学位，1931 年回国后在天津开诊所。1937 年他参加新四军，1941 年加入中共并赴延安，任新四军军医处处长、卫生部部长等职。1956 年第一批中国科学院的学部委员。

20. 《郭沫若在政协第二届全国委员会第三次全体会议上的发言》，《人民日报》1957 年 3 月 20 日，第 3 版。

21. 新华社《集中力量研究防治血吸虫病，聂荣臻向医学界提出建议》，《人民日报》1957 年 4 月 18 日，第 7 版。

22. 中国协和医科大学编：《中国协和医科大学校史（1917－1987）》，第 52－53 页。

23. E. B Chain , "Report on Visit to China April 25 th to June 2nd 1961," Advisory Council on Scientific Policy S. P. , Foreign Office Files China, 1949－1980, FO 371／158432, p. 3；中文翻译可参阅（英）钱恩：《访华报告》，张民军、程力 译注，《中国科技史杂志》第 37 卷，第 1 期（2016 年），第 48－63 页。

24. 刘德培、刘谦主编：《邓家栋画传》，中国协和医科大学出版社，2007 年，第 78 页。

25. 张之强：《我的一生》，自印本，出版单位不详，2006 年，第 212 页。

26. 张敏卿：《延安时期中国共产党发展科技事业的思想和政策》，《自然辩证法研究》第 21 卷，第 1 期，2005 年 1 月，第 93－95 页。

27. 《破除迷信，解放思想，使医学教育跨上千里马》，《健康报》1958 年 6 月 21 日，第 2 版。

28. 吴之理：《一个军医的自述》，华夏出版社，2004 年，第 59 页。

29. 中国协和医科大学编：《中国协和医科大学校史 1917－1987》北京科学技术出版社，1987 年，第 52 页。

30. 张之强：《我的一生》，第 223 页。

31. 章央芬：《自豪的回忆》，华夏出版社，2004 年，第 193 页。

32. 中国医学科学院、中国协和医科大学编：《外科医生黄家驷》，中国协和医科大学，2006 年，第 78 页。

33. 中国协和医科大学编：《中国协和医科大学校史 1917－1987》，第 49 页。

34. 中国医学科学院、中国协和医科大学编：《外科医生黄家驷》，第 78 页。

35. 实验形态学系、生理学系、生物化学系、病理学系组成实验医学研究所；由药用植物学系、药物化学系、药理学系组成药物药理研究所；由抗生素学系改建成抗生素研究所；由营养学系改建为营养研究所；由环境卫生学系改建为卫生研究所。

36. 协和医院、阜外医院、日坛医院、整形医院、实验研究所、药物研究所、劳动卫生研究所、抗菌素研究所、流行病研究所、皮肤病研究所、输血及血液学研究所、寄生虫病研究所、放射研究所、儿研所、仪器研究所、病毒研究所、情报研究室、医学中心图书馆、生物研究所、海南云南药物研究站。

37. 中国协和医科大学编：《中国协和医科大学校史（1917－1987）》，第 70 页。

38. 中国医学科学院、中国协和医科大学编：《外科医生黄家驷》，第 79 页。

39. 章央芬：《自豪的回忆》，第 163 页。

40. 章央芬：《自豪的回忆》，第 164－165 页。

41. 中国医学科学院党委会：《中国医学科学院关于筹办"中国医学院"的初步议案（1959 年 4 月 22 日）》，中国医科大学教务处档案，协和医学院档案馆，案卷号 3。

42. 中国协和医科大学编：《中国协和医科大学校史（1917－1987）》，第 59 页。

43. 董炳琨：《协和育才之路》，第 278 页、第 33 页。.

44. E. B Chain，"Report on Visit to China April 25th to June 2nd 1961"，p. 2，Foreign Office Files China（1949－1980），Marlborough Adam Matthew Digital Ltd，FO 371/158432.

Establishing and Strengthening the Chinese Academy of Medical Sciences (1956 – 1966)

Jiang Yuhong

Jiang Yuhong, associate professor of the School of Humanities and Social Sciences of Peking Union Medical College, Fulbright Research Visiting Scholar. She translated a number of books about the history of Peking Union Medical College, the history of China Medical Board and China's medical history, and a number of articles on the history of the PUMC.

Most research in the history of medicine, disease and health during the early era of People's Republic of China focused either on the research of specific diseases i. e. the eradication of schistosomiasis, and the prevention and control of other infectious diseases, or into specific phenomena or policies in the health care system, such as the "barefoot" doctors of the three-tiered rural health system. Few historical research focused on the development, evolution and complexities of the field of academic medical research in the People's Republic era. This article presents an in-depth exploration of the emergence of the Chinese Academy of Medical Sciences (CAMS).

Founded on August 11th, 1956, CAMS consolidated with Peking Union Medical College (PUMC) in 1957, thus positioning itself as China's top medical research institute. This paper is an investigation into how this top medical research institute came into being within the ideological environment of the 1950s in China which reflects the view of modern western medicine from both the top leaders in China and the medical community perspective. The investigation utilized pretinent Chinese newspapers and publications and drew on records from the Rockefeller Archive Center and those at Peking Union Medical College, including published memoirs of key people involved in the formation of CAMS.

The "Soviet Model", "Centralization" and "Central Planning" on Research Mechanism

Strengthening the system using a centralization strategy in the scientific research in China began in February 1956. This was led by Premier Zhou Enlai (周恩来) and, Vice Premiers; Chen Yi (陈毅), Li Fuchun (李富春) and Nie Rongzhen (聂荣臻). The Chinese Communist Party (CCP) formed a national planning committee for the scienceo. In the months that followed, the committee summoned over 600 scientists and technical specialists from different parts of the country and after many discussions and over the course of many meetings, the committee worked out the long-term plan for the development of science and technology between 1956 – 1967. In terms of medical and health research, the official plan stipulated specific goals, such as; research and development of new antibiotics and medical equipment, advancing the theory and practice of Traditional Chinese Medicine (TCM), to strengthen hygiene, and to develop protective and comprehensive measures as well as carry out prevention and treatment of the major illnesses that related to labor and toxicology.

Believed to be of primary importance in strengthening the health system was the eradication and prevention of parasitic and infectious diseases which significantly added to the burden of disease and threatened people's lives on a daily basis, such as; schistosomiosis, malaria, kala-azar, filariasis, hook-worm, encephalitis, plague, smallpox, venereal diseases etc. Centralized planning at this time emphasized the principle that scientific research in China must follow CCP's direction. It commented that, "with the greatest resources, strengthen the Chinese Academy of Sciences, making it the train ahead, a leader upgrading the scientific level of the whole country and training new man power. "[1]

Establishing first-class scientific research institutions at a national level, required all scientific research to be directly controlled by the CCP following the original Soviet Union Model. China adopted this strategy and the 'one-sided' policy during the early 1950s, when the Soviet Union and China had become allies. Therefore, with the exception of government agencies and the military, the CCP executed a top-down policy of learning from the Soviet Union in aspects of culture, education and scientific research. Xue Gongzhuo （薛公绰）, president of Beijing Medical College in 1954, and later vice president of Chinese Academy of Medical Sciences recalled that one of the top leaders of CCP, Liu Shaoqi （刘少奇） advised him to learn from the Soviet model, to maintain good relations with Soviet specialists; and if the relationship went wrong, the Chinese people in charge of the relationship （justified in their actions or not）, will always be punished. [2] So PUMC, which had enjoyed "Gold standard" research at that time, had to follow suit.

PUMC mirrored the Soviet model, forming teaching and research offices and developing curricula and teaching plans identical to that delivered across the Soviet Union. In 1953, in order to master the Russian Language, the entire institute held 7 intensive training classes to learn Russian, each lasting for 20 days. A total of 622 faculty members and research fellows attended. In addition, 12 departments were involved tirelessly in translating Soviet medical journals from Russian into Chinese. [3] From 1956 – 1957, 12 senior Soviet scientists with advanced academic standing, including the director of Institute of Antibiotics were sent to CAMS as experts. At the same time, CAMS sent 38 research fellows to the Soviet Union for advanced training. [4]

Before 1956, the only medical research institute at the top national level that still bore the "centralized" name was the National Institutes of Health, based in Beijing. The precursor of the institute was the Central Health Experiment Institute (中央卫生实验院) of the Republic era in Nanjing. After the foundation of People's Republic, the institute was taken over by the CCP. In 1950, the Ministry of Health of China held the First National Health Conference and made decisions to enhance medical research. Approved by the central government, the institute moved the headquarters from Nanjing to Beijing and consolidated with the Beijing branch. In October, it was officially named the Central Health Research Institute, with only two affiliates remained elsewhere: the Parasite Institute remained in Nanjing and the Malaria Institute in Hainandao Island.

In 1954, eight research institutes were established and affiliated with the Central Health Research Institute. The remaining six were in Beijing, including: Department of Nutrition, Department of Microbiology, Health Engineering Department, Pharmacology Department, Pathology Office, and TCM Medical and Pharmacology Research Institute. There were 207 professional staff at that time, thirty of whom were research assistants or higher. " In addition, there were 13 extramural specialists from related institutes of higher learning and research institutes conducting research here. "[5] From February 23 to 25, 1956, the institute held the first academic workshop. Fifty articles were submitted, and over three hundred people attended, including professionals and Soviet specialists in Beijing. [6] As a kind of token from the top leaders, the Health Daily on the same day published an editorial entitled, ' Marching Toward Science', which gave special mention to the Central Health Research Institute answering the call from central government to drive science. In order to catch up with innovative scientific standards from around the world, the Central Health Research Institute revealed some achievements. [7]

In August 1956, the central government realized the development of Chinese medical science ought to catch up with international advanced levels, as soon as possible. In order to strengthen the scientific research workforce, the government renamed the Central Health Experimental Institute the Chinese Academy of Medical Sciences[8], which was again modeled on the Soviet model of nationalising medical science research. The Soviet Academy of Medical Sciences was founded in 1944. The predecessor was the National People's Health Care Research Institute and the National Institute of Experimental Medicine established by the Soviet People's Health Committee. On October 15, 1932, the Soviet People's Health Committee decided to reorganize the National Institute of Experimental Medicine as the Soviet Union's Experimental Medicine Institute. Then, the Soviet Academy of Medical Sciences consolidated all medical research institutes scattered around the Soviet Union and as the world's largest high-end medical science research institution, fell under the Soviet government's jurisdiction. This organizational model was adhered to by all the medical research institutions in the union.

In post-war Soviet Union, medical experts and scientists were relatively scarce, and so the Academy trained large numbers of senior staff and improved medical professional skills, which not only ensured their own needs, but also provided the country with a large number of medical and health leaders in a relatively short time. From 1945 to 1946, the Academy established twenty-five research institutes, with 60 full-time academicians.[9] In 1953, when the eighth academic conference was held, there were ninety-nine academicians, 132 correspondence academicians, and over 6,000 full-time scientific researchers.[10] In order to follow the latest trends in the development of medical sciences, the Academy established the Institute of Cardiovascular Surgery in 1956, and planned to establish the first scientific committee for a single disease i. e. the Coordinating Committee for the Study of Malignant Tumors which was formally established in 1959.[11]

The most noteworthy feature of this nationalized medical science research system was the "centralization" authority and "planning".[12] For example, in

1947, the Soviet Academy of Medical Sciences produced a first five year plan for medical science research, and the Academy not only carried out a large number of research projects, but also made further plans, gave guidance and business supervision for the promotion of scientific research tasks throughout the country. Similarly, the Chinese Academy of Medical Sciences effectively implemented planning, controlling and the prioritization of medical science research projects. In Health Daily, there was an editorial by a senior health official who stated, 'We must solve the current problems of industrialization and agricultural collectivization. In medical science, a series of new questions have been raised. The leadership under CCP provides a superior guarantee system.

In comparison, the editorial in the Health Daily pointed out that during the republic era while under reactionary control of Kuomingtang, research institutes of all kinds were incomplete, poorly equipped, and the workforce was dispersed. Although there was no denying that in that era, many scientists were still greatly passionate in scientific research, such a social system could not obtain government support. Sientists were self-governed and conducted research according to their personal interests. This was undoubtedly a way of craftsmanship, however; the result led to a lack of planning and integration. This kind of research is detached from the requirement of the entire society and the needs of the people, hence little was achieved. " [13]

One problem remained which was that even though CAMS was essentially crowned with the 'China' title and therefore represented the nation, CAMS was not sufficiently endowed with influential power to lead and coordinate medical scientific research for the entire country. There was no apparent national leader in terms of research in any specific field and CAMS had a shortage of influential scholars. In October of the same year, CAMS enrolled over 130 graduates from medical schools and comprehensive universities around China, as well as over 90 graduates from professional schools of secondary education level. A news report said that, "It was unprecedented in the history of medical science in our country to have so many people rush into one medical research institute within one year. "[14] As compared to the academic influence of the leadership of Soviet Academy of Medical Sciences, almost all of the leaders were medical experts established in their respective fields of study. The first President Dr. Nikolai Burdenko was the pioneer of neurosurgery in the Soviet Union and had previously been Minister of the Military Health at the Ministry of the Red Army as well as Chair of the Soviet Health Care Medical Science Committee. [15] The President of the Academy in 1956, Dr. Baku Lev, was one of the founders in cardiovascular surgery in the Soviet Union, [16] while at CAMS, there were no equivalent leaders either in terms of academic influence or research areas. [17] As David Lampton put it "No new scholars with the visibility of the older generation have emerged. It is precisely this hiatus that has provided the conditions for the continual re-emergence of elderly academicians and scientist, such as; Huang Chia-ssu (Huang Jiasi), Kuo Mo-jo, Chou P'ei-yuan, and Fei Hsiao-t'ung. "[18]

In order to bolster "centralization" and "central planning", CCP leaders tried to coordinate other national level research institutions to create a CAMS with more academic influence and stronger leadership. On March 20th 1957, Guo Moruo (郭沫若), the then director of Chinese Academy of Sciences (CAS) emphasized in a report the importance of coordination of scientific researches. He thought in medical research, the most significant problems were the coordination between military and civilians, and between TCM and Western medicine. Guo also pointed out that, "Now, CAMS has 15 departments and has done a lot of work, but it lacks backbone leaders and equipment. "[19] One month later on April 16th, Nie Rongzhen, the then Vice Premier who had a marshal rank and was in charge of national level science research, such as nuclear weaponary and man-made satellites, gave a speech. Nie thought that the current medical research should broaden in scope, as there was no concentrated power, no collaboration, and as a result manpower and material resources were wasted, which hindered the implementation of further research. He ordered that it follow the principle of "centralizing the power" and restructure the institutions, as soon as possible. [20] As a specific implementation of the order, initially the central leadership considered that the Chinese Academy of Medical Sciences and Peking Union Medical College be coordinated and cooperate for a period of time before consolidating into one institution.

By the end of July, Nie Rongzhen could no longer wait to change the 'cooperation' strategy, of the two institutions into a full 'merger'. On 3rd August, the Ministry of Health announced the name list of the Preparatory Committee for the consolidation of the two institutions, and wanted to accelerate the process by strengthening the leadership of the Party. On October 18, the CCP Beijing Municipal Committee approved the establishment of an interim party committee to promote the merger of CAMS and China Union Medical College. On November 25th, the Ministry of Health issued an official document[21] confirming the merger. China Union Medical College (now PUMC) discontinued enrolling students, and the newly named "Chinese Academy of Medical Sciences", was to be considered the pinnacle of Chinese medical practice and research.

Soviet Influence, Yan'an Tradition, and the "Old PUMC"

Although CAMS had been established according to the Soviet Model, the collective research model based upon "academic bureaucracy" such as that in the Soviet Union could not be simply copied. The Chinese had access to the Soviet Medical Research model dating back to 1951 when China sent medical students to Soviet Union. At the time, when CAMS was established in 1956, many of students studying in the Soviet Union already finished their studies and returned to China and were actively involved in scientific research. In June 1956, when CAS summoned scientists to develop a 12 year science plan, at least four of the twenty two people involved in the medical group had studied in the Soviet Union. However; Chinese culture inherently dictates a tradition of qualification and length of service deciding the hierarchy and seniority and that of respecting seniors and order. Most researchers at that time were young and emerging assistant researchers with MPhils in their early 30s. So, when facing 50 and 60 year old professors who held either a Ph. D or were research fellows in Europe or US and were already established associate professors or full professors, they were like freshmen students meeting their mentors. The young and emerging scientists had only soft voices with no authority.

The key issue was that the Chinese scholars at that time did not think that Soviet medical research was state-of-the-art, nor was it worth emulating. In 1961, E. B. Chain (1906 – 1979), the British biochemist and Nobel Laureate, invited by CAS and Chinese Medical Association (中华医学会) to visit China, and made extensive contact with professionals from the scientific and medical community in Beijing and Shanghai and exchanged views on Soviet medical science. Chain pointed out that in the past 40 years, the Soviet Union had not invented an important new drug in any of the areas of pharmaceutical chemistry, such as; narcotics, analgesics, thiamines, antibiotics, vitamins or hormones. Chain even said that nowadays the most interesting areas of organic chemistry, such as; high molecular polymer-proteins, nucleic acid and synthetic plastics, and resin research were all developed in the West. In these areas, "the Russian contribution was either completely absent or mediocre quality."[22] Chinese scholars shared this view.

When PUMC fell under the leadership of the People's Liberation Army (PLA) (1952 – 1956), Professor Deng Jiadong (邓家栋) was a member of the Ministry of Defense delegation to visit the Soviet Union. What impressed upon him most of all was that the standard was not as high as he had imagined.[23] Zhang Zhiqiang (1915 – 2005) (张之强), the Party Secretary and the most senior leader at PUMC at that time also recalled: "The Soviet's medical level was not at all higher than that of the PUMC, however; under strong political pressure, PUMC had completely copied the Soviet model."

Zhang also said, "This aroused a serious disturbance among the PUMC professors, although they did not dare say it outright. I think that it is inappropriate to change PUMC this way and I have reported my opposition to the leader of PLA's General Logistic Department and have asked for reconsideration of the decision, but was criticized by them. "[24]

A triumphant side which had overturned the ruling of the National government of Nanjing, CCP, in the process of the seizure of power, had developed their own scientific research model. After the Central Party arrived at Yan'an, the Party, in a very short period of time had made great progress in both medical and healthcare and had established the Central Hospital, Border Region Hospital, Bethune International Peace Hospital, the Eighth Route Army Field Hospital (the hospital directly affiliated to Military Committee), and the reputable Asian Students' Rehabilitation Homes, totaling over 50 medical and health units. These institutions not only served the party and government institutions of the region, providing military services, but also served the local people, and had greatly improved the people's well-being. In addition, in May 1939 the CCP set up the Natural Science Research Institute in Yan'an. In January 1940 it was renamed the Yan'an Academy of Natural Sciences.

At that time, Yan'an was surrounded by the Kuomintang army, so that economic level was low. Although the research institute was the highest CCP academic research unit, it was not competent to carry out advanced scientific research, only making some practical imitation in order to strengthen the struggle against the enemy. Most of the natural science workers who worked in Yan'an at that time took charge in the scientific research after the establishment of the People's Republic. In November 1949, the Chinese Academy of Sciences was established on the basis of the Central Research Institute (Sinica) of the National Government, the Peking Research Institute and the Yan'an Academy of Natural Sciences. "The scientific seeds sown by the CCP in Yan'an period have finally yielded fruit, and the CCP's scientific cause has entered a new stage of development," said a researcher. [25]

In a sense, since 1957, CAMS was built based on this "Yan'an" tradition. Even though the CCP's most senior leaders had emphasized learning from Soviet Union, to cling to "CCP's unified centralized leadership" had been strengthened in every part of lives, serving the Chinese characteristics. The Soviet Union adopted a localized system of control of the communist party. As an institute at the apex of the hierarchy, the Soviet Academy of Medical Sciences elected a president by ballot of votes from academicians. The Communist Party's leadership over the academy belonged to Moscow, and the administrative power the party held was not as important as the president. In addition, the academician policy stipulated that every decision should be made by ballot so that it ensured the autonomy of the scientists in their scientific activities. However, such a model was always likely to be criticized in China.

In Health Daily issued in June, 1958, there was a speech given by Ji Zhongpu (季钟朴) (1913 – 2002), the Director General of Department of Medical Education of Ministry of Health at that time stating "The Soviet has a system in which the president of an institution is in charge, while the Communist Party organization of the institution plays the role of guardian. Also, the academic conferences are predominantly composed of faculty discussing major issues of the institute, and enjoying great power. However, our country is different from the Soviet Union in that they have eradicated the capitalist class and faculties are both politically correct and professional specialized, so that the party leadership is very stable within institutions. [26]

Wu Zhili (吴之理) (1915 – 2008), then the president of Shanghai Second Military Medical University recalled, Soviet specialists recommending that the institution form a faculty committee, and Wu himself liked this idea "However, there was an opposing voice at the meeting of Party Committee, claiming that in the future the party's leadership will be a dummy. "[27] Also, as Zhang Zhiqiang, the then Party Secretary of CAMS and most senior leader in decision hierarchy put it, "At that time, the whole Party was in an era of 'Party Control Everything', whatever the issue is big or small, the Party Secretary would decide. "[28] which also meant that although the Chinese Academy of Medical Sciences had been established based on the Soviet Academy of Medical Sciences model, it's decision-making system and management structure did not completely mirror the Soviet model, and indeed formed its own unique model.

Modern medical research in China can be traced back to the Rockefeller Foundation's establishment of PUMC in 1917. PUMC was built based on the Johns Hopkins education model. With 'Science for humanity' as it's mission statement, PUMC at that time provided the most up-to-date scientific research instruments, equipment, laboratories, library, as well as the superior facilities for living, studying and research, which was not only the best in China at that time, but also in the Far East. During this golden age of the institute from the early 1920s to 40s, a great many leading medical scientists and researchers from America and Europe came to PUMC to teach and research. In addition, PUMC held a few international academic seminars and published many quality research papers, hence PUMC was regarded as the top medical research institute in all Asia. When the Republic government at Nanjing elected the academician of Academia Sinica (中央研究院) in 1948, six of the seven academician elected in the field of medicine were affiliated with PUMC, either faulty or alumni.

In June 1955, when CAS formed its academician department (学部), they had already considered candidates' political and ideological backgrounds, and had selected a few who joined in the CCP's early years' revolutionary efforts and formed a very close relationship with CCP as well as holding leading positions. Among the 16 academicians in the medical division, nine were from

PUMC. This again demonstrates that even after the of founding PRC, the influence of PUMC was still strong. When the central government decided to transfer PUMC from military governance under the Ministry of Health on September 1, 1956, Party Secretary Zhang Zhiqiang reported to Ministry of Health that he was particularly worried about the candidates for the leader of CAMS. Zhang thought that in a new institute consolidated through the merger of various organizations required a leader from the 'Old PUMC'. If not, Zhang thought it would make it hard to convince people of organizational goals which would result in complicated interpersonal relationships and discontent in people's minds. Zhang thought that if the new leader could be "transferred from other institutions who is an outsider, it would make the work less complicated".

Zhang later nominated Huang Jiasi (黄家驷) (1906 – 1984), the then Vice President of Shanghai Medical College to be the new leader of CAMS. [29] Unlike Li Zongen (李宗恩), Huang Jiasi was more likely to follow the political line and to be obedient. In winter 1950, when the Korea War broke out, unlike Li who hesitated and was indecisive about whether China should enter the war, Huang proactively signed up for the Shanghai Volunteer Medical Operation Team and became the Director General of the team and the captain for the second team. In 1952, Huang Jiasi was already middle aged and had therefore already not in the ideal time for foreign languages learning. However, in order to respond to the CCP's call to 'learn from the Soviets', he started to learn Russian from scratch in his spare time. In 1954, he painstakingly translated and published Thoracic Operation written by a Soviet scholar. In 1955, he was appointed a member of CAS, and started to chair work for 12 year Plan for National Science and Technology Development. Huang's personality was more "cautious to everything, avoiding making troubles" [30]. At an era when "fighting with others has endless pleasures" was advocated, Huang, even though he was already in a very senior position, had never overtly blamed anyone. In 1961, he chaired an academic meeting and invited scholars to introduce professional theories that were perhaps considered politically incorrect and had been totally rejected, and endeavored to "correct the wrong inclination of a partial misunderstanding that confused learning from the Soviet academic ideas with political standpoint". [31]

The Arrangement and Operating Model of "One Institute, Two Names"

Huang was a graduate of class of '33 PUMC, and his appointment at CAMS marked the emergence of the 'Old PUMC' at the top medical research arena in China. After all, at the beginning of the founding of PRC, when the relationship between Sino-US governments had deteriorated and the two countries had become enemies, PUMC was labeled "The Fortress of American's Cultural Aggression to China" and was therefore marginalized. PUMC was forced to stop recruiting students, then fell under the control of the military, and started to admit extramural trainees, responsible for training the old carders of those who joined communist revolutionary activities when they were very young' however; many held only very low level of education. In addition, in order to strengthen the military's medical capacity building, a large number of the PUMC clinicians and specialists of basic medicine were transferred to establish the NO. 301 PLA Hospital. This was given as a direct order from the CCP's higher authority, and also to other medical institutes.

At that time, even though scientific research had not ceased at PUMC, due to constant leadership and priority changes, most of the research targeted meeting the needs of clinical diagnosis and solving applicable problems. Statistics show that "In 1955, among the 361 research topics accumulated from various departments, 7.5% were directly related to military troops, 4.1% related to TCM and herbal medicine, 14.6% were research into advanced neurological movements and theory, 52.2% were for clinical diagnostics and treatments, 21.6% of others." [32] When Huang Jiasi became the President of CAMS, he made a thorough investigation into the research projects and activities of the affiliated institutes, and was keen on the revival of the advanced medical scientific research of the 'Old PUMC'. He pointed out that CAMS "must do research to answer cutting-edge questions. It is an issue of the present tasks and tasks for tomorrow. "[33]

To achieve the vision of strengthening the national priority set in scientific development agenda, CAMS began institutional consolidation in order to strengthen its capacity by absorbing other institutes into CAMS. Therefore, from January to June 1958, by the arrangement of the Ministry of Health, the following research institutions became affiliates of CAMS; Beijing Institute of Dermatology/Beijing Epidemic Research (the predecessor of Institute of Dermatology at Nanjing), Beijing Hospital, and Beijing Second Hospital which had been approved by Vice Minister Nie Rongzhen. Beijing Chest Hospital also merged with the Beijing Second Hospital and then changed its name to "Fuchengmenwai Hospital" which is the precursor for the China Cardiovascular Research Center – Fu Wai Hospital as it is known today. The Plastic Surgery Hospital, and The Blood Transfusion and Hematology research Institute (The former People's Liberation Army thirteen military medical school), Labor Protection Scientific Research Institute and the Ministry of Health's Labor Hygiene Institute consolidated were also absorbed by CAMS.

On August 16, the Ministry of Health also ordered that the original ten departments of CAMS be consolidated and converted into five research institutes. Until October 1962, the Chinese Academy of Medical Sciences formed the so-called "national team" in advanced medical research, including the top four hospitals of China i. e. PUMC hospital, Fuwai Hospital, Ritan Hospital (the precursor of Cancer Hospital of CAMS), as well as Institutes specialized in basic medicine research, hygiene and public health, antibiotics, epidemics, skin diseases, blood transfusion and hematology, parasitic diseases and bio engineering, covering almost all the major research areas in medicine.

A large number of the teaching faculty were transferred to research institutes, aiming at strengthening the power of scientific research. Except the Institute of Medical Instruments and Equipment (Tianjin) established in 1958 and Institute of Radiation Medicine (Tianjin) which were initiated by CAMS, all other institutes being absorbed into the CAMS were done so through a top-down decision from the Ministry of Health and was geared toward consolidating CAMS as a complete package with staff and facilities. This reflects the ethos of the era of "gathering all the forces together to do great things" and under the mechanisms embedded by the government strategy of "using the power of the whole nation", from 1958 to 1966, CAMS focused on scientific research which aimed at solving China's medical and health problems.

Of particular note during this period was that in November 1958, Medical Biology Institute, located in Kunming made great effort at the development of polio vaccine. On January 10, 1961, Premier Zhou Enlai inspected the institute and asked detailed questions about vaccine production and scientific research, and examined the whole experimental production process. In 1963, the institute successfully developed the first oral pill formulation of live attenuated polio vaccine and put into mass production and usage. In addition, CAMS succeeded in carrying out leprosy epidemic research, China's first heart mitral valve insufficiency repair operation and successful treatment of choriocarcinoma. At the same time, the CAMS also established China's first cytogenetic research group, and initiated China's human cytogenetics and tumor cytogenetics research.

Meanwhile, another important task for CAMS, or more accurately for the "old PUMC", was to promote medical scientific research and medical teaching to complement one another. Initially, the CAMS leadership and administrative structure had no specific administrative department designating for teaching. Most staff engaged in scientific research and were almost never involved in teaching. The question was whether CAMS should run a medical school, and there were of course contradictory opinions. A great number of people in leadership positions were against running a medical school. As early as 1957, when he served as Director of the Department of Internal Medicine of PUMC Hospital, Zhang Xiaoqian (张孝骞), proposed to restore the 'Old PUMC' s' long-term medical education program and wrote a letter to the relevant government departments. In his letter, Zhang expressed concern that the talent pool was depleted after PUMC ceased enrollment in 1953. Zhang said that, resuming the medical school with the related duties such as teaching and mentoring would not weaken the research strengths. Zhang stressed: "Frankly speaking, teaching is a burden ……but teaching and learning do not contradict research, but rather they are complementary. This is why scientists at CAMS are happy to teach in colleges and universities. "[34]

In addition to Zhang Xiaoqian, Huang Jiasi held the same opinions and tired to advise senoir leaders of the Central Committee of the CCP. Huang never thought that the study of clinical medicine should be confined to clinical observation or case analysis, rather it should include the objective theoretical research so as to conduct innovative work. Huang also made it clear that when running the 8-year curriculum program, CAMS should "commit to the mutual promotion of teaching and research, and enrich the scientific research system through the establishment of the medical school, while the growth of medical students and graduate students can strengthen the scientific research force of CAMS. "[35] As a result of these efforts, the second Standing Committee meeting of CAMS held on May 5, 1959 passed a protocol for the "Preliminary Plan for the Preparation of the Chinese Medical University (PUMC)", and appointed Huang to lead the project and the Preparatory Committee. Then, with the support of the Vice Premier Lu Dingyi as well as other senior leaders of the Party Committee of Ministry of Health, the Party Committee of Beijing Municipal Government and the Party Committee of the Chinese Academy of Medical Sciences engaged in discussion and finally agreed that the Chinese Academy of Medical Sciences should make preparations based on the original PUMC model, and would therefore resume the eight year medical program but rename the school as 'China Medical University'. Huang Jiasi was to serve as concurrent president.

Eventually, on June 20 and August 8, the Ministry of Health and the State Council approved the plan, respectively. On September 5, 1959, China Medical University held a founding ceremony and school opening ceremony at Dong Dan San Tiao Auditorium, marking a new milestone in the history, the co-operation of CAMS and PUMC, which meant that clinical education and advanced research would be conducte under a single organization. This unique arrangement of the mechanism of the Institution, with one leadership team (party), one set administrative body, but with two names, and dual tasks.

This duality of purpose actually created a lot of problems during the initial period of CAMS & PUMC. At the time, the newly established medical school enrolled 60 new students who had attained high scores in the national college entrance examination. New students went to Biology Department of Peking University to study a premedical curricula for three years. Then, from the biology departments of five comprehensive universities: Peking University, Fudan University, Nankai University etc. 30 undergraduate students were enrolled to the newly established medical school to study basic medicine for four years. The Party Committee simply allocated these students to the Institute of Experimental Medicine, without first establishing a permanent full-time teaching department. Teachers at that time were all part-timers, their main duties were in research rather than teaching. Logistics was a problem and teaching laboratories were borrowed from research institutes, while the teaching equipment had been moved from one institute into the other. Teachers handed out the teaching materials during or after class. As a result, less than two months after opening the "new" school, students had begun to complain and many asking to return to their original universities. [36]

In fact, the Party Committee of CAMS had not reached consensus as to whether it should run the medical school, let alone on how to run the school, effectively. Most party leaders paid more attention to scientific research rather than teaching. At weekly routine meetings held on Wednesdays and Saturdays, the party committee only discussed problems that the 13 research institutions encountered. Teaching was never on the agenda for discussion and only in rare cases was teaching mentioned because most of the committee members did not know what happened to the medical program, they found it difficult to express their views. Fortunately, Zhang Huifen who had served as vice president of Shanghai Second Medical College, was appointed Dean of medical education in 1961, and became a member of the Standing Committee of the Party at CAMS, so that another leader entered into the leadership in addition to Huang Jiasi. Both set organizational goals for the education program at CAMS & PUMC. Working very well together, Huang Jiasi and Zhang Huifen persuaded the leadership to agree on setting up a personnel department for the medical school.

Gradually, the leadership approved establishing an independent president's office for the school and agreed on setting up a full-time administrative and logistic departments, specifically for the medical school which included; teaching materials office, printing department, photography workshop, student library, and canteen management office.

Then, in spring of 1963 the medical college building was completed and all students, offices for teaching and research had finally relocated. Teaching standards and quality greatly improved. In 1964, Ministry of Health organized an evaluation for teaching quality of the National Key Medical Schools, and PUMC's medical students were the best. In 1965, the school held a meeting to exchange and summarize teaching experiences which was highly valued by the Ministry of Health and affiliated schools. The school planned to make it a prerequisite for students to be mentored and guided by a specific professor. Students were to carry out an independent medical research project at the final year of their studies. Given that China was in alliance with the Soviet Union and other Eastern European socialist countries, the planning made a commitment that outstanding students would be sent to some allied socialist countries for advanced training. Also, it was the first time that planning proposed that "individuals can also be sent to the capitalist countries to study."[37]

Conclusion

From 1959, the organization consisting of two institutions with two recognizable seals, shared the same administration, under one Central Committee of the CCP. The co-existence of the Academy with the University was favorable for strengthening scientific research and the training of graduate students. In addition, as the "national team" under the direct leadership of the Ministry of Health, it also strengthened the leading position of CAMS and PUMC as China's medical education and scientific research authority, while at the same time greatly promoting the improvement of China's medical and health undertakings.

Indeed, it was the establishment of CAMS that initiated an advanced medical professional community in China. Due to the joint efforts of "Old PUMC" and other distinguished scientists coming back from the Soviet Union, such as Gu Fangzhou" (顾方舟), (the former president of CAMS & PUMC and the inventor of oral polio pills), the institution contributed to many breakthroughs in China's medicine and well-being. CAMS & PUMC have laid a solid foundation for the evolution of the new type of institution up until the 1980s but also right up until today.

Of course, the Chinese always say that 'advantages and disadvantages coexist'. If we should learn from the lessons of merging and establishing CAMS

& PUMC, we can find that the administrative power of the day was too strongly embedded in scientific research and teaching processes. It inevitably caused some 'spur of moment', According to Dong Bingkun (董炳琨) who joined the communist revolution in 1939 and worked in the No. 120 health division of the Eighth Route Army, and later serving as vice president of the Chinese Academy of Medical Sciences, the decades of experiences demonstrates that the Intitution's "one body with two names" arrangement made it hard for a complete education program for undergraduates. In his view, "This loose federal management system could not concentrate on teaching tasks, not to the execution of PUMC's advantages and no demonstration of PUMC's characteristics, it was even more difficult ..."[38]

During this period, China's great achievements in the atomic nucleus explosion, artificial satellite, insulin synthesis, hybrid rice, and even the Nobel Prize in 2010 - artemisinin and other projects were made in the same manner which was, in the shortest time using the power of the entire country. Organizing the "General Assembly War" to solve challenges related to the practical application in national defense and therefore people's lives. However, some of the most original discoveries in medical research, such as DNA double helix structure, genetic code, oncogene, gene regulation in development, apoptosis, learning and memory mechanisms almost all originated from individual's curiosity and accidental discovery in basic scientific research, which is analogous to "just sow without asking about the harvest". In contrast, the idea of establishing CAMS and the merger with PUMC, emphasized the collective co-ordination of the broader system and the central government's will might result in a certain human and material waste, while largely ignoring the cultivation of innovative researchers.

When the British Nobel Laureate visited China from April to June 1961, he pointed out that regarding to the scientific institutions he visited in China, what impressed him most was the high standard of researchers' intellect and knowledge, which demonstrated a vast contrast to the extremely low level of innovative research work. To him, "even some scientists I would call brilliant, the subjects people worked in were mostly of applied nature, but of a low level."[39] When considering the current situation from this perspective, learning from the establishment, as well developing an understanding of the early organizational dynamics between CAMS & PUMC is necessary in order to embed medical innovation and develop strategic planning to meet the needs of the Chinese population, now and in the future.

Bibliography

1. "Long-term planning of Science and Technology development 1956 – 1967" (Amendment Draft), http://www.most.gov.cn/ztzl/gjzcqgy/zcqgylshg/200508/t20050831_ 24440. htm

2. Peng Ruicong (彭瑞聪): *Remembering of Xue Gongzhuo at Beijing Medical University* (《回忆薛公绰在北医》) (Xue Gongzuo Memorial Collection edited by Xu Shouren (徐守仁), Beijing, Beijing Science and Technology Press, 2008, p. 77.

3. *The History of Peking Union Medical College* (1917 – 1987) (《中国协和医科大学校史 (1917 – 1987)》, compiled by Peking Union Medical College, Beijing Science and Technology Press, 1987, p. 49.

4. Shen Qizhen (沈其震), "Appreciate Soviet Union, Learn from its Advanced Experiences, Realize the Great Leap in Medical Science Work" (《感谢苏联援助, 实现医学科学研究工作的更大跃进》), *CAMS Newspaper* (《中国医学科学院院报》), Nov. 5, 1958, p. 1.

5. Shen Qizhen, "Four-Year's Working Report of National Institute of Health Since its Establishment" (《中央卫生研究院成立四年来的工作概况》), *Science Bulletin* (《科学通报》), October 1954, p. 33.

6. "Central Health Research Institute's first Academic Seminar" (《中央卫生研究院举行第一次学术论文报告会》), *Health Daily* (《健康报》), Mar. 2, 1952, p. 1.

7. Marching toward Science (《向科学进军》), *Health Daily*, March 2nd , 1956, p. 1.

8. The Ministry of Health Decided to Strengthen the medical science research power. The former Central Health Research Institute changed its name to Chinese Academy of Medical

Sciences, Health Daily, August 5th, 1956, p. 1.

9. Henry E. Sigerit, Soviet's Medicine and Health Care, translated by Gong Naiquan（宫乃泉）, Huadong Medical Workers Life's Society（华东医务生活社）, 1950, p. 282 – 286.

10. The Eighth Academy of Medical Conference, Science Notification Report, January of 1954, p. 67.

11. Shi Zhongdao（施忠道）, The Forty Years of the Establishment of the Soviet Academy of Medical Sciences, Foreign Medicine（Social Medicine Volume）, vol. 3（1987）, p. 128 – 185.

12. George C. Guins, "The Academy of Sciences of the U. S. S. R. " *The Russian Review*, Vol. 12, No. 4（Oct. 1953）, p. 269 – 278.

13. "Speed Up Science Research Work"（《迅速开展科学的研究工作》）, *Health Daily*, Mar. 30th, 1956, p. 1.

14. Zhu Xiying, " The Fresh Troop in the Battle Front of Medical Science"（《医学科学战线上的生力军》）, *Health Daily*, Oct. 9th, 1956, p. 1.

15. Henry E. Sigerit, Soviet's Medicine and Health Care, p. 286.

16. Shi Zhongdao（施忠道）, The Forty Years of the Establishment of the Soviet Academy of Medical Sciences, Foreign Medicine（Social Medicine Volume）, vol. 3（1987）, p. 128 – 185.

17. Shen Qizhen（1906 – 1993）was the first President of the CAMS. He attended the Tongji University School of Medicine, and Sun Yat-sen University School of Medicine. In 1927 he studied in Japan at the Tokyo Imperial University School of Medicine and obtained a MD. In 1931, he worked in clinic in Tianjin. In 1937 he joined the New Fourth Army, and became a member of the Communist Party of China in 1941 and went to Yan'an. There , he served as director of the New Fourth Military Medical Department, Minister of Health and etc. In 1956, he was one of the academicians of Chinese Academy of Sciences.

18. David M. Lampton's（1978）"Performance and the Chinese Political System: A Preliminary Assessment of Education and Health Policies"（*The China Quarterly*, No. 75, Sep. , 1978, p. 536 ）

19. "Guo Moruo's Speech on the Third Plenary Meeting of Second Congress of Chinese People's Political Consultative Conference"（《郭沫若在政协第二届全国委员会第三次全体会议上的发言》）, *People's Daily*（《人民日报》）, Mar. 20th, 1957, p. 3.

20. Xinhua News Agency, Centralize the power in Schistosomiasis Research, Nei Rongzhen Raise Suggestions to the Medical Society（集中力量研究防治血吸虫病，聂荣臻向医学界提出建议）, People's Daily, April 18th, 1957, p. 7

21. PUMC Press, The History of Peking Union Medical College（1917-1987）, p. 52 –

53.

22. E. B. Chain, " Report on Visit to China April 25th to June 2nd 1961. " Advisory Council on Scientific Policy S. P. Foreign Files China, 1949 – 1980, FO 371/158432, P. 3 – 4.

23. Liu Depei, Liu Qian, *Deng Jiadong's Biography in Photo* (《邓家栋画传》), Peking Union Medical College Press, 2007, p. 78.

24. Zhang Zhiqiang, *My Life* (我的一生), Self printed, no record of press, 2006, p. 212.

25. Zhang Minqing (张敏卿), During the period of Yan'an the Thoughts and Policy of Development of Science and Technology of the Chinese Communist Party (《延安时期中国共产党发展科技事业的思想和政策》), Research of Dialectics of Nature (自然辨证法研究), Vol. 21, No. 1, Jan 2005, p. 93 – 95

26. "Eradicate Superstitions, Literate Thoughts, Push Medical Education Mount on the Swift Horse" (《破除迷信, 解放思想, 使医学教育跨上千里马》), *Health Daily*, June 21st, 1958, p. 2.

27. Wu Zhili, *A Military Doctor's Self Statement* (《一个军医的自述》), Huaxia Publishing House, 2004, p. 59.

28. Zhang Zhiqiang, *My Life*, p. 223.

29. Zhang Zhiqiang, My Life, Self printed, no record of press, 2006, p. 223.

30. Zhang Yangfen (章央芬), *Memory of Pride* (《自豪的回忆》), Huanxia Publishing House, 2004, p. 193.

31. CAMS/PUMC Editor, *Huang Jiasi-A Surgeon* (《外科医生黄家驷》), PUMC Press, 2006, p. 78.

32. *The History of Peking Union Medical College* (1917 – 1987), p. 49.

33. CAMS/PUMC Editor, *Huang Jiasi-A Surgeon*, p. 78.

34. PUMC, The History of PUMC 1917 – 1987, p. 70.

35. CAMS PUMC, Surgeon Huang Jiasi, p. 79.

36. Zhang Yangfen, Pride Memory, p. 163.

37. PUMC archive file 3, Party Committee of CAMS: CAMS Preliminary Proposal for the Preparation for Establishing the China's Medical College, April 22, 1959.

38. Dong Binkun, PUMC's Road to Talents (协和育才之路), PUMC Press, p. 278, p. 33.

39. E. B. Chain, "Report on Visit to China April 25th to June 2nd 1961, p. 2. Foreign Files China, 1949 – 1980, Marlborough Adam Mathew Digital, Ltd, FO 371/158432.

收归国有之后的北京协和医学院（1949－1985）

白玛丽（Mary Augusta Brazelton）

白玛丽，剑桥大学历史与科学哲学系科学、技术与医学全球研究中心讲师。她是现代中国科学和医学史学家，从耶鲁大学获得历史博士学位。

1951 年 1 月，中华人民共和国将协和收归国有。协和一直是中国西方生物医学的标志性机构，而当中国共产党（CPC）掌权时，协和也被当作美帝国主义的象征。1949 年后，中国共产党切断了其与美国及其他西方国家的外交关系，公开谴责这些政府在中国的"帝国主义"活动。[1]在全国各地的医学院校当中，有许多院校都与美国的创办者及资金资助有很密切的关系，这引发了一场紧急的冲突：在意识形态上，是否有可能将西方医学从西方文化和社会观念中区分开来？

历史学家高敏（Miriam Gross）和方小平阐明，尽管存在以下普遍认知，即中国共产党主要推崇中国医学传统，但是事实上，西方生物医学仍然对中华人民共和国早期的卫生政策、卫生运动和实践产生过重要影响。[2]然而，对于这些传统和影响在医学教育领域里的相互作用的探讨非常欠缺。[3]尽管协和停办了几次、更名几次，但在整个 20 世纪 50 年代期间，协和依然是一所高端医学教育与研究机构，这主要归于中国人民解放军的军管。本文揭示了在中华人民共和国早期，西方生物医学在协和存续下来的运行机制。大卫·M·兰普顿（David Lampton）认为，在 20 世纪 50 年代初期，中国卫生部对西方医学的支持，是重要的政治基础。[4]从 1952 年到 1956 年中国人民解放军在军管协和的期间，通过课程及政治改革等方式，其在保留协和的西方医学教育上发挥了至关重要的作用。在关键性的转折时期，协和为中国军事医学提供了人力、培训和资源。为了实现这些目标，中国人民解放军维护了协和的西方医学教育标准。

在本文中，本人调查了 1949 年至 1966 年间协和的教育和政治变化状况，并重点关注了 20 世纪 50 年代初期的关键阶段，此时也正好是这些变化开始时的时期。除了鼓励协和人参与抗美援朝和开展短期高级课程之外，中国人民解放军在协和开展了"三反"运动，同时也开展了思想改造、教师肃反等。在进行这些改革中，中国人民解放军把协和纳入不断壮大的军事医学研究与教育的基础建设中，其中协和的工作人员及其毕业生发挥主导作用。这些机构性的改变重塑了协和，使其在意识形态和政治上与其外国起源区分开来，但是依然在本质上致力于保持了西方生物医学的标准和实践。本文分析了学者们和西方观察者对协和的回顾性陈述、中国共产党机关出版发行的宣传资料以及学院教授撰写的文章。这些文件表明，在西方生物医学向公立机构转型过程中，协和保留着其代表国家级西方生物医学的标杆作用。

1952 年至 1956 年，中国人民解放军领导的巨大变革

中国教育部在 1951 年 1 月 20 日将协和收归国有，几乎没有遭到任何反对。但是，随着中华人民共和国建立全新的卫生政策和行政体系，协和同美国的联系以及其精英身份很快就成为政治问题。[5] 作为一所培养精英医学研究人员的著名学府，协和在卫生方面与平民主义的方式明显不匹配。后者强调服务群众，预防为主，中西医结合。[6] 国有化后，教育部副部长钱俊瑞鼓励协和的工作人员"彻底切断他们与美帝国主义的关系"，强调节俭和大众教育。[7] 卫生部和教育部在协和推进反美语境，但没有开展重大改革。例如，1933 年的协和毕业生邓家栋 1951 年在《人民日报》上发表文章称，协和的美国管理"充满了毒药"，试图"奴役人民"。[8] 在同一年，卫生部教育部将协和的教学语言从英文改为中文，并且，在 1951 年，卫生部将协和改名为中国协和医学院（以下亦简称为"协和"——编者注）。[9] 但总体来说，协和的教育内容在学院归国有化的第

一年没有大的变化。

1952 年，中国人民解放军从卫生部和教育部手中接管协和。[10]在接下来的四年中，中国人民解放军实际上对协和进行了军事化管理，引进了一些苏联和中医的医疗模式；为了提供进修课程而更改课程，改变了其附属医院——协和医院的病人结构。在同一时期，中国共产党为巩固其政权，在全国各地开展了一系列全国政治运动。[11]在协和，除了在很大程度上保留了西方医学的行政改革以外，中国人民解放军贯彻了国家的"三反"运动和思想改造运动，以在政治上控制医学精英。因此，中国人民解放军的改革确立了对协和的军事控制，同时在那里保留了西医教育，又使其从业人员在政治上调整方向，与中国共产党保持一致。

在接管协和之后，中国人民解放军迅速将协和整合到国家军事医学基础设施机构当中，招募教师和学生。[12]中国人民解放军坚持从协和获得其非常需要的人力、培训课程和研究能力，为军队提供朝鲜战争（抗美援朝战争—编者注）医疗队，为创建其精英北京 301 医院和解放军胸科医院从协和调来人员，为其医学研究工作提供了基础。作为西方医学研究的主要场所，军事部门把协和当作为其提供必要的专业知识、改进和"科学化"军事医学的地方，即使他们在协和对科学医学进行军事化管理。在更大的范围实施安全措施，学校遵循军事部门的严格路线。瑞士国籍的何博礼（Reinhard Hoeppli）这样写道："如果是外来人，在门口会被拦下并询问访问对象或访问目的，否则不准许进入"，他直到 1952 年都一直留在协和担任寄生虫学系的负责人。[13]何博礼补充说，"所有的走廊都是人头攒动，有男也有女，其中大部分人身穿黄绿色的军服。"[14]因此，军队按照军事部门的规矩，规范了学院人员的关系，与协和之前更为非正规的美国式管理相反。[15]

中国人民解放军使协和直接参与了军事行动。协和派遣了一支由教师和学生组成的外科医疗队到朝鲜战争的前线。中国的医学院校派出这样的医疗队到朝鲜和中国东北地区接种疫苗，喷洒滴滴涕以及开展其他卫生工作。[16]被派往长春和朝鲜的协和教师和员工给伤兵提供外科治疗，其中也包括外科学系主任吴英恺。[17]中国人民解放军还将协和医院变成了军队医院，从前线撤离的士兵可以在这里治疗伤病。[18]护校学生为部队提供照顾，学校教职工和学生给士兵献血。[19]这一进程既完成了协和的军事化，又预示着医学教育在全国范围内得以更广泛地军事化。

作为抵制西方对协和的影响的一部分工作，中国人民解放军鼓励医学教育的新模式。20 世纪 50 年代初，在全国都要"学习苏联"的指导思想下，1953 年，协和的每个系别都设立了教研室，研究苏联的教育组织、课程和教学法。协和也开始教授俄语课和巴甫洛夫条件反射原理。[20]医院党委书记张之强鼓励无痛分娩、电疗法以及其他苏联盛行的临床方法。[21]然而，这些方法没有成为严格的规定得以执行，似乎也没有大大改变协和的医学教育。[22]总的来说，到 1954 年，中国人民解放军医疗队发现苏联式的重组工作普遍来说没有奏效。[23]

与苏联教育研究同时进行的，是持续中西医结合的尝试。1954 年，中国人民解放军将协和作为第一批接受中医实习医师的主要医院之一。[24]然而，在协和医院行医的医生还是以西医医生占主导。将传统医学纳入协和人的工作中最大范围的工作是对传统药物的药效和有用性的科学解释的研究。一篇于 1956 年发表的报纸文章详述了这一整合两个医疗体系的工作，声称协和的药学系发现人参属（ginseng panax）———一种传统治疗疲劳的草药，对治疗糖尿病也有用，因为它对血糖水平会有影响。[25]在这种情况下，与大多数类似的研究一样，医生和研究人员根据最终占主导地位的西方医学原理和标准，证明了中草药的疗效。对中药科学价值的关注，也符合中国人民解放军的首要任务——利用西方医学教育以加强其军事医疗工作。

隶属于中国协和医学院的教学医院成为军事改革的重要场所。中国人民解放军在那里的改革显示出保留协和作为中国的西方生物医学的象征这一动机，同时也符合强调群众健康的新政策。1952 年之后，医院建立了晨会和综合责任的工作制度，根据这一制度，医生要每天 24 小时听班。[26]1954 年，军管的饶正锡批评长期以来协和坚持的以对医学生产生的教育价值为接受病人的标准的政策。[27]饶正锡解释说，这项政策忽视了中国人民解放军医疗机构所面临的一个重要问题：残疾退伍军人问题。在

1949 年前后中国二十多年的武装冲突之后，许多在战斗中受伤的士兵和干部面临永久丧失劳动能力的问题。这些人员中的很多人在 20 世纪 50 年代初期四处寻求医治，但由于他们的病理已经延续了很长时间成为慢性病，他们被禁止进行住院治疗。[28] "因为协和在国内的声望非常高，凡是在当地的地方医院治不好的病，都会把协和作为最后的求助地，"饶正锡说，他觉得，禁止退伍军人进入协和（住院治疗）可能导致社会动荡。饶正锡声称，如果病人由于其疾病缺乏教育价值或被归类为慢性病而不能入院治疗是非常不好的。因此，医院必须接收一些退伍军人，即使他们的病例是慢性的，也没有临床价值。饶正锡在关于协和医院治疗退伍军人的新军事重点的总结中指出，"这样做也是中国协和医学院解决全军疑难病症的责任所在"。[29]

中国人民解放军还改变了学生的构成，并在协和专门为军医学生开设定制的特别课程，即便课程本身仍然非常专业。1952 年，中国人民解放军关闭了协和本科生和医疗专业，取而代之为需要学习当代手术和急诊医疗方法的军医提供研究生课程。[30] 其目标是通过教育"优质、合格的教师"改进军军事医学。[31] 课程限制在一年内，由系组织并专注于特定的分科。[32] 这一研究生"进修"课程使协和与其他军事医学大学、中国人民解放军军事医学科学院和军队医院保持一致。[33] 协和也成为中国人民解放军发展自己专有医学研究计划的主要部分。1954 年，中国人民解放军招收了第一批军事医学生，其中 12 人已经开始在位于上海的新的中国人民解放军军事医学科学院上课，41 人在中国协和医学院开始上课。[34] 历史学家朱克文、高恩显和龚纯均表示，这些课程促进了部队内部临床基础和研究能力的关键性发展。[35]

"打老虎"行动和承认帝国主义：中国人民解放军领导下的政治改革

部队给协和带来了爱国主义，但是协和过去与美国的关系一直挥之不去。例如，1952 年，中国人民解放军在北京故宫办了一场关于协和历史的展览，对协和的历史进行了最深刻的批评。这次展览展出的图片和文字宣称，美国在协和虐待中国学生和病人。[36] 即使中国人民解放军的改革很大程度上保留了协和以研究为基础的西方生物医学教育，在课程长短与学生构成上进行了变革，但是协和的党的领导公开批评那些负责教育的教授。协和的政治运动，特别是"三反"运动和思想改造，将那里的医学实践同其西方起源区分开来。这些进程恢复了协和在中国人民解放军领导下的政治合法性，允许它继续作为西方医学教育的象征，并准许其毕业生有可能返回到精英的职位。

"三反"运动从 1951 年 12 月到 1952 年中期席卷了中国的官僚和教育机构。该运动找出了先前国民政府、政治和行业官员，并就其贪污、浪费和官僚主义开展了"三反"。[37]作为美国对中国医学科学影响的典型，协和是一个突出的靶子。"三反"运动将协和的贪污、浪费和官僚主义与美国颠覆性的影响联系起来。1952 年《人民日报》文章声称，"在协和的绿色宫殿屋顶下，是一大堆腐朽之物。"[38]党对协和的攻击也是针对腐败与贪污。他们挑出了"老虎"，像李维纲，急诊的护士长，据说偷走绷带、注射器，甚至是已故病人的衣服；或者药剂师王希尧，据说偷窃可待因，在工作时发给病人由淀粉和葡萄糖制成的假药。[39]除了在报纸上攻击这些对象之外，党委还纠出一些人，如"高射炮"张承平，一名工程部门领导，据说从学校偷走水管和其他机器设备运到了改造地。[40]一篇发表于 1952 年的文章称，员工偷了总计 37 亿人民币，大约相当于今天的150 万美元，大约是学校 1949 ～1950 年年度运行预算计划 60 万美元的四分之一。[41]

虽然在"三反"运动期间对协和的意识形态批评强烈，但他们却没有针对协和的西方医学课程。党关于腐败的批判暗示其对医学研究的默认，宣称医学研究也遭受贪污之痛。例如，一篇《人民日报》的文章指责罗氏驻华医社（CMB）的腐败，因为协和的医学教育未达到科学标准。这位匿名的作者写道："协和有一位教授着手写一篇论文，要能够达到'协和标准'和'国际水平'。"作者声称，这位不知名的教授在一个研究中故意使用已经被污染的绵羊血样。[42]通过批判医学研究上的腐败行为，该文的作者暗里认为基于定量生物研究的西方医学是最理想的。党声称支持西方医学教育的普世标准，并使用这一标准批评达不到标准的医生。

　　虽然"三反"运动针对的是协和的管理者和工作人员，思想改造针对的却是作为知识分子的医生和医学研究者。[43]受苏联模式启发，思想改造反对英美影响、利己主义和精英主义。从 1951 年开始，协和党代表 —— 通常是学生 —— 引进了自我批评，并指导校领导来推动各部门的思想改造。结果，许多学者在报纸上发表文章，承认他们受到西方影响，存在精英主义和利己主义的错误。[44]知识分子的自我检讨遵循统一的模式，在协和也一样。检讨书都是自传式的，举出意识形态错误的具体例子，结尾则是对阶级斗争和党的反美主义表示衷心拥护。[45]在协和，1952 年有三篇报纸文章介绍了个人思想改造过程，讲述了政治上自我批评的方法，[46]作者分别是当时的校长李宗恩、药理学家周金黄和妇科医生林巧稚。[47]这些文章的共同主题暗示了具体的方法，用这些方法，对党的意识形态的个人认可将西方生物医学再次纳入到中国共产党的行政结构和逻辑中。这些包括作者对他们的阶级背景的讨论，承认他们的教育已经腐蚀了他们，并使他们成为利己主义的精英，并且宣誓，从今以后利用自己的技能为中国人民和军队的利益服务。虽然美国和中国的观察家在思想改造期间对自我批评的真实性表示怀疑，[48]但这些文章反映了他们在写作时中国的社会力量。可能无法推测这些自我批评背后的真实意图，但这些文件仍然是当时的政治压力的证明，且从中可以看出党对待医学专家的态度（原文如此。——译者注）。

　　林巧稚、李宗恩、周金黄的文章都强调自己清白出身以及青年时期被西方教育的腐蚀。例如，林巧稚强调说，她在福州清贫的出身，而所受的教育改变了她的生活。[49]然而，年轻学生的天真让他们容易受到外国的影响，导致他们早年在协和盲目接受美国文化帝国主义。林巧稚写道："我开始充分认识到美国帝国主义在'协和'进行的文化侵略，"叹息到自己当初的无知："我这么多年都被愚弄了。"[50]周金黄指出，虽然协和培养他成为一名有理想抱负的科学和学术上的专家，"在这个理想背后还隐藏着另一个：加入崇拜美帝国主义的个人主义的行列"。[51]李宗恩暗指美国人开办的协和的氛围鼓励了他的利己主义和精英主义。[52]这些自我批评的辞令表明，是协和的西方学术文化 —— 但不一定是李宗恩或他的同事的实际研究 —— 腐蚀了这些人。

一旦作者承认他或她在美国影响下自己犯了错误被其腐蚀，则其声称已经历了一场从其精英意识、资产阶级观点到拒绝西方"文化侵略"的民族主义者和对党的意识形态表示认同的道德转变。这些陈述的作者把这些转变描写为独立于他们的实际的医学实践活动。例如，林巧稚揭示自己一个具体事例，说在她参观了控诉美国军队在朝鲜进行细菌战争的展览之后，她"清楚地看到美国帝国主义侵略中国的狼子野心"。[53]作者描述了其拒绝美国式教育并接受中国共产党毛泽东思想的转折点。周金黄意识到，他的协和教育以美帝国主义和文化侵略的意识形态的形式毒害了他。而他下定决心，"今天，我必须彻底批判旧协和的一切"。[54]

虽然这些医生与其接受的西方医学教育斩断关系，但这并没有阻止他们继续给中国学生教授西方医学。他们接受新的信仰保护了西方科学医学在中国的地位，因为这发生在深深的个人层面。因为作者们从主观的、个人道德及观点层面来描述他们的转变，同时他们也能够明确表示，其反对的是在学习美国科学医学过程中的文化和社会背景，而不必反对医学体系本身。1951 年，记者浦熙修声称这些自我揭发使得整个学校实现了道德转化。她写道："协和回到中国人民的怀抱后精神上全面复苏。"[55]当协和的医生们脱离罗氏驻华医社（CMB）而公开转向忠于中国共产党时，他们的医学实践工作也发生了转向。在 1952 年至 1956 年中国人民解放军领导期间，"三反"运动、思想改造和军事化运动使协和变成了一所军事机构，为军队医学生提供专门的西方医疗培训。这些过程改变了协和的西方医学教育的政治背景和接受者身份，也允许这种西式教育体系再次融入中国社会。

革命、改革与再造：西方医学教育的坚持

1956 年中国人民解放军管理结束，协和再次成为高水平医学专业的

摇篮。1956 年 4 月，军队委托外科学系主任吴英恺开设了一所新的胸外科专科医院。新的中国人民解放军第 309 医院是中国第一所胸科专科医院，不仅带来了吴英恺，也带来了协和的整个胸科。[56]在吴英恺的带领下，胸腔医院开创了中国右心导管术、心血管疾病诊断和血液动力学研究的发展。[57]协和继续为中国提供医疗领导力量——不过是通过部队，而不是通过民间研究机构。

中国人民解放军还确保在协和医院内为高干患者设立了病房，由此中国人民解放军得以为军队领导和外国客人提供西方医疗。1953 年 10 月，协和第二临床学院成为一所独立的医院，用来治疗解放军高级军官；1954 年 7 月，它成为独立的 301 医院（即中国人民解放军总医院——编者注），并成为解放军系统中声誉最高的医院。[58]虽然党的高层领导人都是去北京医院治疗，但是协和校园内的 301 医院和中国医院也都为高层政府官员服务。[59]1951 年 2 月，中央政府将中国医院与中国协和医学院合并起来，属于中国人民解放军总后勤部的卫生部，并重新命名为中国协和医院。[60]饶正锡指出，医院除了医治军队内部的疑难疾病之外，其目的也是"接受和治疗国际友人"。[61]1956 年 5 月和 6 月，协和向 301 医院和其他军事医疗单位输送了大量的往届毕业生及在职的教授，给其进一步技术支持。[62]例如，汪月增，协和 1957 年校友，20 世纪 90 年代担任血液科主任医生、教授和研究员。[63]匡培根，一位著名的神经病学家，曾在协和神经学系任教，担任 301 医院的神经病科的主任，1954 届协和毕业生曹起龙也曾担任过这一职位。[64]因此，协和帮助中国人民解放军建立了顶级的临床机构。

在中国人民解放军于 1956 年结束其对协和的军管之后，协和开始了新一轮的去西化改革、随后紧跟着政治批判的行政管理循环，这种循环直到 20 世纪 80 年代为止重复了好几轮。1957 年，中国医学科学院把协和纳入辅助的研究机构。1959 年，协和以"中国医科大学"的名义再次招收学生。到 1961 年，学院重新位于中国医学院校和研究中心的领导地位，[65]它又恢复了八年制的课程，每年只接受 60 名学生[66]。到 1967 年，隶属于学院的协和医院，当时还被称作"北京协和医院"，就已经成为医学科学的主要中心，并获得了大量的国家生物医学研究资助。

　　看起来直到"文革"开始之前，"协和"与其1949年之前一样占据很大的成就。在20世纪50年代末和60年代初期，许多协和的毕业生和教师再次在中国生物医学中占据突出的地位。他们很多人在中华医学会以及《中华医学杂志》担任领导职务。[67]例如，林巧稚和1927年协和毕业生胡传揆都是该协会的副会长，还有钟惠澜也在1950年至1965年间主持《中华医学杂志》的编辑工作。[68]自从中国医学科学院与协和1957年合并后，协和的毕业生们很快成为新机构的领导者也就不足为奇了。[69]1933年的毕业生黄家驷，1959年至1983年任院校长；1983年至1984年其继任者则是1942年的毕业生吴阶平。1960年在中国进行了第一例肾移植的吴英恺先生，1995年被美国泌尿外科学院（American Academy of Urinary Surgery）选为唯一的外国荣誉会员。[70]

　　对1933年的班级的一个调查显示，许多协和毕业生在中华人民共和国的医疗机构中占据突出位置，这表明协和的学术资质的价值超过了其政治困境。例如，陈国桢成为岭南大学医学院副教务长，黄家驷成为中国医科大学的校长兼中国医学科学院的院长，周寿恺成为中山医学院的副院长。[71]林巧稚成为协和妇产科的主任，她在国家卫生机构中担任各种高级职位，也是英国、比利时和法国的"友谊使者"。[72]而周金黄在抗美援朝期间参加军事医学研究后，1958年加入中国人民解放军军事医学科学院，并因此获得了二等功。1963年，他加入中国共产党。[73]然而，李宗恩的职业生涯及其生活却因他所面对的政治批评而永久改变。李宗恩在1957年党清除异己时被打成右派之后，于1959年被下放到昆明，并成为昆明医科大学的研究工作者。在1962年，他在那里去世，死因不明；卫生部在他死后将他的名字划入"被错误打成右派的人"。[74]

　　在"文革"期间，自我批判的历史循环又一次重演。红卫兵将教学医院的名称更改为"北京反帝医院"。[75]1968年11月，英文版的中国共产党刊物《中国建设》发表了一篇关于协和的文章，标题为"以友谊为伪装的美帝国主义文化侵略"。作者重复了过去的批判，控诉精英以及美国文化帝国主义对中国患者的折磨。[76]虽然医学院在1970年关闭，但是其附属的协和仍然继续运行。1971年，当《纽约时报》记者詹姆斯·雷斯顿（James Reston）访问北京并在协和医院做了紧急阑尾切除术时，这成为全球新闻头条。雷斯顿生动地记录了其手术过程，包括手术后为了缓解疼痛而进行的针灸以及医院的政治积极性的各种细节，为美国读者提供了中国医学的一瞥。[77]1979年，协和以"中国首都医科大学"的名字复校，1985年更名为"北京协和医学院"（这里指恢复了其英文名称 Peking Union Medical College，中文名字为中国协和医科大学——编者注）。[78]在那一年，中国官员也公开道歉，道歉之前指控美国人在医学院对中国病人施以酷刑，并声称这些言论是"邪恶的谎言"。[79]

本文显示，协和不仅过去与现在都远远不只是一个于1949年结束的慈善项目。而更是西医在中国确立的象征，是在美国式管理、在中国人民解放军和中国共产党的领导下，协和成为西方医学与知识的中国化和军事化的标志。解放军在协和复兴过程中的突出作用表明在改造非军事医学方面，部队扮演着强有力的角色。20世纪50年代初，协和成为中国新医学的首个标志之一，它标志着在中国，国家特别是军事力量在其领土之内对西方医学教育实施着管理权。

参考书目

1. Warren I. Cohen, *America's Response to China*：*A History of Sino-American Relations* (*New York*：*Columbia University Press*, 2000)；and Chen Jian, *Mao's China and the Cold War* (Chapel Hill, NC：University of North Carolina Press, 2001).

2. Miriam Gross, *Farewell to the God of Plague*：*Chairman Mao's Campaign to Deworm China* (Oakland：University of California, 2016)；Xiaoping Fang, *Barefoot Doctors and Western Medicine in China* (Rochester, NY：University of Rochester Press, 2012)；and Kim Taylor, *Chinese Medicine in Early Communist China*, 1945 – 63：*A Medicine of Revolution* (London and New York：Routledge Curzon, 2005), 151 – 53.

3. 对于中国的讨论，见朱潮和张慰丰：《新中国医学教育史》（北京：北京医科大学，中国协和医科大学联合出版社，1990 年）。以及马伯英、高晞、洪中立：《中外医学文化交流史》（上海：文汇出版社，1993 年），第 573 – 84 页。

4. David M. Lampton, *The Politics of Medicine in China*: *The Policy Process*, 1949 – 1977 (Boulder, CO: Westview, 1977).

5. Ruth Rogaski, *Hygienic Modernity*: *Meanings of Health and Disease in Treaty-Port China* (Berkeley and Los Angeles: University of California Press, 2003), 285 – 87; and Gross, *Farewell to the God of Plague*.

6. Taylor: *Chinese Medicine*, 33.

7. "中国和美国：卫生部接管北京协和医学院（新华社，1951 年 1 月 20 日）", *Survey of China Mainland Press*, no. 52 (19 – 20 January 1951): 3.

8. Bullock, *American Transplant*, 193, 211; Deng Jiadong (Teng Chia-tung), "Let Us Examine the P. U. M. C. of the Past," Folder 4, Box 1, FA044, Mary E. Ferguson Papers, Rockefeller Archive Center, Sleepy Hollow, NY (hereafter cited as RAC). 最初出版是以邓家栋的名义：《我们要批判过去 "协和" 的一切》，《人民日报》，1951 年 11 月 16 日; The Research Committee of the Chinese Union Medical College, "Why Did American Imperialism Establish the Peking Union Medical College [?]," translation, Folder 4, Box 1, FA044, Mary E. Ferguson Papers, RAC.

9. Bullock, *American Transplant*, 211; 孙玉珊：《人民政府接管协和医学院的前前后后》，于《话说老协和》，（北京：中国文史出版社，1987 年），467。

10. 吴阶平：《协和育才之路》（北京：中国协和医科大学，2001 年），30。

11. Julia Strauss, "Morality, Coercion and State Building by Campaign in the Early PRC: Regime Consolidation and After, 1949 – 1956," *The China Quarterly*, no. 188, The History of the PRC (1949 – 1976) (Dec 2006): 897.

12. Gu Fangzhou, ed. , *Commemorative Pictorial of Chinese Academy of Medical Sciences* (30th Anniversary 1956 – 1986) and Peking Union Medical College (70th Anniversary 1917 – 1987) (Hong Kong: Hong Kong Novelact, 1987), 22. （顾方舟等，《中国医学科学院中国协和医科大学画册》）

13. Bullock, *American Transplant*, 208; and Reinhard Hoeppli to Harold H. Loucks, October 3, 1952, Folder 10, Box 1, FA050, Harold H. Loucks Papers, RAC.

14. 出处同上。

15. Ferguson, *China Medical Board*, 209.

16. Peking Film Studio of China and the National Film Studio of Korea, "Oppose Bacteriological Warfare," 1952, ARC 1630600 ／ LI 263. 1006, National Archives and

Records Administration, College Park, MD. Available online at https://archive.org/details/gov.archives.arc.1630600；蔡景峰，李庆华，张冰浣主编：《中国医学通史（现代卷）》522－26。

17. Gu, *Commemorative Pictorial*, 21－22；Laurence O'Neal ed. Translator Hou Chi Suen, Victoria Hong Gao Wu Yingkai, *Dr. Wu Yingkai's Memoir: Seventy Years* (1927－1997) *of Studying, Practicing, and Teaching Medicine*, ed. Laurence O'Neal, trans. Hou Chi Suen and Victoria Hong Gao (Beijing: China Science and Technology Press, 1997), 48.

18. 孙玉珊：《人民政府接管协和医学院的前前后后》，于《话说老协和》，（北京：中国文史出版社，1987 年），466－467。军队的入驻发生于 1951 年 6 月。

19. 出处同上。

20. 方生主编，《北京卫生史料：1949－1990》，（北京：北京科学技术出版社，1993 年），209。

21. 北京协和医院与湘雅医学院，《张孝骞画传》（北京：中国协和医科大学出版社，2007 年），125。医生用电疗法对患者头部施加小电流以治疗失眠。

22. 出处同上。

23. 朱克文、高恩显、龚纯：《中国军事医学史》（北京：人民军医出版社，1996），410。

24. Taylor, *Chinese Medicine*, 76.

25. Lois Mitchison, "Chinese Doctors Research Into Traditional Chinese Medicine," January 1, 1956, Folder 5, Box 1, FA044, Mary E. Ferguson Papers, RAC.

26. 北京协和医院与湘雅医学院，《张孝骞画传》，125。

27. 汤少云主编，《饶正锡》，于《开国将帅》（太原：陕西人民出版社，2005 年），197－98；饶正锡：《在中国协和医学院全体工作人员会议上的讲话（节录）》，于《中国人民解放军医学教育史》，王冠良，高恩显主编（北京：军事医学科学出版社，2001 年），368－69。

28. 出处同上。

29. 出处同上。

30. 董炳琨、杜慧群、张新庆：《老协和》（河北：河北大学出版社，2004 年），214。

31. 出处同上。

32. 中国人民政治协商会议浙江省鄞县委员会文史资料研究委员会，张才丽，于鄞县文史资料第六辑：当代鄞籍国内人物专辑之一（鄞县：政协浙江省鄞县委员会文史资料委员会，1993 年），105；朱克文，高恩显，龚纯：《中国军事医学史》，

434 – 35。

33. 朱克文，高恩显，龚纯：《中国军事医学史》，434 – 35。

34. 出处同上，434。

35. 出处同上，629。

36. "U. S. Imperialist Crimes Bared at PUMC Hospital Exhibition," Folder 5, Box 1, Mary E. Ferguson Papers, RAC. Originally published in Shanghai News, June 24, 1952.

37. Theodore Hsi-en Chen and Wen-Hui C. Chen, "The 'Three-Anti' and 'Five-Anti' Movements in Communist China," *Pacific Affairs* 26, no. 1 (Mar 1953): 4 – 5.

38. "Anti-Corruption Campaign Vigorously Conducted in China Union Medical College," translation, Folder 4, Box 1, FA044, Mary E. Ferguson Papers, RAC. Originally published as Bai Sheng, "Zhongguo xiehe yixueyuan jiji kaizhan fan tanwu yundong (The China Union Medical College Actively Conducts an Anti-Corruption Campaign)," *Renmin ribao*, March 12, 1952.

39. "Anti-Corruption Campaign" and "Former American-Operated Institutions in China: The Dark Side of PUMC," New China News Agency (Xinhua), Beijing, March 21, 1952, translation, Folder 4, Box 1, FA044, Mary E. Ferguson Papers, RAC.

40. "Anti-Corruption Campaign" and Hoeppli, Singapore, to Loucks, New York, 22 November 1952, Folder 10, Box 1, RG IV 2A32. 1, FA050, Harold Loucks Papers, RAC.

41. "Former American-Operated Institutions;" Ferguson, *China Medical Board*, 212.

42. 出处同上。

43. Bullock, *American Transplant*, 220.

44. Suzanne Pepper, *Radicalism and Education Reform in 20th Century China* (Cambridge: Cambridge University Press, 1996), 169 – 70.

45. Theodore Hsi-en Chen, Thought Reform of the Chinese Intellectuals (Hong Kong: Hong Kong University Press, 1960), 59 – 60.

46. Pepper, Radicalism, 164 – 75.

47. Li, "P. U. M. C. and I;" Lin Qiaozhi (Lim Kha-ti), "Open the 'PUMC' Window and Take a Look at the Motherland," translation, Folder 5, Box 1, FA044, Mary E. Ferguson Papers, RAC, originally published as Lin Qiaozhi, "Dakai 'Xiehe' chuanghu kan zuguo (Open the Window of PUMC and Look at the Motherland)," *Renmin ribao*, September 27, 1952; and Zhou Jinhuang, "Chedi chanchu chongbai mei diguo zhuyi de sixiang (Totally Eradicating the Ideal of American Imperialism)," *Renmin ribao*, November 24, 1951.

48. Aminda Smith, *Thought Reform and China's Dangerous Classes：Reeducation, Resistance, and the People* (New York：Rowman and Littlefield, 2012), 7；Theodore Hsien Chen, *Thought Reform of the Chinese Intellectuals* (Hong Kong：Hong Kong University Press, 1960), 71.

49. Lin, "Open the 'PUMC' Window."

50. 出处同上。

51. Zhou, "Chedi chanchu."

52. 出处同上。

53. Lin, "打开协和的窗户."

54. Zhou, "彻底铲除."

55. 浦熙修：《接管之后的北京协和医学院》

56. Le-Tian Xu and Qi Miao, *Cardiothoracic Surgery in China：Past, Present, and Future*, eds. Song Wan and Anthony P. C. Yim (Hong Kong：Chinese University of Hong Kong, 2007), 170 – 71.

57. 朱克文、高恩显、龚纯：《中国军事医学史》, 691。Richard A. Lange and L. David Hillis, "Cardiac Catheterization and Hemodynamic Assessment," in *Textbook of Cardiovascular Medicine*, ed. Eric J. Topol (Philadelphia：Lippincott Williams and Wilkins, 2007), 1245.

58. 中华人民共和国日史编委会,《中华人民共和国日史》, 第 44 卷（成都：四川人民出版社, 2003 年）, 227。

59. Li Zhisui, *The Private Life of Chairman Mao：The Memoirs of Mao's Personal Physician*, translated by Tai Hung-chao (New York：Random House, 1994), 414.

60. 北京协和医院与湘雅医学院,《张孝骞画传》, 125。

61. 出处同上。

62. 北京高等教育志编纂委员会主编,《北京高等教育志》[北京高等教育志, 第 2 卷] 北京：华艺出版社, 2004 年, 872。

63. 中国就医网, 中国医师协会, 中国医师爱心工程工作委员会联合主编：《血液病名医名院》（北京：中国医药科技出版社, 2006 年）, 18。

64. 中国就医网, 中国医师协会, 中国医师爱心工程工作委员会主编：《神经内科名医名院》（北京：中国医药科技出版社, 2006 年）, 14 – 16；计毅主编：《中华人民共和国享受政府特殊津贴专家、学者、技术人员名录》1992 年卷第 3 分册（北京：中国国际广播出版社, 1996 年）, 903。

65. R. V. Christie：《交流：中国医学与中国医学教育》,《医学教育杂志》第 42 卷（1967 年 5 月）：463 – 66。

66. 出处同上，465。中国大约 80 所医学院校中，大多数提供五年或者六年的教学，并且每年接受大约 2000 名学生。

67. Bullock, *American Transplant*, 216.

68. 出处同上。

69. 出处同上。

70. Song Yuwu, *Biographical Dictionary of the People's Republic of China*（McFarland, 2013），325.

71. Bullock, *American Transplant*, 222.

72. Wolfgang Bartke, "Lin Qiaozhi," *Who Was Who in the People's Republic of China*（Berlin：Walter de Gruyter, 1997），270.

73. 孙文治主编：《东南大学校友业绩丛书第一卷》（南京：东南大学出版社，2002 年），508 – 509。

74. 贵阳市政协文史与学习委员会编：《筑人行迹：贵阳历史文化人物传略》（贵阳：贵州人民出版社，2011 年），150。

75. 中国医学院革命委员会：《以友谊为伪装的美帝国主义文化侵略》，《中国建设》第 17 卷，第 11 期（1968 年）：44 – 48。

76. 出处同上。

77. James Reston, "Now, About My Operation in Peking," *New York Times*, July 26, 1971.

78. Paul F. Basch, *Textbook of International Health*（Oxford：Oxford University Press, 1999），47.

79. "Peking Hospital Takes Back Pre-1949 Name," *New York Times*, June 9, 1985.

Peking Union Medical College After Nationalization, 1949 – 1985

Mary Augusta Brazelton

Mary Augusta Brazelton is a university lecturer in Global Studies of Science, Technology, and Medicine in the Department of History and Philosophy of Science at the University of Cambridge. She is a historian of science and medicine in modern China, and received her PhD in History from Yale.

In the early twentieth century, Beijing's Peking Union Medical College (PUMC) stood as a prominent symbol of Western medical science and education in China. After the People's Republic of China was established in 1949, the People's Liberation Army (PLA) took control of the College between 1952 and 1956. This chapter suggests that the endurance of PUMC as an institute of scientific, Western biomedicine in China was largely contingent upon reforms that the PLA instituted there. Drawing on Chinese accounts, as well as the observations of North American and European physicians, it asserts that political campaigns under Army leadership decried American influences on the College but avoided direct criticisms of Western medical science itself. This dynamic politically legitimized the Western medical education that the College embodied. It also permitted PUMC to contribute to the development of Chinese military medicine, suggesting a significant connection between civilian and military medical education in the early People's Republic, as well as the lasting impact of the College in educating and shaping China's medical elite.

In January 1951, the People's Republic of China nationalized Peking

Union Medical College. The College had been a landmark establishment of Western biomedicine in China, but when the Communist Party of China (CPC) took power, it assigned new meanings to the school as a symbol of American imperialism. After 1949, the CPC had severed diplomatic relations with the United States and other Western nations, denouncing these governments' "imperialist" (帝国主义) activities in China. [1] At medical schools across the nation, many of which identified closely with American founders and sponsors, these events set up an urgent conflict: was it possible to ideologically distinguish Western medicine from cultural and social concepts of the West? New policies and administration called into question the research-oriented, biomedical focus of Western medicine at PUMC.

Historians Miriam Gross and Xiaoping Fang have demonstrated that despite the common perception that the CPC primarily championed Chinese medical traditions, Western biomedicine in fact remained an important influence on health policies, campaigns, and practices in the early People's Republic of China (PRC). [2] However, the interaction of these traditions and influences in the field of medical education remains largely unexplored. [3] Despite periodic closures and name changes, Peking Union Medical College (PUMC) remained an institution of advanced medical education and research throughout the 1950s, largely due to the administration of the People's Liberation Army (PLA). This chapter reveals the mechanisms by which Western biomedicine endured at the College during the early PRC. David Lampton has asserted that the Ministry of Health was a primary basis of political support for Western medicine in China during the early 1950s. [4] But at PUMC the PLA, which oversaw the school from 1952 to 1956, played a critical role in preserving Western medical education at the school via curricular and political reforms. PUMC contributed manpower, training, and resources to Chinese military medicine during a crucial transition period, and in service of these ends, the PLA maintained standards of Western medical education at the College.

In this chapter, I survey educational and political changes at PUMC between 1949 and 1966, focusing on the key period in the early 1950s when these transformations began. In addition to fostering participation in the Korean War and implementing short-term advanced courses, the PLA launched the Three-Antis Campaign (三反运动), as well as the political rehabilitation of faculty via thought reform (思想改造), at PUMC. In implementing these reforms, the PLA enfolded the school into a growing infrastructure of military medical research and education, one in which College staff and alumni played leading roles. These institutional changes recast PUMC as ideologically and politically distinct from its foreign origins, but committed to essentially the same standards and practices of Western biomedicine. I analyze retrospective accounts of PUMC from students and Western observers, propaganda that CPC organs published, and articles written by College professors. These documents demonstrated that PUMC retained its symbolic role as a national icon of Western biomedicine throughout its public institutional transformation.

Radical Reforms under the People's Liberation Army, 1952 – 56

When the Chinese Ministry of Education nationalized PUMC on January 20, 1951, it encountered little opposition. But the American connections and elite identity of PUMC soon became politically problematic as the PRC established novel health policies and administrations. [5] As a prominent school that trained elite physician-researchers, PUMC was an obvious mismatch with new populist approaches to health that stressed serving the masses, putting prevention first, and combining Chinese with Western medicine. [6] Upon nationalization, the Vice-Minister of Education, Qian Junrui (钱俊瑞), encouraged College staff to "sever completely their relations with American imperialism" and to emphasize austerity and popular education. [7] The Ministries of Health and Education promoted anti-American discourse at PUMC, but did not enact major reforms. For instance, Deng Jiadong (邓家栋), a 1933 graduate of the

College, wrote in a 1951 People's Daily article that the school's American administration had been "full of poison" and sought "enslavement of the people."[8] In the same year, the Ministries changed the language of instruction at PUMC from English to Chinese, and in 1951, the Ministry of Health renamed the school the China Union Medical College（中国协和医学院）, or CUMC.[9] But in general, the content of education at PUMC did not change substantially during the first year of the College's nationalization.

In 1952, the PLA took control of CUMC from the Ministries of Health and Education.[10] Over the following four years, the PLA effectively militarized CUMC, introducing some Soviet and traditional Chinese medical programming, changing the curriculum to provide refresher courses, and revising the patient makeup of the College-affiliated hospital. During the same period, across the nation, the CPC launched a series of nationwide political campaigns to consolidate its power.[11] At CUMC, in addition to administrative reforms that largely preserved Western medicine, the PLA implemented the national Three-Antis and thought reform campaigns to gain political control over medical elites. The PLA reforms thus established military control over CUMC while also preserving Western medical education there, in addition to politically re-orienting its practitioners to align with the CPC.

Upon taking control at CUMC, the PLA quickly integrated the school into the national military medical infrastructure, enlisting all faculty and students.[12] The PLA stood to gain much-needed manpower, training programs, and research capacity from CUMC, which provided the Army with Korean War treatment teams, staff to create its elite 301 Hospital and PLA Thoracic Hospital, and a foundation for its medical research programming. As a major site of Western medical research, military authorities saw CUMC as providing the expertise necessary to improve and "scientize" military medicine, even as they militarized scientific medicine at the College. Security became much more extensive, and the school followed strict lines of military authority. "No outsider is allowed to enter without being stopped at the gate, questioned whom he wishes to see or for what other purpose he comes," wrote Reinhard Hoeppli, a Swiss national who remained at CUMC as head of Parasitology until 1952. [13] Hoeppli added, "All corridors are swarming with people, males and females, most of them in yellow-green military uniform." [14] The Army thus formalized relationships between its personnel along lines of military authority, in contrast to the much more informal previous American administration of the College. [15]

The PLA involved CUMC in direct military action when it sent a surgical team of faculty and students to the front lines of the Korean conflict. Medical schools across China sent such teams to Korea and northeast China to give vaccinations, spray DDT, and carry out other hygienic work. [16] The teams of CUMC faculty and staff sent to Changchun and Korea, including chief of surgery Wu Yingkai (吴英凯), gave surgical care to wounded soldiers. [17] The PLA also turned the CUMC teaching hospital into an Army infirmary where soldiers evacuated from the front lines could receive treatment for their injuries and illnesses. [18] Nursing students provided care to the troops, and College faculty and students donated blood to the soldiers. [19] This process both completed the militarization of CUMC and suggested that medical education had militarized more broadly across the nation.

As part of its rejection of Western influences on CUMC, the PLA encouraged new models for medical education. Following a nationwide imperative to "learn from the Soviets (学习苏联)" during the early 1950s, in 1953 each department of CUMC set up a teaching and research section to study Soviet educational organization, curricula, and pedagogy. CUMC also began to teach Russian-language classes and on Pavlovian conditioning. [20] The hospital's Party Secretary, Zhang Zhiqiang, encouraged painless childbirth, electro sleep therapy, and other clinical practices popular in the USSR. [21] However, these methods were not implemented as rigid regulations and did not seem to substantially transform medical education at CUMC. [22] In general, by 1954, the

PLA medical corps found Soviet reorganizations to be generally ineffective. [23]

Accompanying the study of Soviet training was a continuation of attempts to join Chinese and Western medicine. In 1954, the PLA made CUMC one of the first major hospitals to accept traditional Chinese medicine practitioners as interns. [24] However, the medicine that doctors practiced at the school's hospital remained predominantly Western. The most extensive incorporation of traditional medicine into the work of College staff was the development of research on the scientific interpretation of traditional medicines' effects and usefulness. A 1956 newspaper article detailing this effort to integrate the two medical systems claimed that the College's department of pharmacology had discovered that ginseng panax （人参属）, a traditional herbal treatment for fatigue, was also a useful treatment for diabetes because of its effect on blood sugar levels. [25] In this case, as with most similar research, doctors and researchers demonstrated the efficacy of Chinese drugs according to ultimately predominant Western medical principles and standards. Such a focus on the scientific value of Chinese drugs suited the priorities of the PLA in using Western medical education to bolster its military medical endeavors.

The teaching hospital affiliated with CUMC became an important site of military reform. PLA reforms there revealed motives to preserve CUMC as a national symbol of Western biomedicine, while also accommodating new policies that stressed health for the masses. After 1952, the hospital established morning rally meetings and a comprehensive duty program in which doctors were to be available 24 hours a day. [26] In 1954, military medical administrator Rao Zhengxi （饶正锡） decried a longstanding policy of accepting patients according to the educational value they provided to medical students. [27] Rao explained that this policy overlooked an important problem facing PLA medical organizations: the issue of disabled veterans. Following over twenty years of armed conflict in China before and after 1949, many soldiers and cadres wounded in battle faced permanent incapacitation. Many of these personnel sought medical treatment in the early 1950s, but as their pathologies had become chronic, they were barred from in-hospital services. [28] "Because CUMC's prestige within the country is very high, in local places where treatment has not worked, all are entrusted to it as a last resort," explained Rao, who suggested that barring entry of veterans to CUMC might cause social unrest. Rao claimed it would be highly undesirable if patients were not admitted because their pathologies lacked educational value or were classified as chronic. Therefore, the hospital must accept some veterans, even if their cases were chronic and not of clinical interest. "This also conforms to the responsibility of China Union Medical College to resolve the difficult illnesses of the whole army," explained Rao, in a statement that reflected the new military focus of the CUMC hospital in treating veterans. [29]

The PLA also changed the student body and tailored the curriculum at CUMC to accommodate military medical students, although the courses themselves remained specialized. In 1952, the PLA closed the school to undergraduates and medical students, instead offering graduate-level courses for Army medical officers who needed to learn current methods of surgery and emergency care. [30] The goal was to improve military medicine by educating "high-quality, qualified teachers." [31] The courses were limited to one year and were organized by department to focus on particular medical specialties. [32] This graduate "refresher" coursework aligned the CUMC with other military medical universities, the PLA Academy of Medical Sciences (中国人民解放军医学科学院), and military hospitals. [33] The College also became a major part of PLA plans to develop proprietary medical research. In 1954, the PLA accepted its first class of military medical research students. Twelve began classes at a new PLA Academy of Medical Sciences in Shanghai, but most – 41 – began classes at CUMC. [34] Historians Zhu Kewen, Gao Enxian, and Gong Chun have stated that these courses fostered critical development of basic clinical and research competence within the armed forces. [35]

Hunting Tigers and Confessing Imperialism: Political Reforms under the PLA

The armed forces provided CUMC with patriotic work, but the school's American past haunted it. For instance, in 1952, the PLA delivered its most trenchant criticism of this history when it opened an exhibit on the history of CUMC at the Forbidden City in Beijing. The exhibit featured pictures and texts that asserted American abuses of Chinese students and patients at the College. [36] Even as PLA reforms largely preserved research-based Western biomedical education within CUMC, instead implementing changes in the duration and student makeup of courses, Party leadership at CUMC publicly vilified the professors responsible for that education. Political campaigns at CUMC, notably the Three-Antis Campaign and thought reform, distinguished the medicine practiced there from its Western origins. These processes restored the political legitimacy of CUMC under the PLA, allowing it to continue as a symbol of Western medical education and permitting its graduates to return, eventually, to elite positions.

The Three-Antis Campaign swept Chinese bureaucratic and educational institutions from December 1951 to mid-1952. The movement identified former Nationalist government, political, and industry officials and accused them of the titular "three antis" of corruption, waste, and bureaucratism. [37] As an exemplar of American influence on Chinese medical science, CUMC was an obvious target. The Three-Antis Campaign linked corruption, waste, and bureaucratism at CUMC to subversive American influences. A 1952 People's Daily article alleged, "Under the 'green-tiled roof of the palatial CUMC' is a huge pile of rotten stuff." [38] Party attacks on CUMC also targeted graft and embezzlement. They singledout "tigers" like Li Weigang (李维纲), a head nurse in emergency services who allegedly stole bandages, syringes, and even the clothes of deceased patients, or pharmacist Wang Xiyao (王希尧), who was said to steal codeine and in its place dispense counterfeit medicines made from starch and glucose. [39] In addition to attacking these targets in the press, Party committees sent people like "Archie" Zhang Chengping (张承平), a head engineer who allegedly stole plumbing and other machine equipment from the school, to reeducation camps. [40] One 1952 article claimed that College staff stole a total of 3. 7 billion Chinese yuan, roughly equivalent to USD 1. 5 million today, or approximately one-quarter the school's 1949 – 50 planned operating budget of USD 600,000. [41]

Although ideological criticisms of the College during the Three-Antis Campaign were strong, they did not target the Western medical curriculum of the school. The Party's allegations of graft implied a tacit support for the medical research that it claimed had suffered from embezzlement. For instance, one People's Daily article accused the China Medical Board of corruption because medical education at CUMC had not met scientific standards. The unnamed author wrote, "One of the professors here set out to write a thesis which was supposed to be up to 'CUMC standard' and 'international level. '" The author claimed that the unnamed professor had knowingly used contaminated sheep blood samples for a project. [42] By criticizing the corrupted standards of medical research, the article implicitly endorsed Western medicine, based upon quantitative biological research, as an ideal. The Party claimed to support a global standard of Western medical education and used this standard to criticize physicians who did not measure up.

Although the Three-Antis Campaign targeted administrators and staffers at CUMC, thought reform targeted physicians and medical researchers as intellectuals (知识分子). [43] Inspired by Soviet models, thought reform opposed Anglo-American influences, self-interest, and elitism. Starting in 1951, Party representatives at universities – usually students – introduced self-criticism methods and directed school heads to lead branch committees on thought reform. As a result, many academics published articles in newspapers confessing their crimes of Western influence, elitism, and self-interest. [44] The confessions of intellectuals followed a uniform pattern and were no different at CUMC. They were autobiographical, demonstrated concrete examples of ideological errors, and ended with a passionate committal to class struggle and the anti-American principles of the Party. [45] At CUMC, three 1952 newspaper articles presented personal accounts of thought reforms and demonstrated methods of political self-repudiation. [46] The authors were then president Li Zong'en （李宗恩）, pharmacologist Zhou Jinhuang （周金黄）, and gynecologist Lin Qiaozhi （林巧稚）. [47] Common themes in these articles suggested specific methods in which personal endorsements of Party ideology reintegrated Western biomedicine into the administrative structure and logic of the CPC. These included authors' discussions of their class backgrounds, admissions that their education had corrupted them and made them self-interested elites, and vows to henceforth use their skills for the benefit of the Chinese people and military. Although American and Chinese observers have cast aspersions on the validity of self-repudiations during thought reform, [48] these articles reflected extant social forces in China at the time of their writing. It may be impossible to divine the true intent behind the words of these confessions, but the documents still stand as testament to political pressures at the time and shed light on Party treatment of medical experts.

Lin, Li, and Zhou began their statements by stressing their innocent origins and the corruption of their youth by Western education. For instance, Lin stressed that her education transformed her life from its humble origins in Fuzhou. [49] However, the naïveté of young students had left them susceptible to foreign influence, leading to their early, blind acceptance of American cultural imperialism at PUMC. Lin wrote, "I began to realize fully how U. S. imperialism carried out its cultural aggression in the 'PUMC,'" and bemoaned her ignorance at the time, saying, "I have all these years been fooled." [50] Zhou noted that although PUMC had trained him as an expert with scientific and scholarly ambitions, "behind this ideal lay another: to join together the worship of American imperialism with individualism." [51] Li suggested that the atmosphere of the American-run College encouraged his self-interest and elitism. [52] The rhetoric of this self-criticism suggests that the Western academic culture at Peking Union Medical College—but not necessarily the actual research Li or his colleagues did—was what corrupted them.

Once the author acknowledged the errors of his or her corruption under American influence, he or she claimed to have experienced a moral conversion from his or her elitist, bourgeois perspective to a nationalist rejection of Western "cultural aggression" and identification with Party ideology. The authors of these accounts described these conversions as independent of the actual medicine they practiced. For example, Lin traced this revelation to a specific moment, saying that after she visited an exhibit that accused the American military of conducting bacteriological warfare in Korea, she "saw clearly U. S. imperialism's ambition of aggression on China. "[53] The authors described a turning point in which they rejected their American-style educations and endorsed the Maoist ideologies of the Chinese Communist Party. Zhou realized that his PUMC education had poisoned him with the ideology of American imperialism and cultural aggression. He resolved, "Today, I must thoroughly criticize everything about the old PUMC. "[54]

Although these physicians had rejected their own Western medical educations, their repudiations did not preclude them from continuing to teach Western medicine to Chinese students. Descriptions of this moment of conversion protected the place of Western scientific medicine in China because they occurred on a deeply personal level. Because the authors described their conversions in terms of subjective, individual moralities and opinions, they were able to explicitly reject the cultural and social context in which they had learned American scientific medicine without necessarily rejecting that medical system itself. In 1951, journalist Pu Xixiu (浦熙修) claimed that these personal revelations had achieved a moral conversion for the entire institution. She wrote, "After its return to the fold of the Chinese people, Peking Union Medical College is now resuscitated spiritually. "[55] When the doctors of PUMC switched overt allegiances from the China Medical Board to the CPC, so did the medicine they practiced. During the administration of the PLA from 1952 until 1956, the Three-Antis, thought reform, and militarization movements turned CUMC into a military institution that dispensed specialized Western medical training to army medics. These processes changed the political context and recipients of Western medical education at CUMC, but also permitted the reintegration of this Western-style educational system into Chinese society.

Revolution, Reform, and Renewal: The Endurance of Western Medical Education in Beijing

By the end of PLA administration in 1956, CUMC was once again a source of high-level medical expertise. In April 1956, the military commissioned the chair of surgery, Wu Yingkai, to open a new thoracic hospital. The new 309 PLA Hospital （中国人民解放军第 309 医院） was the first dedicated thoracic hospital in China and brought in not only Wu, but also the entire thoracic department staff of CUMC. [56] Under Wu, the Thoracic Hospital pioneered Chinese development of right heart catheterization, diagnosis of cardiovascular disease, and hemodynamic research. [57] CUMC thus continued to supply medical leadership to China—but via the armed forces, rather than civilian research institutes.

The PLA also ensured a space within the CUMC Hospital for high-profile patients, establishing the PLA as a viable provider of Western medical care for military brass and foreign visitors. In October 1953, the second clinical institute at CUMC （协和医学院第二临床学院） became a separate hospital to treat top PLA officers; in July 1954, it became the independent 301 Hospital （中国人民解放军总医院, or 301 医院） and became the most highly regarded hospital in the PLA system. [58] Although top Party leaders went to the Beijing Hospital （北京医院） for treatment, the 301 Hospital and China Hospital （中国医院）, also on the CUMC campus, served high-level government officials as well. [59] In

February 1951, the central government united the China Hospital with the CUMC Hospital under the Medical Division of the PLA General Logistics Department and the new title China Union Hospital (中国协和医院).[60] Rao Zhengxi noted that in addition to the work of the hospital in treating difficult diseases within the military, its purpose was also to "accept and cure international friends."[61] In May and June 1956, CUMC transferred a considerable number of alumni and professors to the 301 Hospital and other military medical units in order to provide further technical support.[62] For instance, Wang Yuezeng (汪月增), a 1957 alumna of the College, served as chief doctor of hematology, professor, and researcher at the hospital in the 1990s.[63] Kuang Peigen (匡培根), a well known neurologist who had previously taught at the CUMC Department of Neurology, became head of neurology at the hospital, a position that 1954 CUMC alumnus Cao Qilong (曹起龙) also occupied.[64] CUMC thus helped the PLA establish its top clinical facilities.

After the authority of the People's Liberation Army at CUMC ended in 1956, the school embarked upon an administrative cycle of Westernizing reforms followed by political condemnations, which repeated itself several times until the 1980s. In 1957, the Chinese Academy of Medical Sciences (中国医学科学院) absorbed CUMC as a subsidiary research institute. In 1959, the school accepted students once again as the Chinese Medical University (中国医科大学). By 1961, the College had regained its position as China's leading medical school and research center,[65] and it again had an eight-year curriculum that accepted only 60 students per year.[66] By 1967, the hospital affiliated with the College, then called the Peking Union Hospital (北京协和医院), had become a major hub of medical science, receiving the bulk of national biomedical research funding.

It seemed that until the onset of the Cultural Revolution, the old PUMC had become much what it was before 1949. In the late 1950s and early 1960s, many College graduates and faculty once again attained prominent positions in

Chinese biomedicine. They often occupied leading positions in the Chinese Medical Association（中华医学会）, as well as the Chinese Medical Journal（中华医学杂志）.[67] For instance, Lin Qiaozhi and 1927 PUMC alumnus Hu Chuankui（胡傳揆）were both vice presidents of the association, as was Zhong Huilan（钟惠澜）, who was also editor of the *Chinese Medical Journal* between 1950 and 1965. [68] Since the Chinese Academy of Medical Sciences absorbed the College in 1957, it was not surprising that CUMC alumni soon became prominent in its leadership. [69] 1933 alumnus Huang Jiasi（黄家驷）was its president from 1959 to 1983, followed by 1942 alumnus Wu Jieping in 1983 and 1984. In 1995, Wu, who in 1960 had performed the first kidney transplant in China, was elected as the only honorary foreign fellow of the American Academy of Urinary Surgery. [70]

A survey of the Class of 1933 showed that many PUMC graduates took prominent positions in medical institutions of the People's Republic, indicating that the College's academic credentials outweighed its political troubles. For instance, Chen Guochen（陈国桢）became dean of Canton Medical College（南华医学校）, Huang Jiasi（黄家驷）became President of the Chinese Medical University as well as of the Chinese Academy of Medical Sciences, and Zhou Shoukai（周寿恺）became the vice president of Zhongshan Medical College（中山医学院）.[71] Lin Qiaozhi became the chair of obstetrics and gynecology at CUMC. She held a variety of high-ranking positions on national health organizations and was a "friendship delegate" to Great Britain, Belgium, and France. [72] After participating in military medical research during the Korean War, in 1958 Zhou Jinhuang joined the PLA Academy of Military Medical Sciences, where he earned a second-class commendation. In 1963, he joined the CPC. [73] However, Li Zong'en's career and life were permanently changed as a result of the political criticisms he faced. In 1959, Li was sent down to Kunming after being labeled a rightist in the Party's 1957 purges, and became a researcher at Kunming Medical University（昆明医科大学）. In 1962 he died there after an unspecified illness; the Ministry of Health posthumously rehabilitated his name "as one who had been wrongly accused. "[74]

During the Cultural Revolution, historical cycles of self-repudiation repeated themselves. Red Guards changed the name of the school's teaching hospital to the "Peking Anti-Imperialism Hospital (北京反帝医院). "[75] In November 1968, the English-language CPC publication China Reconstructs published an article on the College entitled "U. S. Imperialist Cultural Aggression Disguised as Friendship. " The authors reiterated old accusations of elitism and American cultural imperialism and torture of Chinese patients. [76] Although the medical school closed in 1970, the affiliated teaching hospital continued to function. In 1971, it made headlines worldwide when James Reston, a New York Times journalist, visited Beijing and had an emergency appendectomy there. Reston's vivid account of his procedure, complete with details of post-operative acupuncture to alleviate pain and political activism at the hospital, provided American readers with a glimpse of medicine in China. [77] In 1979, the medical school reopened as the Capital Medical University of China (中国首都医科大学) before reverting in 1985 to its old name, the Peking Union Medical College. [78] In that year, Chinese officials also apologized publicly for allegations that Americans had tortured Chinese patients at the College, saying that they were "vicious lies. "[79]

This chapter has shown that Peking Union Medical College was, and is, much more than a philanthropic project that ended in 1949. Much as the College had been a symbol of the establishment of Western medicine in China under its American administration, under the PLA and CPC, PUMC became a sign of the Sinification and militarization of Western medicine and knowledge. The prominence of the PLA in the rehabilitation of CUMC suggests that the armed forces were a powerful agent in shaping civilian medicine. In the early 1950s, PUMC became one of the first symbols of a new medicine in China, one in which the Chinese state—and especially its military arm—asserted authority over Western medical education within its borders.

Bibliography

1. Warren I. Cohen, *America's Response to China*: *A History of Sino-American Relations* (*New York*: *Columbia University Press*, 2000); and Chen Jian, *Mao's China and the Cold War* (Chapel Hill, NC: University of North Carolina Press, 2001).

2. Miriam Gross, *Farewell to the God of Plague*: *Chairman Mao's Campaign to Deworm China* (Oakland: University of California, 2016); Xiaoping Fang, *Barefoot Doctors and Western Medicine in China* (Rochester, NY: University of Rochester Press, 2012); and Kim Taylor, *Chinese Medicine in Early Communist China*, *1945 – 63*: *A Medicine of Revolution* (London and New York: Routledge Curzon, 2005), 151 – 53.

3. For Chinese discussions, see Zhu Chao and Zhang Weifeng, *Xin Zhongguo yixue jiaoyu shi* (A History of Medical Education in New China) (Beijing: Beijing yike daxue and Zhongguo xiehe yike daxue, 1990); and Ma Boying, Gao Xi, and Hong Zhongli, *Zhongwai yixue wenhua jiaoliu shi* (History of Intercultural Medical Communication between China and Foreign Countries) (Shanghai: Wenhui chubanshe, 1993), 573 – 84.

4. David M. Lampton, *The Politics of Medicine in China*: *The Policy Process*, *1949 – 1977* (Boulder, CO: Westview, 1977).

5. Ruth Rogaski, *Hygienic Modernity*: *Meanings of Health and Disease in Treaty-Port China* (Berkeley and Los Angeles: University of California Press, 2003), 285 – 87; and Gross, *Farewell to the God of Plague.*

6. Taylor, *Chinese Medicine*, 33.

7. "China and the U. S.: Health Ministry Takes Over PUMC (New China News Agency, January 20, 1951)," *Survey of China Mainland Press*, no. 52 (19 – 20 January 1951): 3.

8. Bullock, *American Transplant*, 193, 211; Deng Jiadong (Teng Chia-tung), "Let Us Examine the P. U. M. C. of the Past," Folder 4, Box 1, FA044, Mary E. Ferguson Papers, Rockefeller Archive Center, Sleepy Hollow, NY (hereafter cited as RAC). Originally published as Deng Jiadong, "Women yao pipan guoqu 'Xiehe' de yiqie (Let Us Criticize Everything about the Old PUMC)," *Renmin ribao*, November 16, 1951; The Research Committee of the Chinese Union Medical College, "Why Did American Imperialism Establish the Peking Union Medical College [?]," translation, Folder 4, Box 1, FA044, Mary E. Ferguson Papers, RAC.

9. Bullock, *American Transplant*, 211; Sun Baoshan, "Renmin zhengfu jieguan xiehe

yixueyuan de qianqian houhou（The Events Just Before and After the People's Government Nationalized PUMC），" in *Hua shuo lao xiehe*（Speaking of the Old PUMC）（Beijing：Zhongguo wen shi chubanshe，1987），467.

10. Wu Jieping，*Xiehe yucai zhilu*（PUMC：On the Road to Producing Talent）（Beijing：Peking Union Medical College，2001），30.

11. Julia Strauss，"Morality，Coercion and State Building by Campaign in the Early PRC：Regime Consolidation and After，1949－1956," *The China Quarterly*，no. 188，The History of the PRC（1949－1976）（Dec 2006）：897.

12. Gu Fangzhou，ed.，*Commemorative Pictorial of Chinese Academy of Medical Sciences*（30th Anniversary 1956－1986）and Peking Union Medical College（70th Anniversary 1917－1987）（Hong Kong：Hong Kong Novelact，1987），22.

13. Bullock，*American Transplant*，208；and Reinhard Hoeppli to Harold H. Loucks，October 3，1952，Folder 10，Box 1，FA050，Harold H. Loucks Papers，RAC.

14. Ibid.

15. Ferguson，*China Medical Board*，209.

16. Peking Film Studio of China and the National Film Studio of Korea，"Oppose Bacteriological Warfare," 1952，ARC 1630600 ／ LI 263. 1006，National Archives and Records Administration，College Park，MD. Available online at https：//archive. org/details/gov. archives. arc. 1630600；Cai，Li，and Zhang，*Zhongguo yixue tongshi*，522－26.

17. Gu，*Commemorative Pictorial*，21－22；Wu Yingkai，*Dr. Wu Yingkai's Memoir：Seventy Years（1927－1997）of Studying*，*Practicing*，*and Teaching Medicine*，ed. Laurence O'Neal，trans. Hou Chi Suen and Victoria Hong Gao（Beijing：China Science and Technology Press，1997），48.

18. Sun，"Renmin zhengfu," 466－467. The intake of Army residents occurred in June 1951.

19. Ibid.

20. Shang Feng，*Beijing weisheng shiliao：1949－1990*（Historical Materials on Health in Beijing，1949－1990）（Beijing：Beijing kexue jishu chubanshe，1993），209.

21. Beijing Xiehe Yiyuan and Xiangya Yixueyuan，*Zhang Xiaoqian Huachuan*（A Biography of Zhang Xiaoqian）（Beijing：Zhongguo xiehe yike daxue chubanshe，2007），125. Practitioners of electrosleep therapy applied a small electric current to a patient's head in order to treat insomnia.

22. Ibid.

23. Zhu Kewen，Gao Enxian，and Gong Chun，*Zhongguo junshi yixue shi*（A History

of Military Medicine in China) (Beijing: Renmin junyi chubanshe, 1996), 410.

24. Taylor, *Chinese Medicine*, 76.

25. Lois Mitchison, "Chinese Doctors Research Into Traditional Chinese Medicine," January 1, 1956, Folder 5, Box 1, FA044, Mary E. Ferguson Papers, RAC.

26. Beijing Xiehe Yiyuan and Xiangya Yixueyuan, *Zhang Xiaoqian Huachuan*, 125.

27. Tang Shaoyun, "Rao Zhengxi," in *Kai guo jiang shuai* (Founding Generals) (Taiyuan: Shanxi renmin chubanshe, 2005), 197 – 98; Rao Zhengxi, "Zai Zhongguo xiehe yixueyuan quanti gongzuo renyuan huiyi shang de jianghua (jielu) (Speech [Recorded] at the China Union Medical College United Workers' Assembly)," in *Zhongguo renmin jiefang jun yixue jiaoyu shi* (A History of Medical Education in the Chinese People's Liberation Army), eds. Wang Guanliang and Gao Enxian (Beijing: Junshi yixue kexue chubanshe, 2001), 368 – 69.

28. Ibid.

29. Ibid.

30. Zhong Bingkun, Du Huiqun, and Zhang Xinqing, *Lao Xiehe* (The Old PUMC) (Hubei: Hubei daxue chubanshe, 2004), 214.

31. Ibid.

32. Zhongguo renmin zhengzhi xieshang huiyi Zhejiang sheng Yin xian weiyuanhui wenshi ziliao yanjiu weiyuanhui, "Zhang Caili," in *Yin xian wenshi ziliao di 6 ji: dangdai Yin ji guonei renwu zhuanji zhi yi* (Yin County Materials on Literature and History, vol. 6: A Special Collection of Contemporary Yin Records of Domestic Figures) (Yin xian: Zheng xie Zhejiang sheng Yin xian weiyuanhui wenshi ziliao weiyuanhui, 1993), 105; Zhu, Gao, and Gong, *Zhongguo junshi yixue shi*, 434 – 35.

33. Zhu, Gao, and Gong, *Zhongguo junshi yixue shi*, 434 – 35.

34. Ibid., 434.

35. Ibid., 629.

36. "U. S. Imperialist Crimes Bared at PUMC Hospital Exhibition," Folder 5, Box 1, Mary E. Ferguson Papers, RAC. Originally published in Shanghai News, June 24, 1952.

37. Theodore Hsi-en Chen and Wen-Hui C. Chen, "The 'Three-Anti' and 'Five-Anti' Movements in Communist China," *Pacific Affairs* 26, no. 1 (Mar 1953): 4 – 5.

38. "Anti-Corruption Campaign Vigorously Conducted in China Union Medical College," translation, Folder 4, Box 1, FA044, Mary E. Ferguson Papers, RAC. Originally published as Bai Sheng, "Zhongguo xiehe yixueyuan jiji kaizhan fan tanwu yundong (The China Union Medical College Actively Conducts an Anti-Corruption Campaign)," *Renmin ribao*, March

12, 1952.

39. "Anti-Corruption Campaign" and "Former American-Operated Institutions in China: The Dark Side of PUMC," New China News Agency (Xinhua), Beijing, March 21, 1952, translation, Folder 4, Box 1, FA044, Mary E. Ferguson Papers, RAC.

40. "Anti-Corruption Campaign" and Hoeppli, Singapore, to Loucks, New York, 22 November 1952, Folder 10, Box 1, RG IV 2A32.1, FA050, Harold Loucks Papers, RAC.

41. "Former American-Operated Institutions;" Ferguson, *China Medical Board*, 212.

42. Ibid.

43. Bullock, *American Transplant*, 220.

44. Suzanne Pepper, *Radicalism and Education Reform in 20th Century China* (Cambridge: Cambridge University Press, 1996), 169 – 70.

45. Theodore Hsi-en Chen, Thought Reform of the Chinese Intellectuals (Hong Kong: Hong Kong University Press, 1960), 59 – 60.

46. Pepper, Radicalism, 164 – 75.

47. Li, "P. U. M. C. and I;" Lin Qiaozhi (Lim Kha-ti), "Open the 'PUMC' Window and Take a Look at the Motherland," translation, Folder 5, Box 1, FA044, Mary E. Ferguson Papers, RAC, originally published as Lin Qiaozhi, "Dakai 'Xiehe' chuanghu kan zuguo (Open the Window of PUMC and Look at the Motherland)," *Renmin ribao*, September 27, 1952; and Zhou Jinhuang, "Chedi chanchu chongbai mei diguo zhuyi de sixiang (Totally Eradicating the Ideal of American Imperialism)," *Renmin ribao*, November 24, 1951.

48. Aminda Smith, *Thought Reform and China's Dangerous Classes: Reeducation, Resistance, and the People* (New York: Rowman and Littlefield, 2012), 7; Theodore Hsi-en Chen, *Thought Reform of the Chinese Intellectuals* (Hong Kong: Hong Kong University Press, 1960), 71.

49. Lin, "Open the 'PUMC' Window."

50. Ibid.

51. Zhou, "Chedi chanchu."

52. Ibid.

53. Lin, "Open the 'PUMC Window."

54. Zhou, "Chedi chanchu."

55. P'u, "PUMC After Takeover."

56. Le-Tian Xu and Qi Miao, *Cardiothoracic Surgery in China: Past, Present, and*

Future, eds. Song Wan and Anthony P. C. Yim (Hong Kong: Chinese University of Hong Kong, 2007), 170 – 71.

57. Zhu, Gao, and Gong, *Zhongguo junshi yixueshi*, 691. Richard A. Lange and L. David Hillis, "Cardiac Catheterization and Hemodynamic Assessment," in *Textbook of Cardiovascular Medicine*, ed. Eric J. Topol (Philadelphia: Lippincott Williams and Wilkins, 2007), 1245.

58. Zhonghua renmin gongheguo rishi bian weiyuanhui, *Zhonghua renmin gongheguo rishi, di 44 juan* (Daily History of the People's Republic of China, vol. 44) (Chengdu: Sichuan renmin chubanshe, 2003), 227.

59. Li Zhisui, *The Private Life of Chairman Mao: The Memoirs of Mao's Personal Physician*, translated by Tai Hung-chao (New York: Random House, 1994), 414.

60. Beijing Xiehe Yiyuan and Xiangya Yixueyuan, *Zhang Xiaoqian Huachuan*, 125.

61. Ibid.

62. Beijing gaodeng jiaoyu zhi bianji weiyuanhui 北京高等教育志编纂委员会编, ed., *Beijing gaodeng jiaoyu zhi, zhong* 北京高等教育志, 中 [Beijing higher education gazetteer, vol. 2] (Beijing: Huayi chubanshe, 2004), 872.

63. Zhongguo jiu yi wang 中国就医网, Zhongguo yishi xiehui 中国医师协会, Zhongguo yishi aixin gongcheng gongzuo weiyuanhui lianhe zhubian 中国医师爱心工程工作委员会联合主编, *Xueyebing mingyi mingyuan* 血液病名医名院 (Beijing: 中国医药科技出版社, 2006), 18.

64. Zhongguo jiu yi wang 中国就医网, Zhongguo yishi xiehui 中国医师协会, Zhongguo yishi aixin gongcheng gongzuo weiyuanhui lianhe zhubian 中国医师爱心工程工作委员会主编, *Shenjing neike mingyi mingyuan* 神经内科名医名院 (Beijing: 中国医药科技出版社, 2006), 14 – 16; 计毅, ed., 中华人民共和国享受政府特殊津贴专家、学者、技术人员名录 1992 年卷 第 3 分册 (Beijing: 中国国际广播出版社, 1996), 903.

65. R. V. Christie, "Communications: Medicine and Medical Education in China," *Journal of Medical Education* 42 (May 1967): 463 – 66.

66. Ibid., 465. Most of China's approximately 80 medical colleges provided five or six years of instruction and accepted about 2, 000 students per year.

67. Bullock, *American Transplant*, 216.

68. Ibid.

69. Ibid.

70. Song Yuwu, *Biographical Dictionary of the People's Republic of China* (McFarland, 2013), 325.

71. Bullock, *American Transplant*, 222.

72. Wolfgang Bartke, "Lin Qiaozhi," *Who Was Who in the People's Republic of China* (Berlin: Walter de Gruyter, 1997), 270.

73. Sun Wenzhi, *Dongnan daxue xiaoyou yeji congshu di yi juan* (A Series on the Outstanding Achievements of Southeastern University Alumni, vol. 1) (Nanjing: Dongnan daxue chubanshe, 2002), 508 – 509.

74. Guiyang shizheng xie wen shi yu xuexi weiyuanhui, ed., *Zhu renxing ji: Guiyang lishi wenhua renwu zhuanlve* (Building a Path for Mankind: Biographies of Historical and Cultural figures in Guiyang) (Guiyang: Guizhou renmin chubanshe, 2011), 150.

75. Revolutionary Committee of the China Medical College, "U. S. Imperialist Cultural Aggression Disguised as Friendship," *China Reconstructs* 17, no. 11 (1968): 44 – 48.

76. Ibid.

77. James Reston, "Now, About My Operation in Peking," *New York Times*, July 26, 1971.

78. Paul F. Basch, *Textbook of International Health* (Oxford: Oxford University Press, 1999), 47.

79. "Peking Hospital Takes Back Pre-1949 Name," *New York Times*, June 9, 1985.

第三部分　新生
REVITALIZATION

协和学子：百年回顾

马超

　　马超，1999 年毕业于中国协和医科大学（PUMC 八年制），获医学博士学位。毕业后在北京协和医院外科任住院医师 1 年。2000 年以博士后访问学者身份赴美国耶鲁大学医学院麻醉学系从事慢性痛发生机制的研究，2008 年开始成为助理教授。2011 年底回到母校，任北京协和医学院、中国医学科学院基础医学研究所解剖与组胚学系主任，"协和学者"特聘教授，博士生导师。2015 年 4 月开始担任北京协和医学院教务处负责人。

协和学生的基本情况

　　北京协和医学院自 1917 年建校以来，到 2016 年为止先后共毕业了 20271 名全日制学生，其中包括以下专业和类型：

八年制临床医学

　　自 1917 年建校时开始确定了 8 年制的临床医学教育体系并沿袭至今，开启了我国长学制医学教育的先河。学生入学后需经历医预科 – 基础医学 –临床医学三个阶段的学习，毕业时符合要求者被授予医学博士（Medical Doctor，M. D.）学位。学校曾在 1917 – 1925 年期间自主开办医预科，后来逐步转为由燕京大学等综合大学本科培养预科学生，并按照严格的标准筛选学生进入校本部学习。1924 年首批毕业生仅有 3 名，到

1930 年后逐步增长至 20 名左右。1941 年太平洋战争爆发后学校停办，直至抗日战争胜利后 1947－1951 年期间曾短暂恢复；之后再次停办直到 1956 年复校并开始招生；最后一次停办是 1966－1978 年，1979 年再次恢复招生，每年通过全国高考招生 30 名左右，医预科学生在北京大学生物系（后更名生命科学院）就读。1994 年开始高考招生数量增至 60 名左右，2000 年后进一步增至 90 名以上。自 1995 年开始学校通过 "7 转 8" 计划招收少量国内其他医学院校的 7 年制临床医学专业学生进入 8 年制课程学习，毕业后达到要求者可授予医学博士学位；1995 年还增设了 "MD＋PhD" 双学位计划，在临床医学阶段后增加 3 年的科研课题研究时间，毕业后授予临床医学和理学的双博士学位。2002 年开始与清华大学合作，招生专业为 "清华大学临床医学专业"，医预科学生在清华大学生命科学院就读，每年高考招生数量在 70－90 名之间，此外还有少量名额从清华大学其他专业转系。自建校以来八年制临床医学专业共毕业了 2,888 名学生，其中 1949 年之前毕业了 309 人，之后毕业了 2579 人（包括 256 名 "7 转 8"、36 名 "MD＋PhD" 双博士、和 20 名留学生）。

护理本科

始创于 1920 年开办的协和护士培训学校，1924 年更名为护理学院，是国内第一所开办护理本科的学校，学制 5 年（包括在燕京大学的 2 年预科课程），毕业时授予护理学文凭和燕京大学理科学学士学位。由于要求严格，1924 年首批毕业生仅有 1 名，后逐步增长到 10～20 名。1941 年抗日战争期间，护理学院在当时的院长聂毓禅女士带领下千里搬迁到四川成都，1943 至 1946 年在四川华西联合大学期间招收了三班共 50 名学生，为国家培养了战时急需的护理人才。1946 年护理学院迁回北京正式复校。1951 年学校再次停办。从 1924 年第一届毕业生至 1951 年停办高等护理教育，共毕业 28 个班 264 名学生，毕业生中 1/3 以上曾担任过中华护理学会或各省市护理学会的理事长、副理事长、秘书长，护校校长及医院护理部主任，各种护理专业杂志或护理教科书的主编、副主编等，她们成为新中国成立之初，中国护理事业发展的奠基者、开拓者和创业者。1984 年卫生部和教育部在首届高等护理教育座谈会上决定恢复高等护理教育。1985 年中国协和医科大学护理系正式成立并开始恢复招收本科生，学制 4 年（1988－1994 年期间曾改为 5 年制），每年的招生规模从十多人逐步上升到目前的 90 人。自建校以来护理专业共毕业本科生 1406 名，其中 1952 年之前毕业了 264 人，之后毕业了 1142 人。自 1931 届毕业生王琇瑛成为中国第一个南丁格尔奖章获得者至今，协和护理学院还有陈路德、林菊英、黎秀芳、刘淑媛、吴欣娟等 5 名毕业生先后获此殊荣。

以上两项本科毕业生数量汇总见图 1。

除了八年制临床医学与护理本科之外，北京协和医学院还培养了大批的专科生和研究生，具体情况如下：

护理专科

1920 年北京协和医学院护士学校建立开始即开设了 3 年制的护理学课程，毕业时授予护理学文凭。1950 年全国卫生工作会议决定停办高等护理教育，重点发展中等护理教育。1954 年北京协和医院护士学校开始中等护理教育工作，到 2002 年为止共培养 1，960 名毕业生（不含护理员培训班、职工中专班和职高班），多数人已成为所在医疗机构的骨干力量，还有不少人在医院、学校及国内外的学术团体中担任重要领导职务。1996 年经教育部和卫生部批准，中国协和医科大学护理系与中国医学科学院卫生学校合并成立中国第一所护理学院，开始招收大专生，每年的高考招生规模从约 50 人逐步上升到目前的 70 人左右。从 1999 年至 2016 年共毕业护理专科学生 1，219 名。从 2017 年开始，北京协和医学院将停止护理学专科的高考招生计划，原有的专科招生名额将纳入护理学本科，并增加了助产士和老年护理的培养方向。

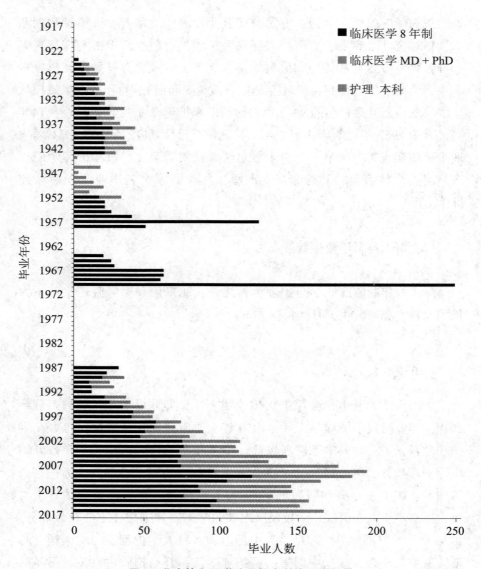

图 1　北京协和医学院历届本科毕业生数量

注 1：所有数据均按照实际毕业年份统计；

注 2：1941 年底由于太平洋战争爆发，学校被迫关闭之前为 1942 届的临床医学和护理学院的毕业生举行了临时毕业典礼。1943 届的临床医学八年制毕业生在校外授予了学位；

注 3：1963 – 1965 年入学的医学生在 1970 年同时毕业。

实验技术专科

1986 年开始学校开设了实验技术专科教育，学制 3 年，每年招生数量开始为 20 名左右，后增加到 40 名，1998 年后停止招生。从 1989 年到 2001 年共毕业了实验技术专科学生 421 名，毕业生大部分就职于生物医学研究机构或相关企业。

研究生

北京协和医学院的研究生教育始于 1954 年，截至 1965 年共招收培养研究生 210 余人（无学位）。"文革"期间，研究生教育被迫中断达 10 年之久。1978 年院校恢复研究生招生，是国务院首批批准可授予博士、硕士学位的单位，也是实行单独考试和可面向港澳台招生的院校之一。1982 年组成了第一届院校学位评定委员会，并于 1982 年首次授予硕士学位，1985 年首次授予博士学位。1986 年 7 月成立研究生院，统一领导院校的学位与研究生教育工作，1996 年 10 月顺利通过国务院学位办对 33 所研究生院的合格评估并正式挂牌。在此期间，1993 年护理学院被确定为硕士学位授权点。1996 年招收了第一名护理学硕士研究生。2004 年护理学院与美国约翰·霍普金斯护理学院启动中国首个护理学博士研究生联合培养项目，2005 年开始招收博士研究生。目前学校的研究生教育覆盖理学、工学、医学、管理学和哲学 5 个学科门类。培养研究生的研究领域包括基础医学，临床医学，生物学，药学，公共卫生与预防医学，中西医结合，口腔医学，公共管理，生物医学工程，图书馆、情报与档案管理，科学技术与哲学等。截至 2016 年 9 月，学校已获得生物学、基础医学、临床医学、护理学、药学、公共卫生与预防医学、中西医结合、生物医学工程 8 个一级学科博士学位授权点。学校共有一级学科国家重点学科 2 个、二级学科国家重点学科 8 个、三级学科国家重点学科 2 个、国家重点培育学科 1 个；一级学科北京市重点学科 1 个、二级学科北京市重点学科 3 个、三级学科北京市重点学科 1 个；并拥有国家级重点实验室 6 个、部委级重点实验室 9 个。从 1978 年到 2016 年毕业全日制博士研究生 7,281 名，硕士研究生 7,056 名，共计 14,337 名。

除了上述全日制学生之外，北京协和医学院自建立以来就开设了继续教育课程，培养来自全国各地的进修生。学校于 1984 年成立了职工教育办公室开展继续教育工作，1998 年成立成人教育学院，2003 年更名为继续教育学院，举办专科起点的本科层次学历继续教育，目前开设有护理学、医学影像技术、医学检验三个专业。在非学历继续教育方面，除了各附属医院和研究所的进修生外，还举办了"乡村医师培训班"、"基层医生培训班"、"全科医生师资培训班"、"北京市住院医师规范化培训"等授课活动，取得了良好的社会效益。

协和八年制医学生的培养模式

医预科课程、基础医学课程和临床医学课程概述

政府接管后的协和八年制教育可根据两次中断而分为 3 个时期，即 1951 – 1957 年、1959 – 1970 年和 1979 年至今这 3 个时期。政府接管北京协和医学院以后，北京协和医学院停止招生，但原 1945 – 1949 年入学燕京大学医预科的学生则继续完成后几年的学业直至毕业，因而这一时期至 1957 届协和毕业生毕业结束。第 2 个时期始于 1959 年中央同意重新建立长学制医科大学而重建协和医学院（当时更名为"中国医科大学"），至"文革"开始高校瘫痪而结束，全部医学生最迟于 1970 年离校。第 3 个时期则是 1979 年再次复校一直到现在。但无论哪一时期，八年制课程始终按照医预科阶段、基础医学阶段和临床医学阶段进行培养，坚持与老协和在培养模式上基本保持一致，学生的基础知识宽广而扎实，这一点在全国医学院校是非常独特的。

（1）校名的变更

协和校名经历过多次变更，自民国时期就已开始，随着各种政治和社会因素，已经使用过 5 个校名，更改 7 次；但英文校名 Peking Union

Medical College 已经是多年未曾改变了。协和建校之初的名称为"北京协和医学院",在 1928 年北伐战争胜利以后,因北京改名北平,遂按照国民政府要求,改称"北平协和医学院"英文名称也由"Peking Union Medical College"改为"Peiping Union Medical College"。至 1949 年新中国成立,将"北平"改回"北京",则中英文校名悉数改回原名称。1951 年解放军接管协和以后,将"北京协和医学院"改为"中国协和医学院"。1959 年协和复校,校名改为"中国医科大学",一直用至"文革"期间。至 1979 年再次复校时,校名使用了"中国首都医科大学"。至 1986 年,学校校名恢复"协和"字样,改校名为"中国协和医科大学",此校名在建国后使用时间最长,达 20 年。至九十年代后期,全国大学合并在教育部主导下蔚然成风,北京医科大学改为北京大学医学部,上海医科大学改为复旦大学医学部,清华大学也有意合并中国协和医科大学,经多年洽谈后,最终签订的是合作办学协议;2006 年,"中国协和医科大学"改称"北京协和医学院",同时挂"清华大学医学部"的牌子。

总之,历经多次变更以后,协和的校名回归了建校之初的第一个校名"北京协和医学院",也是一个不错的选择吧。

(2) 预科学校的变更

在老协和办学之初,罗氏驻华医社(简称 CMB)曾经考察了当时中国的主要大学,发现它们都未能达到作为协和预科学校的标准,因而自行建立了预科学校,老协和的前 10 届医学生均在该预科学校学习。至 1926 年以后,燕京大学在司徒雷登校长的管理下渐入佳境,CMB 将协和医预阶段的学习改在了燕京大学理学院生物系,而同时协和也停办了预科学校,预科学校的设备、图书等全部捐给燕京大学,师资也大部分直接进入燕大理学院。此后多数协和医学生的医预科阶段均在燕京大学度过,但其他著名教会大学的优秀学生通过考试也有可能进入协和医学院学习。如金陵女子大学的郁采蘩、东吴大学的宋鸿钊、清华大学的黄宛(清华大学是个特例)等。这一模式一直延续至 1951 年协和被军管之时。1952 年，燕京大学在全国院系调整中被撤销，当时已经读到三年级的医预科学生继续读完所需课程进入协和，成为这一阶段的最后一届协和医学生。

第二阶段始于 1959 年。当时得到上级支持以后，协和以"中国医科大学"新校名，迅速开始招生，预科在承接了燕京大学多数理学学系的北京大学开设。但是，招收医学生等不及预科培养了，于是从北京大学生物系的三年级直接招收了一批学生，开始基础医学的学习。此后两年也是如此。而直接报考"中国医科大学"的学生，则是 1962 年才从北京大学生物系医预科进入协和的校门。

第三阶段则从 1979 年开始，协和学生的第一站是进入北京大学生物系医预科就读，这种状况一直持续到了 2002 年。此后协和的预科改设在清华大学生物系，一直沿袭至今。

总之，1951 年以后的医预科教育，是由初期的燕京大学，沿袭至北京大学，在新世纪以后改至清华大学。

（3）医预科、基础医学和临床医学阶段课程的各自目标

洛克菲勒基金会创建协和医学院的最初目的，就是要建造一个可媲美欧美的高水平医学院，教学模式是精英教育，因而一切是按照高标准来要求的，从自建医预学校这一点就可以看出来。对医预科教育的要求，长期以来基本未曾改变，就是放在综合性大学的理学院里，充分学习科学的思维过程，以便进入医学院以后可以用科学的思维来理解、来研究人类身体的奥秘，也为未来的医学研究打下基础；另一方面，在综合性大学能够接触许多人文学科，对将来行医时与病人交流大有裨益。因此，医预科的课程往往与生物系学生并无区别，协和也并不干预医预科学生的学习。因此，无论在五十年代、六十年代还是在"文革"后，医预科的总体教育目标是非常明确并且一脉相承的。

　　基础医学的教育在老协和时期是由各基础医学的学系如解剖学系、生理学系承担的，在解放军接管协和后继续沿袭了各自的任务；在1952年协和不再招生后，各学系的重点转向研究，直至1959年协和复校。而在文革，几乎所有的基础医学学系都跟着实验医学研究所迁往四川简阳，直至"文革"后再次迁回北京。1979年复校以后，基础医学研究所（简称"基础所"）已经在实验医学研究所的基础上成立，医学生的基础医学阶段就由基础所负责，基础所也成为学校的基础医学院。此后传统课程均由相关专业的研究室负责，但并无专门教学机构。在上世纪八十年代，学校曾聘请了一批刚刚退休的美籍华裔科学家担任教学工作，一般均为英语授课，很长时间内对协和医学生的专业英语能力提高大有帮助。九十年代后，这批教授陆续返回美国，又因为教学经费不足，基础医学阶段的训练一度处于非常困难的境地。这种状况在近年来得到了改观。北京协和医学院成为国家6所"小规模特色高校"之一，教学经费大幅改善，基础医学院的教学工作也逐渐得到学生们的好评。基础医学阶段的学习是为临床医学打好知识基础，同时要掌握一定的实验能力；这一目标，即使在最困难的时期，也未曾有过动摇。

　　临床医学阶段的教育一直由北京协和医院承担。在政府接管协和以前，医学院和医院实际上是一体的；但此后医学院停止招生而医院却承担了越来越重要的任务，尤其是领导人的保健任务，医学院和医院的作用就逐渐有所分离，即便"文革"时期医学院彻底关闭了，协和医院还挂着"反帝医院"的院牌继续营业，并且在社会上有着重要地位。但作为协和医学院的临床医学院，医院对医学生的培养目标也非常明确，即必须培养未来的优秀临床医生。因为协和医院有着最多的协和毕业生，临床医学的教学往往能够通过言传身教而传承下来，一直保持着一种独特的教学传统。

八年制临床医学课程简介

（1）八年制始末

八年制医学教育实际上来源于美国医学教育革命。二十世纪初，弗莱克斯勒报告出炉以后，霍普金斯大学医学院成为全美医学教育的典范，为"4＋4"模式，即医学院必须在综合性大学毕业生中招收医学生。这种模式被认为当时是在最先进的医学教育模式，因此同属洛克菲勒基金会资助的北京协和医学院，也必须采用最先进的教学体系，根据中国实际情况，修订为"3＋5"模式，即3年医预科加上5年医本科的学制。

1917年，北京协和医学院正式成立。这所医学院，根据洛克菲勒基金会的宗旨，按照霍普金斯大学医学院的标准来招聘教员和设立课程；洛克菲勒基金会保证足够的运营资金。而反观国内同时期的其他医学院校，绝大多数在为捉襟见肘的办学经费和极为匮乏的师资发愁。因此，在成立之初，协和的教学体系和教育质量就远远优于其他医学院校，国内医学界对于北京协和医学院的教学质量和地位也是极为推崇的。

其实洛克菲勒基金会的主流观点一直受到各方面的质疑。基金会内部部分资深管理层对协和医学院的庞大预算开支感到不安，而中国政府以及诸多社会名流认为协和医学院如此优越的各种条件应该尽可能多地培养足够数量的医生。协和医学院生理学系主任林可胜教授就持有这种观点：中国人需要医生数量的缺口巨大，协和的资源应该用于大量培养医生造福于中国社会。因此，放弃严苛的八年制，而采取速成并相对节约的短学制，是另一种办学的声音，从未停止。尽管如此，以第一任校长麦可林为代表的主流观点所主张的"精英教育"，仍然被坚决地执行下去了。

1947年，协和在日军洗劫后的校舍复校。虽然建筑并未破坏，但实验室硬件已经不复存在。洛克菲勒基金会再次捐赠了巨款以确保协和的运营，但是声明这是最后一笔捐赠，此后将靠协和自行造血来解决学校和医院运营了。即便如此，八年制教育依然是牢不可破的教育体系，继续被坚持到政府接管协和。

1950年10月，中国人民志愿军越过鸭绿江，抗美援朝正式开始，中美关系进入冰点。1951年1月20日，政府正式接管协和，接下来6年进入军管状态，以服务军队为主。协和医学院作为美帝国主义的"文化侵略"的代表机构，遭到了全方位的批判。而八年制医学教育作为被洛克菲勒基金会长期坚持的教育模式，更是成为批判的重点，扣上了"培养为资本家服务"的人大帽子，因此停办也就是情理之中的事了。但此前已入学的医学生，则继续学习至毕业，成为那一阶段八年制医学教育的尾声。这批医学生里，后来也出现了罗慰慈、史轶蘩、卢世璧、吴宁、孙燕等医学界的一代宗师。

1957年，经周总理的安排，协和由解放军交付卫生部。当时以张孝骞为首的一批老专家提出要重新开设长学制医学院，但是因为种种原因未能成功。到1959年，一批老专家再次上书中央，要求开设长学制医学院。这次在周总理支持下得以成功，协和以"中国医科大学"的名称再次复校，1933届协和毕业生、时任上海医学院院长的黄家驷出任校长。当时从上到下的一致认为的教育指导方针是"党的领导＋旧协和"，因此所有课程设置实际上是沿袭了老协和的传统模式。这一点后来也在"文革"中被大加鞭挞，《血泪斑斑旧协和——彻底砸烂中国医大八年制》书名就说明了八年制和老协和之间的紧密联系已经被当时师生所公认。1959年第一届医学生实际上是直接从北京大学生物系三年级挑选入学，同时在北京大学生物系招收医预科学生，每届60人。这一阶段结束于1966年，虽然此后1970年最后几届医学生才最终一起离校，但实际上在"文革"开始后便不再有学习的机会了。

1979年，协和以"中国首都医科大学"的名称第三次复校，仍然坚持了八年制的医学教育，每届招收30人。这种学制一直延续至今，未曾改变。与1959年复校所不同的是，第一届招收医预班学生时，并未考虑从北京大学生物系高年级招生直接进入医学院，因而第一届毕业生出现在1987年。此后的八年制教育在此基础上有过一定的改动，但框架体系一直未出现大的变化。

总的来说，协和八年制是老协和教育的标志之一，开始争议颇多，但后来已经为广大协和教职员工所认可，一直坚持到了今天。按照玛丽·布洛克的话来说，"协和医学院对维持学院顶尖地位的'八年模式'极为珍视并抵制一切想要加以修改的努力"。当前"5 + 3"硕士培养联合规范化培训已经被国家确定为医学教育主流，传统八年制教育体系已经面临新的挑战。但新的挑战往往也意味着新的机遇，严峻形势对协和传统教育体系的改革也许恰恰有促进的作用。

（2）预科课程简介

北京协和医学院预科学校在 1917 年开始正式授课，于 1926 年并入燕京大学。预科学校也接受其他医学院预科学校转学而来的学生，如后来内分泌的著名教授刘士豪教授就是在 1919 年由长沙湘雅医学院预科学校转入协和预科的。

1926 年，预科学校并入燕京大学，自此协和医预科即主要在燕京大学理学院开设，直至 1952 年燕大撤销。课程设置总体来说变化不大，因而 1953 ~ 1957 届毕业生所学课程与此前较为相似。

1954 届毕业生、后来著名的血液病学家张之南曾经回忆了预科课程设置：

> 作为协和的医学前培养基地，对学生的业务要求极高，目的是为今后学医和从事医务打好坚实而宽阔的基础，所以，除了数、理、化、生物学之外，还要学人文科学。三年内要学完下列课程：普通生物学（教师林昌善）、无脊椎动物学（博爱理，Miss Boring）、脊椎动物学（胡经甫）、普通遗传学普通化学（许鹏程）、定性分析化学、定量分析化学、有机化学（Wilson）、物理化学；普通物理学（储圣林）；微积分（徐献瑜）。英文读两年，社会学读一个学期（严景耀）。因为必修课程多，所以选修课少，我一直选读心理学，一年级是普通心理学（沈乃彰）及心理卫生学（夏仁得，Sailor）、二年级是儿童心理学（清华大学的孙国华）、三年级是工业心理学（也是清华老师教）。不同的课分别在不同楼不同教室上，课间要在校园里赶，所以大多数同学都有自行车。生物、物理、化学都有实验，要认真、仔细、准确，都要出报告，生物实验要绘图，全靠自己的真功夫。尤其是定性、定量化学的实验，每次拿到未知标本都很紧张，就怕做不出来

或结果不对。教学效果并不完全取决于教师的学术资历，我的微积分没学好，一部分原因是教师不善于教书，我当时非常担心会考不及格；普通心理学的收获也远不理想。而徐、沈两位老师却都是刚刚从美国深造回来的教授。社会学是二门每个医预学生都要学的课程，因为与文科学生同堂上课，人数很多，最后要自选二个题目，交一篇论文。由于学生多，大家估计论文没人看，戏称凭运气得分，不过听完这门课，对社会学有了一个大体的认识。教我英文的教员都是美国人，同学在中学都有一定基础，到大学就是多听、多练习交流……

1959 ~ 1965 阶段的协和医预科教育在北京大学生物系进行，3 年预科和生物系学生完全在一起，除了多了政治课程以外，其余和生物系其他专业的基本相似，和老协和在燕京大学的课程也颇为相似。1963 级医学生沈悌对此的体会是"思维方法能够得到熏陶"，有利于以后的临床工作。1959 级医学生吴兆苏还能记起当年入学时黄家驷校长对设置医预科的解释：

> 按照黄家驷开学典礼说的，为什么我们要办协和八年制，正常 5 年出来就能挣钱养家了呀。你们跟别的医学院最大的差别就在于基础科学要比其他医学院扎实。地基越好房子造得越高，我们很信服。老协和就是这么办下来的，他们觉得这个方向是对的。后来慢慢体会了，越学到需要物理化学基础的时候越觉得当初应该学。如果从来没学过不可能的，要是学过就可以回去翻书……

1979 年开始，协和重新复校后仍然由黄家驷出任校长。1979 - 2002 年，协和医预科教育仍然设在北大生物系（后改称生命科学院）。课程设置包括普通生物学、比较解剖学、微生物学、遗传学、生物化学、高等数学、物理学、无机化学、分析化学、有机化学、物理化学、计算机语言、普通心理学、大学英语、马克思主义哲学。这些课程并非完全一成不变，经常因北大生物系的课程改革而出现相应变动。比如，1991 和 1992 级医学生在医预科学习时，原本 1 学年的普通生物学课程就取消，改为植物学 1 学年、动物学 1 学年的学习。但总体来说，以生物学为主的打基础的教学思想贯穿始终。至 2003 年，协和医预科因种种原因，开始放在清华生命科学院进行，但除了没有专门的动物学、植物学和脊椎动物比较解剖学等课程之外，课程设置风格仍然保持一致。

(3) 基础医学课程简介

1953～1957 届协和毕业生的医学基础课仍然由老协和的基础学科承担。总的来说，因为外国教授的离去本身对协和教学力量的损失并不算太大，因为当时已经仅有生物化学系主任窦威廉由于是外国人而离开，而接任的刘士豪教授在生物化学方面也造诣极深。

张之南教授对这一阶段的学习有着清晰的记忆：

> 协和的前两年是临床前基础课。第一年是解剖、生理、生化三门。是最难的一年，这三门都有同学不及格，特别是神经解剖和生化。第一堂解剖课，张鋆教授即严肃地说念不好解剖学就没有资格作医生。于是，同学都日夜紧张地看书、看尸体、背、记，开夜车是经常的事，有的女同学为了提神也学会吸烟。我和同屋孙瑞龙都不会晚睡觉，冬天就到街上买冰冻的柿子，出去吸凉气，回来又吃冻柿子，可以提精神，但作用短暂，过一会儿又困了，干脆睡觉。上解剖课先要过一个心理关，天天要与尸体为伍，尤其是晚上，谁也不敢一个人呆在实验室，谁也不敢最后一个走，所以常常是几个同学一起最后离开。…听说在抗日战争时期，上海医学院的学生为了上解剖课，师生要在半夜到附近的歌乐山盗墓偷尸，而我们上课就有尸体，两人一具，没有感到困难。现今尸体的来源很难，是本人或家属自愿献出，对医学教育是极大的支持和贡献，所以学校师生都要举行仪式对捐献者致敬和致谢，而我们当年缺乏对尸体尊敬的应有教育是一个缺陷。张教授用英文讲课，他可以用左右手在黑板上画图。教科书是《Gray's Anatomy》和 Cunningham《Regional Anatomy》。解剖学考试出的题目很活，譬如一个枪弹从左大腿外某点以 45 度角打穿，问可能损及什么肌肉、筋膜、血管和神经。神经解剖学是请北京医学院的臧玉诠教授来教，要熟记的内容很多，同学大都感到很难…和解剖学一起上的还有张作干教授教的组织学和胚胎学，张教授虽然留学美国，但口音很重，组织学每人一台显微镜、一套片子，直观的东西多，比较容易学。胚胎学则不然，当年没有

什么模型，课又常常放在下午第一堂，尤其是关灯放幻灯片时，实在犯困，学习效果欠佳。当年解剖科还有史济纶讲师、穆家圭助教。生理学是张锡钧教授执教，他曾在美国得到 Ph. D. 和 M. D. 双博士学位，对乙酰胆碱有较好的研究成果，曾见过许多著名的生理学家 [包括 Pavlov（巴普洛夫）]，这两件事使他倍感得意。但是他的英语发音和口才不好，讲课欠精彩。好在课堂上课较少，很多时间用于实验。课本是 Fulton 的《Physiology》。当年，观察肌肉、神经等的活动还是用记纹鼓较多，要学会熏鼓。对脏器功能的了解是看切除后的变化。若用鼠、蛙做实验，每个学生可有一份，用兔子则有时两个人一只，用狗时是四个人一组，林从敏、张德树两位讲师和刘伯春技术员对动物实验很有经验，给我们很大帮助。生物化学由 Adolph（窦威廉）教授授课和指导实验，李佩珊任助教。Dr. Adolph 的工作服比别人的短，浆得特别挺，样子特帅。他讲课前常常给每人发一个纸条，问一两个问题，学生迅速答完上交，他就有针对性地讲课，有时在讲完课之后，每人发块小纸，问二个课时讲过的有关问题，考查讲课效果，第二天上课再作补充。他讲课时愿意当场做些小实验（大都是有关物理化学方面的）。平时重视安排学生的实验内容和方法，期末前要让学生自己想个问题、自己设计、自己完成、写出论文、当众报告…整个过程实际上就是一个小型的科研，是一种很好的训练。第一年结束时，有两名同学两门不及格，按学校规定一门不及格要留班，两门不及格要退学，在我班全体的请求下，从轻给予留班处理。

"协和第二学年是学药理学、病理学、细菌学、寄生虫学。这些课都很有吸引力……我最有兴趣的是病理课由胡正祥教授主讲，王德修讲试管实验，后来刘永教授自美回国，也讲过几堂课。指定参考书是 Boyd 的《Textbook of Pathology》，实际上学生经常读的是胡正祥与秦光煜合写的《病理学》内容简练、概念清楚，胡教授用英文讲课，也是简单明了尤其是实验课，每人台显微镜，一套片子，有王德修老师细心辅导，有时看大体标本，更多时间是自己看片，印象很深，记得牢固，对以后的临床学习大有帮助。药理学是周金黄教授主讲，以后协和毕业生雷海朋医生从加拿大多伦多大学研修药理学完毕回到协和，他给我们讲了维生素和内分泌药理此外，当时在协和药理学系进修的朱颜先生也讲过几课。用的教科书是美国 Goodman & Gilman 合编的。周教授很有学问、在我国很知名，后来也支持和从事中西医结合工作，对我很器重，曾邀我参加他主编的《Recent Advances in Chinese Herbal Medicine》（英文本）和中文的《衰老、抗衰老、老年病》……但是，我仍坦言药理学的整体教学效果不够理想，不像想象的那样引人入胜，我在学生时代和进入临床之后都感到药理学很重要，然而必要的知识实际上是在用的时候才学到的。细菌学由谢少文教授主讲，霉菌部分请郭可大教授来校讲授，当年细菌科还有张宽厚、张乃初两位副教授，没有给我们上过课。谢少文教授是医学院毕业生，曾在协和作到总住院医师；他是一位知识渊博而且十分用功、善于捕捉新信息的学者，较早地涉足免疫学。他提倡基础医学联系临床，并且以身作则，经常参加内科大查房发表意见；他要求学生就一些问题看资料、写综述。寄生虫学由协和瑞士籍教授何博礼（Dr. Reinhard Hoeppli）主讲，在我国政府与瑞士未正式建交前，他还代理瑞士有关领事事务。另外，冯兰洲教授也是该科主要成员，当时的技术员是曹兴午。寄生虫学条理清楚，加上有大量实际标本可看，学习不难，但是期末考试厉害，特别是口试，显微镜下给你一张标本片子，问是什么，或是给你看一条蚊子腿、一只翅膀，问是什么科目的蚊子。何教授还算和蔼，总是给你一些引导，一步一步让你接近正确答案，而在冯教授面前则是完全靠自己，一句话决定对或错，同学都把这种考试叫做"鬼门关"！

张之南教授对两年医学基础课的印象极为深刻，他认为学习这些基础课对理解临床课大有裨益：

> 协和最初两年的临床前基础课确实对临床学习很有帮助，进入临床后，疾病的表现、诊断、治疗都要联系临床前基础课的内容去理解。

1956 年 8 月，中国医学科学院在原中央卫生研究院的基础上成立。1957 年，中国医学科学院与协和医学院合并，并在 1958 年成立了 5 个研究所，实验医学研究所（现在的基础医学研究所）就是其中之一，主要任务是基础医学研究。

至 1959 年，八年长学制的中国医科大学重建。在黄家驷校长的主持下，实验医学研究所的部分人员被调去支持恢复教学工作，先后重建和新建了解剖学、组织胚胎学、药理学、微生物学和免疫学、寄生虫学、公共卫生学和流行病学、统计学等教研室。因此，1959 - 1965 级医学生的医学基础课阶段，就均由这些教研室负责，尽管受政治运动一定影响，但还是为同学们打下了很好的基础。

1969 年 10 月 26 日，中共中央发出《关于高等院校下放问题的通知》（林彪"第一号通令"），多所高校陆续外迁。1969 年底，实验医学研究所也全部迁移至四川省简阳县，并入医科院四川分院；1973 年后，原中国医大基础各教研室也被缩编调整，一半教学人员及仪器教材调往原卫生部北京中医学院，其余教职员工成立基础教学组，直属医科院。混乱局面一直延续至"文革"后。1978 年，经国务院批准，原实验医学研究所迁回北京，与基础医学组教学人员合二为一，成立基础医学研究所。1982 年基础医学研究所和医科大学基础部（1993 年称基础医学院，2006 年改称基础学院）正式成为双名一体的机构，基本按学系/教研室建制延续至今。自 1982 年始，协和学生医学基础课的教育就在基础医学研究所进行。课程设置仍然与此前相似。在讲授课程结束后，曾经设置 4 个月的基础医学科研训练课程，后来自九十年代初开始和临床医学课程中的临床医学科研训练课程合并，成为一门科研训练课，学生既可选择基础医学的导师、也可选择临床医学的导师进行科研训练，成为协和八年制医学教育的一个新的特色，将在下文单独介绍。

（4）临床医学课程简介

对于 1953 ~ 1957 届毕业生来说，虽然协和医学院停止招生，但已入学医学生仍可继续上学至毕业，临床教学又高度重视实践，因此所受影响虽然较大，但是仍然能够完整地完成学业。但是许多细节方面实际上还是受形势影响，改动了不少的；比如 1954 届毕业的学生在实习阶段只能选择内科、外科或妇产科进行专科实习，以至于后来成为中国工程院院士的内分泌学教授史轶蘩回忆起学生生涯时仍对未能在外科妇产科实习感到非常遗憾。

张之南教授对此也有非常详实的回忆，在《成长与经历》里仔细描述了当时的学习状况。

首先描述的是这一阶段第一年的课程：

> 从第三年起进入临床学习，以诊断学基础、实验诊断学、治疗学总论开始，逐渐进入内科学、外科学、妇产科学讲课，并且分为三组，分别到内科、外科、妇产科作见习生（extern），在导师的指导下接触病人。诊断学基础由邓家栋教授主讲，主要内容是物理诊断方法和原理，当时由于病人少，一些特殊的体征如麻疹、猩红热、伤寒、斑疹伤寒的皮疹、麻疹口腔黏膜的 Koplic 斑等要到传染病院去看，某些少见的体征要到其他医院去看。实验诊断学主要讲血、尿、粪三大常规和一些常用的血液生化检查，三大常规要每一个学生亲自操作并掌握．另外，也上一些 X 线诊断学的课和示教性读片活动。治疗学总论讲药物治疗的概念和原则、物理治疗、营养治疗浅介。这些课都是为以后讲对疾病的认识和诊治打下基础。

接下来的课程中，内科学、外科学、妇产科学的顶尖泰斗们亲自授课，异彩纷呈；医学生的收获是巨大的。

> 内科学是一门大课，不同系统的病由不同专长的教授分头讲授，每位都有各自的风格、特色，张孝骞教授讲课一如其人，严谨认真，一字一句地仔细斟酌；刘士豪教授从容不迫、挥洒自如；朱贵卿教授诙谐幽默、听后不忘；张学德教授讲课内容丰富、有条不紊；钟惠澜、黄宛、张安等都有自己的特点。临床医生讲病好像面前有个患者，常常能讲得生动自然、栩栩如生、易懂好记。外科学是曾宪九教授主讲，像他的手术一样，一板一眼、条理分明。妇产科学由林巧稚教授主讲，葛秦生教授帮助讲妇科、王文彬教授帮助讲产科，他（她）们的讲课效果都很好。

这一时期同时开始见习，传统的导师制就是指在这一阶段的学习中采用的教学方式。

> 作见习生是学会接触病人、进入临床最重要的阶段。全班分三组，每组也就是七、八个人，分头到三大科，在导师的指导下进行见习。有的同学还计较指派谁作自己的导师，譬如在内科，分到朱贵卿老师门下就高兴，因为他年资高又风趣；分到张学德老师也得意，因为张老师讲的多。当时担任导师的大都是教授、副教授，而指派给我的是年轻的方圻讲师，他是

我的入门老师，他为人谦虚、和蔼，做事认真细致，对病人无微不至，有一颗善良的心，所以在他的一生中充满了光辉的业绩和绝佳的口碑。他作为我的启蒙老师，以身垂范，是我的幸运，他的表率作用也影响了我的为人和医学生涯。我的见习生学习阶段始自内科，内科导师不仅指导我如何采取病史、体检、化验和进行正确分析，我认为更重要的是教导我如何对待病人、接触病人。病人是我的学习对象、知识来源，学生反复问病史、查体，其实不是医疗的必要内容，而是病人对学生的贡献，是牺牲自己的精神、体力为学生的学习提供条件，因此，学生应该把患者视为恩人，在向他们学习的同时，尽量为他们做些力所能及的事，更不能因为患者的一些不耐烦而抱怨。还有一个问题应该提到当给一位异性病人做体检时，特别是患者一般愿意隐蔽的部位，需有其家属或是导师或第三者在场，暴露的范围越小越好，这是对患者的尊重。端正了对患者的认识和态度，能以换位思维去分析和处理问题，能理解患者、对患者有同情心，是日后医学活动中医德、医风的根本要求。由吴蔚然大夫带领我们小组，观察、分析、讲解病人的病情、手术适应证以及手术和手术后的注意事项，观看如何作术后观察、换药、伤口愈合情况、拆线等等。为弥补不能亲自动手的缺陷，特设动物手术实验课，让学生在动物身上学习如何选择切口、切开、止血、结扎、缝合等基本手法。到妇产科见习时，我的导师是印尼归国华侨曾绵才教授，他的国语不太好，要我用英文写病历，他用英文给我改和讲。后来，科里怕我将来不会写中文病历，又请谭蕴涛讲师作我的副导师，足见科里对一个学生的学习多么负责！在妇科由导师带领去看妇科检查，在产科由导师带领或应病房呼叫去看产妇生产的全过程，学生没有动手的机会。每看一件事都有讨论，由导师或当场的医师讲解，印象还是很深的。

其后一年的临床学习包括了前一年未涉及的几乎所有科室，教学风格相似，但已经不能采用一对一的导师制来教学了，而以小组教学的形式为主，也非常注重实践。

协和的第四年主要是内、外、妇以外的课，包括眼、耳鼻喉、皮肤、神经精神、放射诊断学、儿科等。这一年除讲课外，大都是跟着各科医生看病人，一般以小组为学习单位，不再是每人一位导师。这学年涉及的病种很多，各科的授课老师都非常善于讲课，眼科的罗宗贤、张晓楼、劳远秀教授讲课清楚，而且后两位还有一手在黑板上画示意图的本领，用笔如神，一气呵成，几乎用不着涂擦修改。皮科的李洪迥教授和蔼可亲、风趣幽默，在他与病人或患儿家长的对话中，学生不仅可以学到疾病的治疗和预防知识，并且可学习如何有效地与患者交流，譬如他用诙谐的口吻指责湿疹患儿的父母育儿不当，这些语言和情景令人终身难忘。儿科的周华康教授又高又大，但是小孩子都不怕他可是我们作为他的学生却对他有点敬畏，因为他有一个独特的教学法，他对你提问，一个问题接一个问题，一问到底，有时已经说出了正确答案，他还要问下去，试探你是否真认定了这个答案，神经精神科由冯应琨、许英魁教授主讲，然后到当时8楼三层神经科和地窨子的精神科病房看病人，主要是学接触和检查病人的方法。放射诊断学也以学习读片方法为主。记得一次考试中，同学拿到一张片子，看来看去没有什么不正常，结果是个右位心，看片时未注意持片先看左右！在进入临床学习阶段，跟着老师看了各种各样的病人，男妇老幼、精神状态正常的和不正常的、脾气好的和不好的、合作与不合作的、文化水平高的和不高的、表达清楚的和不清楚的等，要学会如何接触不同的病人，争取他（她）们的合作，是一项十分重要的基本功。与病人沟通有态度问题也有技巧方法，想做一名好医生需终身磨练，我在作实习医师和下乡医疗活动过程中都有深切的体会。

张之南教授对"学生临床病理讨论会"这样一种教学形式印象极为深刻，认为教学效果相当满意。

　　在协和的临床学习阶段还有一种特殊形式的教学活动，就是学生临床病理讨论会（Student CPC），由病理科老师选择适当病例，请一位学生写出病历摘要（不包括病理结果），事先分发给同学，由一位同学任主要发言人，分析诊断及治疗中的问题，两三位同学被指定参加讨论，另外一些同学自由发言，然后由一位同学报告病理解剖结果，最后由老师总结生前诊断、对病情的认识与病理所见是否一致，若不相符，原因是什么，治疗方面有无不当，应吸取什么教训。学生仍可继续提问讨论。这种教学方式真实具体，使学生对疾病表现的内在原因、诊断思维的误区、治疗不当的后果，立即明了并且记忆深刻。

实习阶段对医学生的成长十分重要，当时的特殊时期采取了专科重点实习的方案，张之南教授对此作了客观的评述。

　　临床学习的最后一年是做实习医师，到临床第一线，在上级医师的指导下，负责所管病人的诊断、治疗和其他有关问题，开始通过亲身经历积累临床经验和获取临床实际工作能力。一些医学院校是内、外、妇产三科轮转实习，而我们当年因形势需要是专科重点实习。专科实习一年的优点是出来就可以直接作该科的住院医师，我感觉最大的缺点是对其他科的临床认识和处理能力太少，在内科重点实习的学生只会内科病的处理，从来都没接过生、没有处理过伤口、不会切开缝合！在以后的工作中深感不足。实习医师受住院医师带领和指导，因此实习医师的最直接的导师就是上级住院医师，我深切感到住院医师对实习医师的作用和影响。在内科时期，带我的住院医师先后是黄大显和何培琨（黄大夫后来去解放军总医院，曾任心内科主任。何大夫后来去了积水潭医院，后到香港，在港开业多年，有两个诊所，现在美国洛杉矶，已退休，但仍在社区看病人）。这两位虽都不是协和毕业生，但在环境的熏陶下，均有良医风范，为人正派，医术精湛，有良好的教学意识。他们手把手地教我操作中的一些技巧和窍门。

　　对于 1959～1965 年入学的医学生来说，仅有 3 届医学生真正完成临床医学课程。即使如此，由于当时的政治形势变化，包括"反右"、"四清"等运动，在一定程度上都干扰着教学。这一批医学生毕业后几乎都分配去了西藏、新疆、青海等大西北地区，对于低年级学生非常不利，后来他们的临床能力在"回炉"中得到提高，后来文革结束后大多考研究生回到协和，实现了更高层次的突破。

　　1979 年后的临床医学课程也一直秉承老协和的观念，讲授课程精炼而临床实践和床边教学多。强调最多的常常是第一门课——诊断学，几乎历年来教学工作都在强调诊断学是整个临床医学的基础，要求内科每个专业组和内分泌科、神经科各派出 1 名专职教师负责小组教学，保证每个医学生的查体基本功过关，并且有每日听课的义务；这一传统沿袭至今。自二十世纪九十年代末，整个临床教学又作了一次较大的改革，将原本内科、外科及其他科室的精华课程围绕器官系统进行整合，设置为综合课课程，而其余内容整合入见习阶段学习中。见习 1 年结束后，学习眼、耳鼻喉、口腔、中医等不列入常规见习实习轮转的课程。此后是实习 1 年。这一模式自 1999 年延续至今，细节仍在不断改进中。临床医学课程还是卓有成效的，但偶然性也很大，教学效果与病房主治医生及住院医生的能力和教学意识息息相关。

（5）科研训练

在 1979 年复校以后，前几届医学生完成基础课程学习后，有 4 个月基础医学科研训练；而后续临床医学课程结束以后，再有 4 个月临床医学科研训练。在 20 世纪 90 年代初的教学改革中，二者合二为一，医学生可选择跟随基础医学的导师或临床医学的导师进行科研训练。这一阶段在国内各医学院可以算绝无仅有，而效果也因人而异，在下一步教学改革中何去何从，也尚未可知。

众所周知，老协和的医学教育体系中并不包括单独的科研训练课程，而国外其他医学院一般也未设置这一训练课程。这一阶段的学习实际上从培养方式来看，和 PhD 非常相似；但是时间上来说，比 PhD 要短得多，因此像 PhD 那样出成果也是非常不现实的。所以这一课程被视为医学博士和理学博士的混杂产物，对医学生的影响究竟如何，尚有争议。

一方面，国外医学教育界对科研训练课程的认同度并不高，因为临床医学的课程非常需要时间，要以实践为主。而另一方面，8 个月的科研训练往往不足以发表论文，也很难在工作以后以科研训练的成果作为工作基础。因此，对科研训练课程的教学改革，下一步到底如何发展，仍然是众说纷纭。

协和八年制校友问卷调查结果

为了撰写本文，笔者在 2016 年 9 月至 11 月期间通过互联网（Email、微信和网页问卷）在 1956－2008 年入学的协和八年制校友中进行了问卷调查，调查结果汇总如下：

基本情况

截至 2016 年 11 月 21 日，本调查共收集到来自 1956~2008 年入学的北京协和医学院八年制校友的有效问卷 511 份（为便于统计，未包括七转八和留学生校友），问卷总回收率为 26.4%（511/1932）。按照入学年份统计，各年代的校友问卷回收率如下：

- 1956~1965 级八年制问卷回收率为 14.1%（49/347）；

- 1979~1989 级八年制问卷回收率为 29.2%（105/360）；

- 1990~1999 级八年制问卷回收率为 43.6%（207/475）；

- 2000~2008 级八年制问卷回收率为 20.0%（150/749）；

回答问卷的 511 名八年制校友中，共有女性 240 人，男性 271 人。各年代回答问卷的校友性别构成见图 2。（注：本文以下各图内的横坐标均为入学年份。）

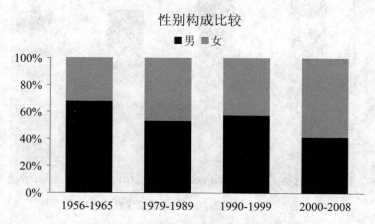

图 2　回答问卷的八年制校友性别构成比较

工作情况

　　根据问卷回答的结果，大部分协和八年制校友都从事医学临床、教育和生物医学相关的科学研究工作（图3），也有少数从事其他工作，如卫生管理部门、制药企业或投资机构等。从工作性质的比例而言，从事临床医学工作的毕业生在近30年来呈逐步上升趋势，近10年的毕业生90%以上都选择了临床工作。

　　校友的工作地点也呈现出显著的年代特征（图4）：上世纪50－60年代入学的校友多数（84%）在国内工作；上世纪80年代受"出国潮"的影响，出国学习工作的校友超过了一半，主要是去美国（63%）；随着中国经济和社会的变化，出国的校友比例逐年下降，近10年的毕业生93%都在国内工作。

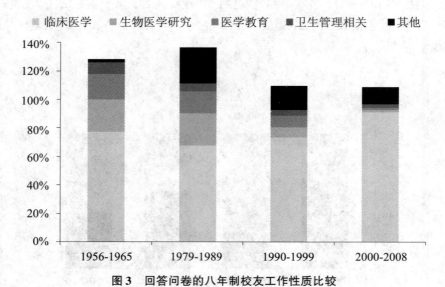

图3　回答问卷的八年制校友工作性质比较

工作地点比较

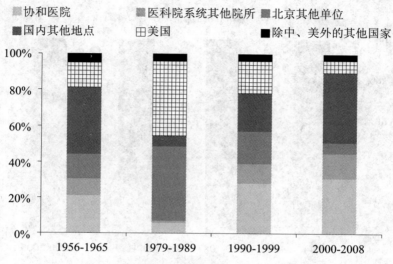

图4　回答问卷的八年制校友工作地点比较

职业发展情况

我们还统计了校友的学术职称（图5）和行政职务（图6）情况，作为职业发展情况的参考：上世纪50～60年代入学的校友，留在国内工作的90%以上获得了高级职称（在国外行医的未统计职称），且大部分具有行政职务；1979～1989年入学的校友也大致如此；1990年之后入学的校友尚处于职业发展期，高级职称比例不到30%，大部分还没有行政职务。

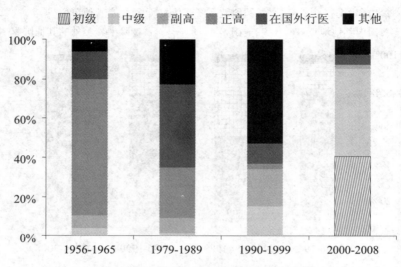

图5　回答问卷的八年制校友学术职称比较

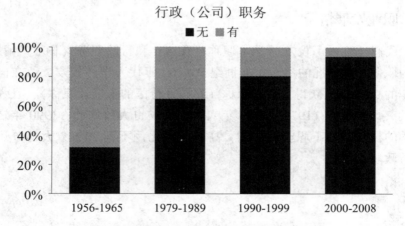

图6. 回答问卷的八年制校友担任行政职务比较

（注：包括在学术机构或公司担任的行政职务）

留言反馈

这份问卷的最后一个问题是个开放式问题（open question）：从母校

学到最重要的东西是什么？对于这个问题，校友们各自给出了自己的答案。其中包括校训中的"严谨、博精、勤奋、奉献"等词汇频繁出现在各个年龄、地区和性别的校友答案之中。这些共同点也早已成为了"协和精神"的内涵。

以下列举了部分校友对这个问题的回答，从中可见鲜明的时代特征和贯穿始终的协和精神传承：

1959～1965 年入学的校友：
"正直做人，专心做事，全心全意为病患服务"
"全心全意为病人，技术精益求精"
"严谨、务实、全心全意为人民服务"
"清清白白做人，认认真真做事"
1979～1989 年入学的校友：
"协和毕业生必须做开拓者的意识"
"开拓精神，独立思考"
"批判性思维、知识、严谨的态度、仁爱"
"敬业精神，对自己的病人尽心尽力"
"老教授老医生们对医学的无私奉献"
"精诚行医，学无止境；如临深渊如履薄冰"
1990～1999 年入学的校友：
"以人为本的人文关怀、放眼全球的国际视野、终身学习的自我完善方法、持之以恒坚持不懈的人生态度"
"有独立思考的能力，也有团结合作的精神"
"认真对待每一位患者的严谨态度"
"专注、坚持、敬业"
"坚守，不忘初心"
"人文底蕴"
2000～2008 年入学的校友：
"自主学习的能力，求真求实的态度"
"钻研的精神与社会责任感"

"终身学习，拼搏进取"
"自学能力和医学情怀"
"从医理念与敬业精神"
"医者仁心"

马　超（1991级八年制临床医学生）
李乃适（1992级八年制临床医学生）
李晗歌（2004级八年制临床医学生）
张婉莹（2009级八年制临床医学生）

PUMC Alumni: A Centennial Review

Mao Chao

Ma Chao, M. D. , graduated from the Peking Union Medical College (PUMC) in 1999 (8-year curriculum program) and then worked at PUMC Hospital for one year. In 2000, he went to the United States and began his post-doc training at Department of Anesthesiology of Yale University School of Medicine engaging in chronic pain mechanism research and became assistant professor there in 2008. At the end of 2011, he came back to PUMC and served as director of Department of Anatomy and Embryology of Institute of Basic Medical Sciences of Chinese Academy of Medical Sciences and was appointed as PUMC's Distinguished Professor, and tutor for doctoral degree candidates. In April 2015, he became the head of the Office of Academic Affairs of PUMC.

A total of 20,271 students have graduated from Peking Union Medical College (PUMC) since it was established in 1917 until 2016. This report provides an in-depth analysis of programs offered at PUMC, demographics and employment after graduation.

PUMC alumni

The following programs and majors are offered at PUMC.

8-year curriculum clinical medicine program

Ever since it began in 1917, PUMC has implemented an 8-year clinical medicine program which continues today. PUMC embedded and initiated the 8 year medical program in China. Enrolled students go through three stages, including: premedical, pre-clinical, and clinical medicine.

Candidates granted MD (medical doctor) status if they meet the requirements at graduation.

From 1917 – 1925, PUMC opened a premedical school, however, this was later closed. At that time, other famous universities such as Yenching University (later Peking University) provided pre-medical education for PUMC and student selection was based on rigorous standards before candidates were admitted to PUMC. The number of graduates steadily increased from 1924 when there were only three until the 1930s when the number of graduates reached around 20 per year.

When the Pacific War broke out in 1941, PUMC closed. Then after the Sino-Japanese War, PUMC was able to resume from 1947 to 1951, then unfortunately had to close once more. In 1956, PUMC resumed enrollment; however, was forced to close once more from 1966 – 1978, only resuming student intake in 1979. Since then, PUMC has enrolled around 30 students through the national college entrance examinations, with the premedical program based in Department of Biology of Peking University, which later changed its name to College of Bio Sciences.

Since 1994, the number of students enrolled reached around 60 through national college entrance examinations, and after 2000, the number increased to over 90. Since 1995, PUMC started a new transfer program in which PUMC admits a small number of students from other medical schools in China which offer a 7-year clinical medicine program to transfer to the 8-year clinical program at PUMC. When they meet the requirements of PUMC at graduation, they are conferred an MD of PUMC.

In 1995, the MD/PhD dual degree program was added to the list of PUMC programs. Candidates following this program will devote 3 additional years to research projects after completing the clinical program. Students from this course are granted both MD and PhD status upon graduation. In 2002, PUMC started to cooperate with Tsinghua University and began to enroll students through Tsinghua under the major of "Clinical Medicine of Tsinghua University". In this instance, pre-medical students from PUMC study are based at the Bio Science College of Tsinghua University, who enroll around 70 – 90 students per year. In addition, a small quota is provided to students transferring from other majors from within Tsinghua University. Since PUMC established the 8-year curriculum over 2. 888 students have graduated. 309 graduated before 1949, and 2, 579 after 1949 (including 256 from the 7 to 8 year program and 36 from MD / PhD Dual Degree Program, 20 of whom have been overseas students.

Nursing Undergraduate Program

Originally the 'Nurses Training School' of PUMC in 1920 which changed name to the 'School of Nursing' in 1924. This was the first nursing program in higher learning in China with a five year course of study at that time. This course included a 2 year pre-nursing course at Yenching University, after which students were granted a nursing diploma from PUMC as well as a bachelor degree from Yenching. Due to the academic demands of the course only one student graduated from the first course in 1924. From 1924 to 1930s, numbers fluctuated between 10 – 20.

During the Sino-Japanese War, the then Dean Nie Yuchan (Vera Nie), led a team from the school to Chengdu in Sichuan Province to reopen the nursing school there. From 1943 to 1946, the school enrolled 3 classes, totaling 50 students when the school relocated at West China Union University, and trained nursing professionals of emergency for wartime China. Then in 1946, School of Nursing moved back to Beiping (Peking, Beijing) and reopened until 1951 when the school was closed once more. From the first graduate class in 1924 until 1951, the school enrolled 28 classes consisting of 264 students.

One third of the graduates from the school went on to become leaders in the nursing profession, including presidents of the Chinese Nursing Association, presidents and vice presidents of national and international health care related organizations, secretary of associations, deans and heads of nursing departments in and around China. Several have also gone on to become chief editors and associate editors of professional nursing journals or textbooks. They were the founders, pioneers and trailblazers of nursing development at the beginning of the People's Republic of China (PRC).

In 1984, Ministry of Health and Ministry of Education decided to resume higher nursing education at the First Conference on Nursing of Higher Learning. Then in 1985, the Nursing Department of PUMC resumed the undergraduate program which implemented a 4 year curriculum. Previously from 1988 to 1994, the course was a 5 year program. The school increased capacity from a dozen students to 90 students today. Since the nursing program was established, 1,406 have graduated, among whom 264 graduated prior to 1952, and 1,142 after 1951. Wang Xiuying, Class 1931 became the first Nightingale Prize winner, and later five graduates of the school also won the great honor of the prize. They are Chen Lude, Lin Juying, Li Xiufang, Liu Shuyuan and Wu Xinjuan.

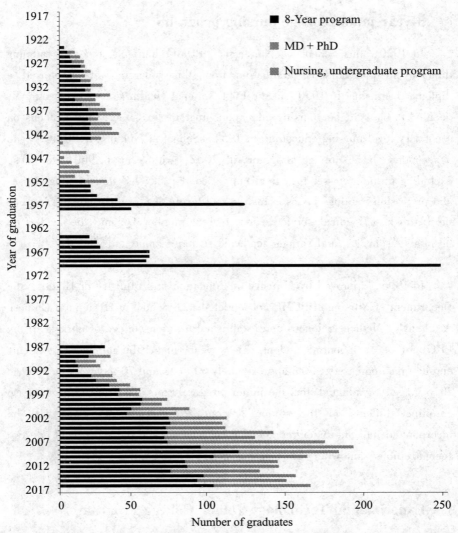

Figure 1. Histogram representing graduate numbers from 1917 – 2017, including;

8-year program, MD/PhD, and undergraduate nursing program histogram

Nate:

1) *All the data based on the actual graduating year*

2) *At the end of 1941 before the Pacific War broke out, PUMC held the special graduation ceremony for the medical class and School of Nursing. The 1943 class of medical program was conferred degree outside PUMC.*

3) *Graduates of Clinical Medical Program of 1963 – 1965 graduated simultaneously in 1970.*

3-year junior college nursing program

In 1920, the School of Nursing at PUMC initiated a 3-year nursing diploma program. Students graduating from this program were conferred a diploma in nursing. In 1950, at the First National Health Conference, officials decided to close higher nursing education programs in China, and to focus on secondary level nursing education. In 1954, School of Nursing at PUMC began a secondary level nursing program till 2002, with over 1,960 graduates, excluding training classes for caregivers, secondary leveled staff training classes and profession training classes of high school level. Most of the graduates became the bedrock of medical service, and a great number became the leaders in hospitals, schools, and various academic societies home and abroad.

In 1996, approved by Ministry of Education and Ministry of Health, the Department of Nursing of PUMC consolidated with School of Hygiene of Chinese Academy of Medical Sciences and established the first college of nursing in the PRC and began to enroll students. Every year since, the number of students enrolled has increased, from approximately 50 to around 70 today. From 1999 to 2016, 1,219 graduated from the junior program. From 2017, PUMC will cease enrolling students to the junior program. The enrollment quota will be incorporated into the undergraduate nursing program and the school will add two specializations; midwifery and aging nursing.

Experimental Technology Junior College Program

In 1986, PUMC began a 3-year course program with annual enrollment around 20 and later reached 40. The program stopped in 1998. From 1989 to 2001, graduates of the program summed 421. Many graduates are now employed in biomedical research institutes and biotech enterprises.

Graduate Program

The graduate program began in 1954 and continued until 1965, having enrolled and trained about 210 students – a non degree program. This program was suspended during the Cultural Revolution for over ten years only to resume enrollment in 1978. At that time, the school was one of the first cohort of universities/colleges approved by the state council to confer doctoral degree and masters degree and were allowed to set up separate entrance examinations and enroll students from Hong Kong, Macao, and Taiwan.

In 1982, the College established the first PUMC/CAMS Academic Degree Assessment Committee and conferred master degrees for the first time in its history. In 1985, the College also conferred its first doctoral degrees. In July 1986, the Graduate School was established by consolidating all the work relating to degree granting and training. In October 1996, after the Academic Degree Office of the State Council made assessment to 33 graduate schools in China, the School passed the assessment and announced what was termed 'official openness' (挂牌). In 1993, School of Nursing was endorsed as the master degree granting institute and the first cohort of candidates for the masters in nursing degree were recruited in 1996. In 2004, the School of Nursing initiated the joint nursing doctoral training program with School of Nursing of Johns Hopkins University, and started to enroll candidates.

Nowadays, courses offered by the Graduate School are classified into five categories: science, engineering, medicine, management and philosophy.

Courses cover: basic medicine, clinical medicine, biology, pharmacology, public health and preventative medicine, integrated medicine of TCM and western medicine, dentistry, public management, bio-engineering, library science, information study and archive management, science technology and philosophy, etc.

Up until September 2016, the Graduate School has been accredited with the ability conferring doctoral degree to 8 first class disciplines, including: biology, basic medicine, clinical medicine, nursing, pharmacology, public health and preventive medicine, integration of TCM and western medicine, and bio-engineering.

Among the disciplines the school offers, 2 disciplines which are regarded as national 1st class key disciplines, 8 disciplines are classified as national 2nd class key disciplines, 2 3rd class key disciplines, and 1 national priority discipline.

At the municipal level (Beijing), 1 discipline is considered 1st class , 3 2nd class level, 1 3rd class, and 1 priority discipline.

PUMC also has 6 national key laboratories, and 9 key ministry laboratories. From 1978 to 2016, the school graduated 7,281 full time doctoral degree student, 7,056 master degree students, with a total number of 14,337 graduates.

Aside from the above full time students, ever since its establishment, PUMC set up continuing education courses and has trained refreshment students from all parts of the country. In 1984, PUMC set up a staff training office responsible for continuing education. In 1998, it was upgraded into the School of Adult Education (成人教育学院) and changed the name to the School of Continuing Education in 2003. The school offers continuing education starting from junior college level up to undergraduate academic training.

Nowadays, the school offers 3 programs including nursing, medical image technology, and medical testing. Apart from the academic training program, the school also offers refreshment training to affiliated hospitals and research institutes and holds courses for rural doctor training, community doctor training, train the trainers for family medicine, and "Standardized training for residents of hospitals in Beijing", all of which provide measurable social benefits.

PUMC's 8-Year Medical Curriculum

After PUMC was nationalized in 1951, the 8-year curriculum was interrupted twice so PUMC's history can be divided into three periods, 1951 – 1957, 1959 – 1970, and 1979 till now. Before PUMC was nationalized in 1951, students enrolled in a premedical program at Yenching from 1945 to 1949, then completed study as usual. However, this program was suspended after the class 1957 graduated.

The second period began in 1959 when central government approved resuming the long-term medical education program and PUMC changed its name to China Medical University. The program continued until the collapse of China's higher learning at the beginning of the Cultural Revolution. PUMC closed its door after the class of 1970.

The third period refers to a time when PUMC resumed the medical education program in 1979 until now. During each period, the 8-Year program maintained the high standards of the 'old PUMC' model, which is sequential training consisting of premedical, preclinical and clinical education. This was embedded so that students would gain a broad and solid knowledge base, unique among medical schools in China.

Organizational name changes

The college has changed its name a dozen times in its 100-year history. In the Republican period, influenced by political and social factors, it used 5 different names, reverting back and forth 7 times. However, the English name of the College – Peking Union Medical College was almost always used to refer to the College. When established, PUMC was called Beijing Xiehe Yixueyuan. However, after the success of the Northern Expedition in 1928, Beijing changed its name to Beiping so PUMC had to also change to "Peiping Union Medical College".

In 1949, when the People's Republic of China was founded, the city changed its name back to Beijing, and so did PUMC. In 1951, when the People's Liberation Army took charge of PUMC, PUMC changed its name to China Union Medical College (中国协和医学院). In 1959, PUMC resumed enrollment and once again change its name to "China Medical University" (中国医科大学) until the Cultural Revolution. When PUMC resumed in 1979, it named itself "China Capital Medical University" (中国首都医科大学). In 1986, the College used Union (xiehe) in its name again and changed the name to China Union Medical University (中国协和医科大学). The name was continually used for 20 years, the longest period after 1949.

After mid 1990s, led by the Ministry of Education, a merger of universities in China prevailed. Beijing Medical University merged into Peking University and became the Peking University Health Sciences Center, while Shanghai Medical University became the Health Division of Fudan University. Tsinghua University intended to merge PUMC. Although after several years of discussion, the two organizations reached a collaborative agreement to run a joint program.

Then in 2006, the college changed its Chinese name back to Beijing Xiehe Yixueyuan i. e. PUMC and another plaque "Medical Division of Tsinghua University" hung over the main entrance of the campus.

Changes of the premedical program

In the beginning when PUMC was established, the China Medical Board (CMB) conducted an investigation into the main universities in China and found that there were no college or university delivered a premedical program up to the PUMC standard. Therefore, the foundation decided to set up its own premedical school, so that PUMC's first ten classes would study at their own premedical school.

Since 1926, Yenching University, led by President John Leighton Stuart, steadily improved the standard to a 'good' university, and as a result the CMB closed PUMC's premed school, preferring to base the premed program at Department of Biology of Yenching University. All the equipment and library of premed school were dedicated to Yenching University and faculty members joined the College of Science of Yenching. Since then, most of the premed students of PUMC studied at Yenching University. However, some outstanding students graduated from premed education in other famous universities in the Republic period were also admitted to PUMC after passing the exams. This arrangement continued up to 1951 when PUMC fell under the military regime. In 1952, Yenching University merged with another university and lost its identity when the PRC restructured higher learning. Those PUMC premed students who had completed 3 years' premed studies continued the study at PUMC and became the last class of this period.

The second period started in 1959 and with support from the authorities, "China Medical University" became the new name for PUMC. PUMC began to take in students at anaccelerated rate and made premed education at Peking University with which the College of Science at Yenching University merged into. However, time was insufficient for training new premed students, so PUMC enrolled students from the Department of Biology of Peking University and started to offer pre-clinical courses for students. During the following two years, this arrangement continued. It was not until 1962 when candidates could directly apply to China Medical University (PUMC) for admission; however students enrolled through the Biology Department of Peking University to the premed program of PUMC.

The third period started in 1979 when PUMC students first entered the premed program with Department of Biology of Peking University and this continued until 2002. From 2002, the premed program was instituted at Department of Biology of Tsinghua University till now.

In sum, the premed education after 1951, first based in Yenching University, continued to Peking University and after the new century, to Tsinghua till now.

Academic goals set out in the three stages of training – premed, preclinical, and clinical respectively

The Rockefeller Foundation's vision of creating PUMC was to build the best medical school comparable with the best in America and Europe, offering elite medical education with the highest standards. This vision was embodied in the premed training ever since it began. The requirements for the premed training remained unchanged for a long time, which was based in the best comprehensive university so that the students study thoroughly conceptualized and practice using advanced scientific thinking, which included gaining the ability to use the scientific reasoning to the study the human body, and laying the foundation for future medical research.

Likewise, comprehensive universities would also be able to offer many humanity courses to students, which enhance communication between future practitioners and patients. Therefore, premed courses are no different from those delivered by the biology department, and PUMC never interfered with courses for the premed students. So, whether it is in 1950s, 1960s or after Cultural Revolution, the overall goals of premed are consistent, and unambiguous.

Preclinical education, for the 'old PUMC' period was undertaken by different departments of basic medicine, such as Department of Anatomy, Department of Physiology, as well as other departments. After the People's Liberation Army (PLA) took over the leadership of PUMC, this arrangement continued. However, after PUMC stopped recruiting students in 1952, all basic medicine departments changed to focus on research, until 1959 when PUMC resumed enrollment.

During the Cultural Revolution, almost all the basic medicine departments relocated to Jianyang (简阳) in Sichuan Province following relocation of the Institute of Experimental Medical Research. Then, the institute relocated back to Beijing after the Cultural Revolution. After, resuming in 1979, the Institute of Basic Medical Sciences (IBMS) was established on the basis of the Institute of Experimental Medical Research, so preclinical education was undertaken by the IBMS, and IBMS became the School of Basic Medicine at PUMC. Since then, conventional courses have been delivered by related departments or research offices. There was no staffing allocated to teaching arrangement.

In the 1980s, PUMC hired a number of American Chinese scientists who had just retired from American universities and they were offered courses mostly in English so that English proficiency was instrumental to the improvement of PUMC's medical students. In 1990s, most of those professors returned to the US due to a lack of funding, leaving basic medical training wanting for funding for long time. This has only recently changed.

Presently, PUMC has been categorized as one of the 6 so-called "Small Scale Specialized Universities/Colleges" by the Ministry of Education, and there has been a big improvement in terms of funding. The teaching offered by IBMS steadily received good feedback from the students. Preclinical training has also developed laying a solid foundation of knowledge for clinical training, while embedding experimental skills for further professional growth. This has always been a PUMC aspiration, even throughout times of political upheaval and social unrest.

Clinical training has always been carried out by the PUMC Hospital. Before nationalization, PUMC and the PUMC Hospital were one entity. However, after nationalization, PUMC discontinued enrollment, while the hospital engaged the workforce in clinical activities. PUMC's hospital was charged primarily with the medical care for the leaders, so the hospital gradually separated from the college. Even during the Cultural Revolution, when the college had been closed, the hospital continued serving the population even when it had been renamed the "Anti – Imperialist Hospital".

PUMC has always been seen as the gold standard in China, placing it in a pivotal role for the country. As the teaching hospital for PUMC, the goal of training is very clearly stated i. e. to train outstanding clinicians for the future. Due to the fact that most PUMC graduates continue at the PUMC Hospital this has developed a unique culture which can pass on clinical traditions and maintain the unique teaching tradition.

Overview of the courses for 8-Year Program

The chronicle of 8-year program

The 8-Year Medical Education program originated from the medical education reform at the beginning of twentieth century. After the publication of the Flexner Report, Johns Hopkins University (JHU) became the role model for all the medical schools in the US with the 4 + 4 education model which means medical schools enrolling students from comprehensive universities. This model was regarded as the most advanced in medical education. Therefore, the PUMC, founded by the Rockefeller Foundation, as the Johns Hopkins of China should adopt the most advanced education model. Based on the Johns Hopkins model, PUMC revised the model into 3 + 5 by adjusting to Chinese societal demands, by shortening the premed i. e. 3 premed + 5 medical education.

When officially established in 1917, PUMC recruited faculty and set up courses based on the JHU medical model and standard, with the Rockefeller Foundation guaranteeing adequate funding for the College. In contrast, most medical colleges in China were struggling with deficiency in funding and extreme staff shortage. Therefore, since inception, PUMC was at a great advantage and superior to other medical schools in terms of teaching programs and quality. PUMC has always stood high in the estimation of medical society in China.

In fact, the vision and main concepts of the Rockefeller Foundation were always challenged. Top leaders of the foundation were always worried and uneasy about PUMC's huge budget, while the Chinese government at that time and many celebrities in society thought that PUMC, with all its advantage should produce more qualified doctors. Lin Kesheng (Lim, Kho-seng, nicknamed for K. S. Robert, the director and professor of the Physiology Department at PUMC held the same view. He apparently thought that there was a huge demand for doctors in China and PUMC should devote resources to train a greater number to benefit the Chinese society. There was another voice that advocated PUMC should give up its demanding 8-Year curriculum and adopt the fast-track, less expensive program. However, the countervailing view, advocated the elite education at PUMC, represented by the first director of the college – Franklin McLean and others who eventually prevailed.

In 1947, PUMC resumed after the Japanese army ravaged the campus. Even though the buildings were not damaged, all the equipment and instruments were gone. The Rockefeller Foundation contributed a huge endowment again and declared that this was the last endowment and that PUMC subsequently had to depend on itself. Even so, the 8-Year program has always been a steadfast and committed program until it was nationalized.

In October 1950, the PLA crossed the Yalu River to Korea and the so-called "Anti-American and Assist Korea" War had begun. At this point Sino-US relations were very tense and on Jan 20th, 1951, the PLA officially took over the leadership and control of PUMC for 6 years. During that time the college turned to serve the army. PUMC as the representative of the "bulwark of the American Imperialist Aggression" was castigated in every aspect. The 8-year program that the Rockefeller Foundation insisted on for a long time was the main target of criticism and was considered a program "to train students to serve the capitalists" so it was discontinued. For those who were admitted to the program, they continued their studies and graduated as the last class for that period. Among those students, there are the very established masters in medicine, such as Luo Weici, Shi Yifan, Lu Shibi, Wu Ning, Sun Yan and others.

In 1957, arranged by Premier Zhou Enlai, the PLA handed over PUMC to Ministry of Health. At that time, some senior physicians such a Zhang Xiaoqian suggested resuming the long-term medical program but failed in his attempt. In

1959, a number of senior scholars filed a request to resume the long-term medical program and with the support of Premier Zhou Enlai, PUMC succeeded and reopened under the new name "China Medical University". Dr. Huang Jiasi, graduate of the class of '33, and president of Shanghai Medical College became the President of PUMC. At that time, the top-down governing guidance unanimously was "The Party's leadership plus Old PUMC", therefore, the course of study followed the 'old PUMC' program.

During the Cultural Revolution the program once again came under attack. From the title of the Brochure "The Bloody OLD PUMC – Destroy thoroughly PUMC's 8-Year Curriculum Program", one can see that all the faculty and students of PUMC identified the 8-Year program with the Old PUMC. In 1959, the first class was selected from the students of the third grade of Department of Biology Peking University and admitted to PUMC. At the same time, PUMC enrolled premed students from Department of Biology of Peking University, 60 students each year. This period ended in 1966. Even though the last classes of this period graduated in 1970 altogether, it was actually impossible to study after the onset of the Cultural Revolution.

In 1979, PUMC resumed to enroll students for the third time under the new name "China Capital Medical University", admitting 30 students each year. It adheres to the 8-Year Curriculum program till now, and never changed. Unlike the resumption in 1959, the first class of this period did not enroll students directly from the senior students of Department of Biology to enter the PUMC premedical training when PUMC resumed the premed enrollment at PKU. So, the first class graduated in 1987. Since then, there have been slight changes for the 8-year curriculum program, but the main structure remains with only minor adjustments.

In summary, PUMCs' 8-Year curriculum is the landmark of the 'old PUMC' education system. It has aroused wide discussion and disputes, but it has been unanimously identified by the faculty and staff of PUMC and lasts until today.

Mary Bullock said, "PUMC maintains the 8-Year model of education of its leadership position and cherishes the program and resists any attempt to revise it. "

Now, the "5 + 3 Training model" which is a master degree based standardized training has been established as the mainstream of medical education model by the Chinese government, the old 8-Year Curriculum program is facing great challenge. However, new opportunities always go hand in hand with challenges. The challenging context now will be able to push forward the education reform at PUMC.

Overview of Premed Courses

The premed school of PUMC started to offer classes in 1917, and in 1926, the program started to be instituted at Yenching University. The premed school also took in premed students transferred from other universities that offered premed courses. For example, Prof. Liu Shihao, an established professor in endocrinology was transferred to PUMC premed program from Hunan-Yale Premedical School in Changsha in 1919. In 1926, the premed started to base in the College of Science of Yenching University till 1952 when Yenching was closed down. The courses of study did not change much which means that classes of 1953 to 1957 studied almost the same courses as did their former fellow schoolmates.

Zhang Zhinan (class of '54), established hematologist, recalled the courses offered for premed[1]:

As the basis for training before medical training for PUMC, the Premed is very demanding, in order to lay solid and an inclusive basis for the students to study medicine and practice medicine. So, in addition to mathematics, physics, chemistry and biology, we had to study humanity courses. We have to complete the study of the following subjects within 3 years: general biology (taught by Lin Changshan), invertebrate zoology (taught by Miss Boring), vertebrate zoology (by Hu Jingfu), general genetics and general chemistry (by Xu Pengcheng), qualitative analysis chemistry, quantitative analysis chemistry, organic chemistry (by Dr. Wilson), physical chemistry, general physics (by Chu Shenglin), calculus (by Xu Xianyu). English courses lasted two years and sociology lasts for one semester (by Yan Jingyao). There were few optional subjects because we had many compulsory courses. I continued studying psychology and studied general psychology (by Shen Naizhang) and psychology health (by Dr, Sailor) when I was a freshman, studied children's psychology (by Sun Guohua from Tshinghua University) when I was sophomore, and industry psychology when I was junior (also taught by teacher from Tsinghua). The courses were taught in different classrooms of different buildings, so most students had to rush to the classrooms by riding bicycles. We had to do experiments at the classes of biology, physics and chemistry and we had to be careful, attentive, and accurate, writing a report. The biology class required drawing, depending on one's own real mastered skill set, especially for quantitative and qualitative chemistry experiment. Every time when I got the unknown specimen, I was very nervous, worrying about the result was not correct. The teaching effect was not totally depended upon the teacher's academic credential. I did poorly for calculus, partly because of the teacher was not skillful in lecturing. I was worried that I might fail the class.

The premed program from 1959 to 1965 period was carried out at the Department of Biology of PKU. There students spent 3 years undergoing premed training together with students of the Department of Biology. Except for the added political subjects, the rest of the subjects they took were almost the same as did the biology majored students, and similar to those of the 'Old PUMC's' premed courses at Yenching University.

Shen Ti, graduate of the class of 63 felt that this has "cultivated the ways of thinking" and beneficial to the clinical work later. Wu Zhaosu enrolled with PUMC in 1959 still remembers President Huang Jiasi explaining the premed program when they were admitted to the college, saying:

> *Huang Jiasi's remarks at the opening ceremony were around why we set up the 8-year curriculum. Usually, after 5 years education, students began to make money to support their families. The biggest difference between you guys and students from other universities is that you will lay a more solid foundation in basic sciences than others. It is analogous to that the stronger the base is, the higher the building could be built. We were all convinced. The old PUMC was run in this way, and they thought this direction is correct.*

At the inception of 1979, Huang Jiasi was the President of PUMC when it resumed. From 1979 to 2002, PUMC's premed program was in the Department of Biology of PKU. The subjects included: general biology, comparative anatomy, microbiology, genetics, biochemistry, advanced mathematics, physics, inorganic chemistry, analysis chemistry, organic chemistry, physichemistry, computer, general psychology, college English, and Marxism philosophy. These subjects did not remain unchanged and often adjusted correspondingly with the curriculum reform of the Department of Biology of PKU. For example, the premed students studied at PKU from 1991 to 1992, the former one year general biology was canceled, and substituted by one year botany and one year zoology. But in general, the teaching philosophy that the courses should be centered on the basis of biology courses was consistently carried out. Till 2003, owing to many reasons, PUMC's premed moved to the College of Biology Sciences Tsinghua University. Except the specialized zoology, botany, and vertebrate animal, and comparative anatomy, all other things in curriculum remains the same.

Overview of Courses of Basic Medicine (preclinical)

The courses for preclinical medicine of classes 1953 – 1957 were conducted by the Departments of Basic Medicine of the "old PUMC". Generally speaking, foreign professors returning home due to a lack of funding did not diminish the teaching capacity of PUMC. This was because that even though one foreign faculty, William Adolph, director of Department of Biochemistry left PUMC due to his citizenship, his successor – Prof. Liu Shihao was very established in biochemistry.

Prof Zhang Zhinan recalled in detail of this period of study,

The first two years studying at PUMC was on preclinical medicine. For the first year, we had three courses – anatomy, physiology, and biochemistry. This was the toughest time for us. Each of the three courses had someone who failed, particularly for courses in neurology anatomy and biochemistry. At the first lecture of anatomy, Prof. Zhang Fang (张銎) said solemnly that if we did not do well in anatomy, we were not qualified as doctors. Therefore, all the classmates studied very hard, reading day and night, studying the bodies, memorizing, keeping notes. Staying up late was very common. Some of the girl students learned to smoke in order to stimulate themselves. For the anatomy class, we had to go through one of the psychology obstacles – to hang around with the bodies every day. Particularly at night, nobody dared to stay in the lab alone; and nobody would be the last person to leave the lab. So, almost always, several students left the lab together. We heard that during the Anti-Japanese war, students of National Shanghai Medical College would go to steal body from the bombs in the Gele Mountain nearby at midnight in order to take the anatomy class. However, at PUMC, the bodies were available for us with one body for two students. No difficulty to get bodies at all. But now, it was difficult to get bodies. They were all dedicated voluntarily by the dead or by his or her relatives, which was a great contribution and support to the medical education. Therefore, every time, the faculty and students would hold a ceremony to show respect and gratitude to the donor.

Prof Zhang Zhinan continued,

In the second year at PUMC, we studied pharmacology, pathology, microbiology and parasitology, all of which were very appealing. I liked these courses very much and my performance was good. I was particularly interested in pathology taught by Prof. Hu Zhengxiang（胡正祥）. Lecturer Wang Dexiu taught test-tube experiment. Later, Liu Yonghui taught a several times after he came back to China from America. We used Boyd's Textbook of Pathology in this course, but the students often read Pathology coauthored by Hu Zhengxiang and Qin Guangyu（秦光煜）, which was succinct and the concepts clearly presented. Prof. Hu conducted the class in English, very concise and clearly presented, particularly for experiment classes. At experiment class, each student had a microscopy and a set of slides. Teacher Wang Dexiu（王德修）assisted us attentively. Sometimes, we observed the specimen of the body, but most time we watched the slides ourselves. It left us with a strong impression and memorized well in our mind, and very helpful in the clinical study later on! Pharmacology was taught by Prof. Zhou Jinhuang（周金黄）. Later, Dr. Lei haipeng（雷海朋）, a PUMC alumnus came back to PUMC to work after he did his fellowship at Toronto University in Canada. He taught us pharmacology of vitamin and endocrine. In addition, Mr. Zhu Yan（朱颜）who did fellowship training at Department of Pharmacology PUMC at that time gave us lectures for several times. We used the textbook coauthored by Goodman & Gilman from the US. Prof. Zhou was very learned and well known throughout the country.

Microbiology was taught by Prof. Xie Shaowen（谢少文）. Prof Xie Shaowen was an alumnus from PUMC and used to be the chief resident at PUMC Hospital. He is knowledgeable and worked very hard. He was sensitive scholar ready to capture new information. He was a pioneer in immunology study. Also, he advocated integrating basic medicine with clinical medicine. He led by example, often attending the ward round of Department of Internal Medicine and giving his opinion. He required the students to consult literature and write review about some specific cases. Parasitology was taught by Swiss Prof. Hoeppi. Before PRC established diplomatic relationship with Switzerland, he also acted as agent for consulate affairs. In addition, Prof. Feng Lanzhou（冯兰洲）was an important member of the department. [4]

Prof. Zhang Zhinan clearly had a extreme deep impression of the two years' pre-clinical training and thought that studying courses of basic medicine benefited tremendously the clinical training. He went on to say that,

> The first two years' preclinical courses on basic medicine at PUMC were instrumental to the clinical training. After we went to do the clinical training, the understanding of the manifestation of the illness, diagnosis, and treatment were based on the related content of preclinical courses.

In August 1956, Chinese Academy of Medical Sciences (CAMS) was established and in 1957, PUMC merged into CAMS. Later, in 1958, five institutes were established under the merged institute, one of which was the Institute of Experimental Medicine Research (Now, known as the IBMS), whose main task was basic medicine research.

In 1959, the 8-year long-term medical education program resumed. Under the leadership of President Huang Jiasi, some of the faculty members of the Institute of Experimental Medical Research were transferred to support the resumption of teaching tasks. So, PUMC rebuilt or initiated the so-called teaching and research offices of anatomy, histology and embryology, pharmacology, microbiology and immunology, parasitology, public health and epidemiology, statistics and etc. Therefore, courses offered for classes 1959 – 1965 were conducted by these teaching and research offices. So in spite of the influences of socio-political movements, the courses offered laid a sound foundation for the students.

On October 26th, 1969, the Central Committee of CPC issued the Notice of Relocating the Institutions of Higher Learning to the Grass root" also referred to as the "NO. 1 Order" by Lin Biao (林彪). As a result, many institutions of higher learning relocated to places outside Beijing. By the end of 1969, the Institute of Experimental Medicine Research was moved entirely to Jianyang (简

阳) of Sichuan Province, and merged into the Sichuan Branch of CAMS. In 1973, the various teaching and research offices of the former Chinese Medical University (PUMC) was consolidated and restructured, with half of the staff and equipment being transferred to Beijing TCM College which belonged to Ministry of Health at that time. The rest of the faculty and staff formed the teaching group for basic medicine under direct leadership of CAMS. This chaos lasted until after the Cultural Revolution.

In 1978, approved by the State Council, the Institute of Experimental Medicine Research moved back to Beijing and merged with the teaching group for medicine and formed the IMBS. In 1993, IBMS was given another name i. e. the School of Basic Medicine (基础医学院) and the name changed to School of Basic Science (基础学院) in 2006.

Since early in 1982, PUMC's pre-clinical training has been conducted at IBMS, with a similar course of study as before. After receiving pre-clinical training, there used to be a four month intensive training period for basic scientific research. Later, at beginning of the 1990s, this training started to be integrated into the research training at clinical stage and became one scientific training course, in which students were able to choose a tutor either from basic medicine or from clinical medicine to do the scientific training. This has become a new feature for the 8-year program of PUMC which will be introduced in the following part of the chapter.

Overview of Courses of Clinical Medicine

For the classes from 1953 to 1957, even though PUMC had stopped enrolling students, those registered could continue their studies until graduation because clinical training emphasizes practicable skills, and discontinuing would have influenced the students, but the students could be able to complete their training without interruption. However, many details in training were in fact affected and revised accordingly. For example, for the class 1954, the students could only choose one from the three-internal medicine, surgery or gynecology for clinical rotation, so that Shi Yifan, professor of endocrine who later became the academician of Chinese Academy of Engineering felt it is a great shame for her not being able to do the rotation at surgery and gynecology when she recalled her student time at PUMC.

Prof Zhang Zhinan recalled in detail of the clinical practice as a PUMC student. In his memoir Growth And Experience, he described in detail the study at that time. [2]

First, he described the courses of study for the first year of this period:

From the third year, we began the clinical training, starting from courses of basic diagnosis, experimental diagnosis, general introduction of treatment, then gradually moved on to lectures on internal medicine, surgery, ob & gyn. We were divided into three groups and went separately to Departments of Internal Medicine, surgery and obstetrics and gynecology to be the Extern. We began to have access to patients under the guidance of the supervisors. Basic diagnosis lecture was conducted by Prof Deng Jiadong who focused on physical diagnosis approach and principle. At that time, because there were not many patients, for some of the special symptoms such as measles, scarlet fever, typhoid, the rash from typhus, Koplic spot on the membrane of mouth from measles, we had to go to the infectious disease hospital; for other symptoms, we had to go to other hospitals to see the patients. For experimental diagnosis course, it focused on the three routine biochemistry testing-blood, urine, and feces as well as some common routine blood biochemistry testing. The major three routine testing were practiced by students themselves and to be mastered. In addition, we were given lectures on X-ray diagnosis and demonstration of reading the X-ray results. General Treatment focused on concepts and principle of pharmaceutical treatment, physical treatment, and brief introduction to nutritional treatment. All those courses laid a foundation for the identification, diagnosis and treatment of diseases in the future.

He continued：

> *The following courses – on internal medicine, surgery and obstetrics & gynecology were taught by established medical masters and were very impressive. The students were benefited a lot from the instruction.*

> *Internal medicine was an extensive course, and diseases of different human systems were taught by different professors who specialized in that particular area, therefore, each had its own style and features. Prof. Zhang Xiaoqian's teaching style was just like the person himself – vigorous, attentive, and careful with details. Prof. Liu Shihao was very composed, steady and conducted the class skillfully. Prof Zhu Guiqing was humorous, instructions of which were easy to remember. Prof Zhang Xuede's lecture included rich information and arranged in good order. Prof Zhong Huilan, Huang Wan, Zhang An and others all had his or her own characteristics. When clinicians taught classes about diseases, they could do it vividly and in a natural way as if there were a patient in front of him or her, so that it was easy to remember. The surgery class was taught by Prof Zeng Xianjiu. He taught the class just as if he were performing an operation, careful with each detail and in good reasoning. Ob & Gyn was taught by Prof Lin Qiaozhi, assisted by Prof Ge Taisheng in gynecology and Prof Wang Wenbin assisted Lin Qiaozhi in obstetrics. They all conducted class in an effective way.*

The clerkship also started simultaneously. The traditional tutorship refers to the teaching methodology at this stage of study.

Professor Zhang, continued：

> *The clerkship is the most important stage of clinical study on how to treat patients. The class was divided into three groups, with 7 or 8 students in each group and the groups went to 3 different departments. Under the instruction of the supervisor, students did their clerkship observation. Some students were picky on the assigned professors. For example, the students were very happy when Prof. Zhu Guiqing was assigned as the supervisor at department of internal medicine, because*

Prof. Zhu was senior and humorous. Also, when the students had Prof Zhang Xuede as their supervisor, they were also very contented, because Prof Zhang gave extensive information. At that time, most of the supervisors were professors, associate professors, but I was assigned a young lecture – Dr. Fang Qi. Dr. Fang was my teacher who led me to medical career. He was modest, amiable, and very dedicated to work. He also cares much of the patients with a kind heart. So, he made great achievements in his career for his whole life and with excellent image. I started my Externship from internal medicine so that the tutors of intern medicine not only instructed me on how to take medical record, do physical checkup, do testing and make correct analysis, but also taught me how to treat patients, and how to communicate with them. The patients are the ones that I have to learn from and they are sources of knowledge. The students repeatedly ask patients questions about history of illness and do the physical checkup, which was not considered the must for the medical care, but it served as a contribution to the students, because the patients sacrificed their time and stamina so as to provide learning opportunities for the students. Therefore, we should regard patients as benefactors. When we learn from patients, we should do what we can to the patients. We should not complain when the patient showed a little impatience. Another concern is that when we examine a patient of the opposite sex, particularly on some private parts, it is necessary to have a third person – either the relative or the supervisor at present with the exposure of body as little as possible. This shows the respect to patients. To have a correct perspective and attitude toward patients ensured that the students can put themselves in the patients' shoes to analyze and deal with problems, understand the patients and have compassion toward patients. It is also the basic requirements for medical ethics and ethos for the future medical care. Sometimes, during physical checkup, students should try to find new discoveries, raise new questions, and asking questions while examining. Students should observe how the supervisor asked questions, how to ask questions about the history of illness. During physical checkup, students should watch the way and technic the supervisor did it, and find out why the supervisor can discover the signs that the students failed to find out. Sometimes, it is only a small tip. When analyzing the conditions using testing results, do not just learn what the supervisor said about the specific knowledge of the disease, but learn from the supervisor about his or her thinking processing of the symptoms, signs, abnormal signs (normal), how to assess the significance using the case, how to integrate the things observed to make holistic judgment; more important is the critical thinking mindset and assessment method.

When I stayed with the Surgery Department, we were supervised by Dr. Wu Weiran to observe, analyze, explain patients' conditions, operation adaptation and precautions for the operation and for post operation, the observation of post operation, administration of medication, the healing of cutting, stitches removing and etc. We had a class of doing operation on animals because we cannot practice operation on humans at this stage. The students learned basic skills of how to choose point for cutting, and how to cut, stop bleeding, ligation and stitch, and etc. When we were at ob & gyn, my supervisor was Prof. Zeng Miancai, a returned overseas Chinese form Indonesia. His mandarin was not good, so he asked me to write case record in English and he made revision and comment on it in English. Later, the department was worried that I might not be able to write in Chinese and asked Dr. Tan Wentao to be my assistant supervisor. It showed how the department paid attention to the students. In Ob & Gyn, the supervisor instructed me to do gynecology checkup, while the obstetric supervisor took me to observe the labor on call. The students could not practice, but they involved in every case study, led by the supervisor or the doctor present, so it left us with strong impression.

The last year of clinical study included all the departments that were not covered in the previous year; the style of teaching was the same, but the mentorship was no longer one to one, but in small groups, and emphasized on practice.

The fourth year at PUMC, in addition to the three major departments of Internal, Surgery and Ob &Gyn, it included departments of eye, ENT, dermatology, neurology and mental health, radiology diagnosis, pediatrics and etc. Apart from lectures, the students had to follow doctors of different departments to see the patients, in either the wards of pediatrics and neurology, or in the out-patient department, or watch teaching films in small groups for the radiology diagnosis. It was usually conducted into small groups instead of assigning each student a supervisor. This year we observed a great variety of illness. The instructor of each department was skillful in teaching. Dr. Luo Zongxian, Zhang Xiaolou, Lao Yuanxiu of the Eye Department presented the class very clearly and the last two doctors had the talent to draw pictures on the blackboard when giving lecture. They were so skillful with the strokes and drew the pictures without much thinking, even without slight hesitation or revision. Dr. Li Hongjiong of Dermatology Ddepartment was agreeable and humorous. In talking with patients or parents of the sick kids, the students not only learned the knowledge of treatment and prevention of the diseases, but also learned how to communicate effectively with the patients. For example, the doctor could point out with witty words to the parents of the kids with eczema that they were wrong in rearing the kid. Those scenes and language was hard to forget in our whole life. Pediatrician Zhou Huakang was a tall and strong person, but the kids, unlike the students, were not intimidated by him. He was intimidating to the students because he has a unique way of teaching by pouring questions on them, one question after another and went all the way to the root. Even though we had answered the questions, but he would continue asking and probing if we were sure about the answer. When recalling this, I think only by this can we gain the knowledge and remember them. After lecture, we went to the underground ward of building No. 8 to observe the mental health patients, mostly for the method of access to patients and examination. To learn to communicate with different patients and win over their cooperation was one of the most important basic skills. It needs technique to communicate with the patients. To be a good doctor, one needs lifelong training. I have deep understanding of this when I was an Extern and when I provided medical care in rural areas."

Prof. Zhang Zhinan obviously had a deep impression on the teaching method of "involving the students in pathology discussion" and thought the result was very satisfactory. Stating that:

At PUMC's clinical training period, there was another special kind of teaching-Student CPC, which the pathologist picked up a certain case, and asked a student to write down an overview of the case (excluding the pathology result), and handed out to the students beforehand. Then, a student would give presentation analyzing the diagnosis and treatment. Two to three students were asked to involve in the discussion, and other students could present their view freely. Then, another student will report the pathology result. Finally, the supervisor would summarize whether the diagnosis and the understanding of the condition was corresponding to the pathology result. If not, what caused that, whether the treatment was appropriate or not, and what lessons should be learned from. The students could continue to ask questions. This method was authentic, specific and made the students immediately realize the root causes, misunderstanding in diagnosis reasoning, or the consequences of mistreatment and led to a deep memory.

The clinical practice of this period is very important to the growth of a medical student. Regarding the adaptation of specialized focused practice of the special period of the era, Prof Zhang Zhinan made an objective comment on it, saying:

In the last year of clinical study, students were interns, doing clinical work under the guidance of a higher ranking doctor and responsible for diagnosis, treatment and dealing with other issues, which we started to accumulate clinical experience and gain competence of working through authentic and real working experience. In some of the medical colleges, students rotated in the three departments of internal medicine, surgery, and Ob &Gyn, while at PUMC, because of our situation at that time, we focused our rotation on one department. Most of students in my class rotated at internal medicine for one year, while some focused on department of anesthesia, ENT, neurology, but again it was one year for one specialized department. The advantage of the one year specialized rotation is that one can be the resident for that specialized department directly after training, whereas the biggest disadvantage of it, I believe, is that we had too little clinical knowledge of the other departments and obtained little competence to deal with the cases of other department. The students who specialized in internal medicine only know how to treat internal diseases, and never dealt with labor or cutting, nor incision or stitch. In the work later on, we can feel it was a big defect. So, my last year's clinical rotation was less than one year. However, it was a real situation learning, so that it was effective and it benefited my whole life. The interns were under the guidance and direction of the residents, so that our supervisors were actually the resident of a higher ranking. I had deeply realized about the role and influence of the residents to the intern.

To the classes entered the PUMC from 1959 to 1965, only 3 classes of students really completed all clinical courses. Even for those students, the political background of that time, such as the "anti-rightist" and "four purge" movements interfered with the teaching at the college. So, all the graduates of the above classes went to remote areas in Northwest China, such as; Tibet, Xingjiang, Qinghai and other places, which was not good for the training of students in junior classes, however; later their clinical skills improved by so called "returning to the furnace". After the Cultural Revolution, most of the students of those classes were admitted as graduate students back to PUMC and made a new beginning in their career.

After 1979, the clinical courses followed the old PUMC model, offering the carefully designed courses and extensive clinical and bedside practice. The primarily focus of course of study is the first course of clinical training-diagnosis. Almost all the teaching since then stressed that diagnosis is the basis for the whole clinical training. Each specialized discipline of internal medicine, endocrine department and neurology department assigns one full time teacher responsible for group teaching to ensure every medical student pass the requirement of physical examinations. Teachers were also responsible to sit in the class every day, which was insisted on and lasts until today.

Since 1990s, clinical teaching has undergone a huge overhaul, integrating key aspects of modern scientific reasoning and high quality delivery which used to be done separately by internal medicine, surgery and other clinical departments then integrated into a comprehensive course which is based on the system of the organs, while the contents of other courses were integrated into the clinical rotation period. After one year in clinical rotation, students will study eye, ENT, stomatology, TCM and etc., which are not included in the clinical rotation. After 1 year's rotation, students take up internships for a further year.

Since 1999, this arrangement continues and is being developed. Clinical courses are effective; however they are still influenced by external factors. Its effect is intimately related to the competence and teaching mentality of the attending of the wards and the residents.

Scientific training

Since PUMC resumed in 1979, the first couple of classes had 4 months of basic medical science training after which they completed the pre-clinical courses, and after the initial clinical training there was another 4 month period of clinical scientific research training. During the teaching reforms in the 1990's, the two training processes merged into one and students can choose a supervisor for their scientific research project training either from the IBMS or clinician. It is very unique among all the medical schools in China, and produces highly skilled practitioners and professional. It is still not known what the next step of teaching reform will be.

It is well known that the 'old PUMC' medical program did not include separate scientific research training, nor do the medical schools in other countries. From the training offered, it is more like training for a PhD candidate. However, it is much shorter than that of PhD training. Therefore, it is not likely to yield the same results as the PhD training, so that it is regarded as the hybrid of MD training and doctoral training for natural sciences. There is still much discussion concerning its influence upon medical students.

The medical education in other countries does not hold scientific training in high regard, because clinical medicine requires mainly for practice. Also, having 8 months to focus on research training is perhaps not long enough to publish a paper, nor will the result of the project be likely to serve as the working basis for future work. As a result, the next step for teaching reform on the scientific research training is under extensive discussion.

Results from Surveys of PUMC Alumni of the 8 year Program

During 2016 a survey was distributed to PUMC alumni enrolled from 1956 – 2008 via email, WeChat and through the online program

Findings are summarized, as follows:

In September 2016, 1932 questionnaires were distributed to alumni from the 8 year medical program at PUMC. In order to maintain precision of findings the survey excluded alumni from the 7 + 1 program.

By November, 511 responses had been received which represents an overall response rate of 26.4%. This overall response rate was further categorized according to stages in PUMC's history and enrollment.

- Alumni enrolled years 1956 – 1965, 14.1% (49/347)

- Alumni enrolled years 1979 to1989, 29.2% (105/360)

- Alumni enrolled year 1990 – 1999, 43.6% (207/475)

- Alumni enrolled year 2000 – 2008, 20.0% (150/749)

Among the 511 alumni who responded to the survey, 240 were female and 271 male. Figure 1. provides a visual representation of gender distribution for each historical period. (Note: The horizontal line of charts 2-6 shows the enrollment year.)

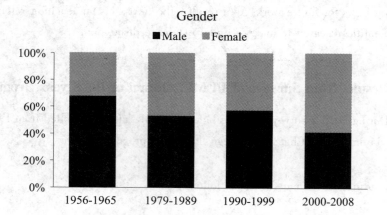

Figure 2：The comparison of the gender distribution of alumni of 8-year program responding to the questionnaires

The status quo of careers of the alumni

According to the results of the survey, most alumni of 8-year program are engaged in clinical medicine, education and bio-medical related research work (see also Figure 3). There are a small number of alumni working in other areas such as health management, pharmaceutical companies or investment corporations. From the proportion of the work type, the alumni engage in clinical medicine showed a gradual upward trend in the past 30 years, and more than 90% of graduates have made clinical work their career in the past 10 years.

Also, the workplaces of the alumni showed a significant era characteristic (Figure 4): most of the alumni (84%) who enrolled in the 1950s and 1960s in China; However, because of the impact of "Going Abroad Trend" in the 1980s, more than a half of the alumni went abroad for further education, primarily went to the United States (63%); With the changes in China's economy and society, the proportion of the alumni going abroad declined year by year, and 93% of alumni of the classes graduated in the past 10 years are working in China.

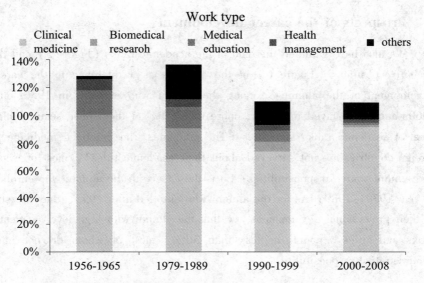

Figure 3：The comparison of the work type of 8-year program responding to questionnaires

（Note：Percentage is above 100 because multiple choices are available）

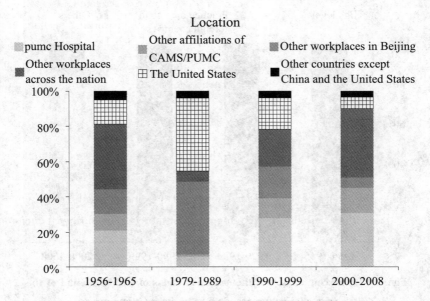

Figure 4：The comparison of the location of PUMC alumni of 8-year Program corresponding to the questionnaires

Prospects of the career development:

We also have gathered the data of the academic ranks (Figure 5) and the executive positions (Figure 6) of the alumni, as a reference to the career development of the alumni: Among the alumni who enrolled in 1950s and 1960s and later stayed in China, more than 90% of them have secured high level of academic ranks and titles (The graduates who practiced medicine in foreign countries are not surveyed about their academic titles), most of whom had administrative responsibilities; So is the case with the alumni who enrolled in year 1979 – 1989; As for the alumni who enrolled after 1990, they are still in their professional development, so that the alumni with high level academic ranks and titles account for less than 30%, most of whom do not have administrative responsibilities.

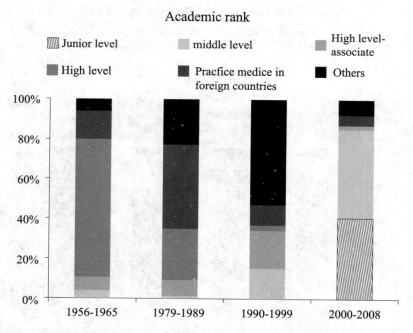

Figure 5: **The comparison of the academic ranks of PUMC alumni of the 8-year curriculum responding to the questionnaires**

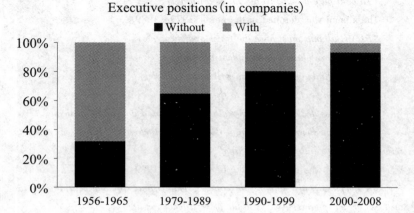

Figure 6: The comparison of PUMC alumni of the 8-year program with administrative responsibilities who responded to the questionnaires

(Note: Both working in companies and in academic institutions are included)

Comments and feedback

The last part in the questionnaire is an open question i. e. what is the most important thing that you have learned from your alma mater? The words such as those in PUMC's motto "rigorousness, excellence, diligence, dedication (严谨、博精、勤奋、奉献)" and etc. are frequently shown in the answers given by alumni from various age groups, different regions and gender. These shared focuses have long been the essence of "PUMC Spirit".

Here are some of answers of the alumni to this question, from which we can see the distinct characteristics of the era and the inheritance of the "PUMC Spirit" throughout the time:

> The alumni who enrolled in the period of 1959 – 1965:
> "*Integrity; concentration, serve the patients wholeheartedly*"
> "*Wholeheartedly for the patients, striving for skill excellence*"
> "*Rigorous, practical, and serve the people wholeheartedly*"

"To be a pure person. To do things attentively"

The alumni who enrolled in the period 1979 – 1989:

"PUMC alumni must have the trailblazer awareness"

"Spirit of trailblazer, independent thinking"

"Critical thinking, knowledge, rigorous attitude, benevolence"

"Dedication, wholeheartedly to their patients"

"The selfless dedication of the senior professors and doctors to medicine"

"Practice medicine skillfully and dedicatedly, lifelong learning; always hold reverence and be caution for everything"

The alumni who enrolled in the period 1990 – 1999:

"A People-oriented humanistic care, global vision, lifelong learning as the methods of self-improvement, Attitude of persistence for life"

"Think independently and teamwork"

"The attentive attitude to each patient"

"Concentrated, perseverance, dedication"

"Persistence, never forget the origin ambitions"

"Humanistic endowment"

The alumni who enrolled inperiod 2000 – 2008:

"The ability of self-learning, the attitude of truth-seeking"

"The spirit of probing and research and the social responsibility"

"Lifelong learning, striving, and improving"

"The ability of self-learning and sensibility for medicine"

"The belief of being a doctor and the spirit of professional dedication"

"The benevolence of doctors"

Contributors

Ma Chao 马超 Class 1999

LiNaishi 李乃适 Class 2000

LiHangen 李晗歌 Class 2012

ZhangWanying 张婉莹 Class 2017

建院以来的主要科技成就及其影响

刘德培

　　刘德培，1986 年毕业于中国协和医科大学生化与分子生物学专业，获博士学位。2001 年 9 月至 2011 年 8 月，任中国医学科学院院长。主要从事基因表达调控、基因治疗与心血管疾病发病机制研究。先后承担国家自然科学基金重大、重点项目、国家 863 重点项目等，国家自然科学基金委 "优秀创新群体" 学术带头人，心血管 973 项目首席科学家。曾任国务院学位委员会委员。现任第十二届全国人大常务委员会委员、中华医学会副会长、国际医学科学院组织主席、医学分子生物学国家重点实验室主任。

　　1956 年中国医学科学院（简称医科院）成立，是我国唯一的国家级医学科学学术中心和综合性医学科学研究机构。1957 年，中国协和医学院（"协和" 当时的名称）与中国医学科学院合并，实行院校合一的管理体制，医科院为北京协和医学院提供雄厚的师资和技术力量，北京协和医学院为医科院培养高层次的人才，相互依托，优势互补，教研相长。院校设有 18 个研究所（以及 5 个分所）、7 所临床医院（含与北京市共建的天坛医院）、6 所下属学院、1 个研究生院。

　　中国医学科学院建院 60 多年来，院校在不同历史时期，始终坚持面向世界科技前沿、面向国家重大需求、面向国民经济主战场，围绕影响人民群众生命健康的重大科技问题，艰苦创业，甘于奉献，勇攀高峰，不辱使命，攻克了一个又一个难题，取得了减毒与灭活小儿麻痹疫苗的研制、生产与应用，全国控制和基本消灭麻风病，化学疗法根治绒癌等一大批重大标志性成果，先后获得 7 国家科技进步一等奖，为防控重大疾病、保障人民健康、推动经济社会发展做出了重大贡献，在新中国医学史上立下了不可磨灭的功勋。

总结分析院校 60 多年以来取得的主要科技成就，有助于提升院校在国内国际的影响力，激励院校广大科技工作者致力于医学科技研究，取得更多的成就，同时为院校的科技管理工作提供经验和借鉴。

重大疾病防控

重大传染病防控

新中国成立以来，面对传染病和寄生虫病肆虐的严峻形势，组织开展了重大传染病和寄生虫病的防控的科研工作，对我国重大传染病的防控起到了重大作用，对我国临床医学的发展起到了引领作用。

脊髓灰质炎是严重危害儿童健康的急性传染病，多数儿童患病后会出现下肢肌肉萎缩、畸形，结果引起终身残疾，俗称"小儿麻痹症"。l955 年江苏南通发生了脊髓灰质炎大流行，此后，其流行日趋严重，上海、济南、青岛等地相继报告发生"脊灰"流行。面对疫情，刚刚成立的中国医学科学院临危受命，于 1959 年在昆明建立医学生物学研究所，向脊髓灰质炎全面宣战。

时任中国医学科学院病毒学系首任脊髓灰质炎研究室主任的顾方舟教授带领课题组开始致力于"脊髓灰质炎"的病原学及预防的研究。研究团队在环境极其艰苦，当时没有冷链运输的情况下，研制成功中国第一个口服组织培养活疫苗、首创"糖丸疫苗"新剂型，提出了有别于其他国家的免疫方案和免疫策略，有效控制和阻断了"脊灰"病毒的传播，缩短了中国消灭"脊灰"的进程。2000 年 7 月经国家消灭"脊灰"证实委员会确认，我国已经成功阻断了本土"脊灰"野病毒的传播，实现了无"脊灰"的目标。这一功在当今、利在千秋的造福子孙后代的伟大业绩，使我国数千万儿童免受脊髓灰质炎侵害，极大地提高了人口素质。

麻风是世界上最早有记录的传染病之一，中医经典《素问》就有相关记载。在人类发展的大部分时间里，由于受到医疗条件的限制，麻风造成大量患者肢体、面部和眼睛残疾。直到今天世人仍对麻风病谈之色变。新中国成立后，人民政府高度重视，卫生部组成了由中国医学科学院皮肤病研究所牵头，相关流行省（市、区）麻防负责单位参与合作的麻风防治大军，从实验、临床、康复、流行病学、社会医学和现场多方位展开了控制和基本消灭麻风的防治研究，取得了骄人成果。上世纪80年代，皮肤病研究所提出"早期发现，联合化疗，化学隔离，在家治疗"的策略，并通过开展 WHO 联合化疗方案试点，建立和推广了适合我国情况的联合化疗方案。麻风防治研究成果，不仅在我国产生了巨大社会和经济效益，而且也成为发展中国家实现消除和基本消灭麻风的范例。

艾滋病是一种危害性极大的传染病，由感染人类免疫缺陷病毒（HIV）引起。1985年6月3日，中国医学科学院北京协和医院感染内科王爱霞教授报道了我国境内发现的首例艾滋病人，由此揭开了中国艾滋病防治序幕。多年来，中国医学科学院北京协和医院开展的"适宜国情的艾滋病抗病毒治疗和免疫重建研究"结合基础研究与临床转化，获得了系列创新性成果：制定并优化出适合国情的效优、价廉、毒副作用低的艾滋病治疗方案，显著降低病死率；首次建立艾滋病综合诊治体系，为降低重要脏器并发症提供科学依据；2005年主持制定我国第一部《艾滋病诊疗指南》，有效规范我国艾滋病诊治，遏制艾滋病蔓延势头。

近年来，中国医学科学院还组织人员开展了"新发突发传染性疾病病原体的发现、治疗和预防研究"，取得了一系列令人瞩目的成就：

建立了国际上首个最为系统的重大传染病的动物模型资源库，从根本上扭转了我国传染病动物模型资源匮乏的被动局面，是国内唯一、国际上最系统的重大传染病动物模型资源库，其中艾滋病模型、流感模型、SARS 模型和 MERS 模型均为国际首创。

创建了新型病原体组合筛查技术体系，基本解决了组合检测已知病原体同时鉴别未知病原体的国际性难题。该技术体系应用于近年来历次重大新发传染病，如 2009 年甲型 H1N1 流感、2013 年人感染 H7N9 禽流感疫情及 2013 年江西省全球首例人感染 H10N8 流感病例的病原体的快速筛查及确诊，系统阐明了我国代表性地区呼吸道病毒的感染谱，发现一批重要新发病毒在我国的流行，为国家防控突发/新发疫情和社会稳定提供了有力支撑。

重大慢性非传染性疾病防治

在 20 世纪 60 年代初期，严重危害妇女健康、又称"癌中之王"的绒毛膜上皮癌，被公认为最凶险的不治之症之一。中国医学科学院北京协和医院妇产科宋鸿钊教授领衔的研究团队，用化学疗法成功的治愈了绒毛膜上皮癌的患者，不仅可保留子宫，而且可保留生育能力。此项成果纯属世界之奇迹，是中国对世界医学的一大贡献。该成果具有重大科学意义和社会价值，曾获 1978 年全国科学大会奖、1985 年国家科技进步一等奖。

恶性肿瘤的防治是我国医学界的最大课题。20 世纪 60、70 年代在李冰院长力主之下，中国医学科学院肿瘤医院在肿瘤防治研究方面，开展了现场（河南省林县）、实验室、临床三结合的最早的大规模人群队列研究。中国医学科学院肿瘤医院在几代研究人员的努力下，对食管癌的综合防治展开了全面研究，取得令人瞩目的成果。建立了我国食管癌规范化治疗模式和关键技术体系，出版我国第一部《食管癌规范化诊治指南》，相关成果荣获了 2013 年国家科技进步一等奖。

　　近 60 年来，随着中国医学科学院阜外医院的创建和发展，我国心血管疾病的救治水平和防治体系发生了翻天覆地的变化。阜外医院几代人对建立心血管疾病救治体系进行了大量开创性工作。1974 年，郭加强教授率先在阜外医院完成了我国首例冠状动脉搭桥手术，标志着我国冠脉外科的开端，开启了外科血运重建治疗冠心病的先河。随后，高润霖院士在阜外医院开展了国内最早的冠脉内溶栓治疗急性心肌梗死和第一代金属裸支架治疗冠心病，大幅降低了心肌梗死急性期的住院病死率和冠脉介入治疗再狭窄率等难题。胡盛寿院士率先在我国组织了复合技术（Hybrid）治疗冠心病的平台，并在国内广泛推广"中国人冠心病外科风险评估模型"。朱晓东院士牵头在阜外医院研制了我国第一代牛心包人工生物瓣膜（简称 BN 瓣），并率先应用于临床及推广至全国。如今，中国医学科学院阜外医院逐渐发展为综合性国家级心血管疾病防治中心，逐渐构成了完整的心血管疾病治疗体系，彻底改变了我国心血管病技术救治体系和局面。

　　中国医学科学院血液病医院是中国最大的国家级科研型血液病医疗机构，是中国血液病诊疗和血液学研究由弱到强的实证。1986 年，严文伟教授成功实施中国第一例自体造血干细胞移植。此后，韩忠朝教授等首创自体外周血干细胞移植治疗下肢缺血性疾病的新技术，两项临床治疗技术的成功实施和推广，惠及众多患者。近几年来，程涛教授牵头"造血干细胞维持、衰老与再生的调控机制研究"等多个国家重大研究项目的开展，许多成果发表在世界顶级杂志，代表中国造血干细胞基础研究与国际接轨，在造血干细胞在损伤或疾病状态下的反应机制及其再生策略等研究领域发挥引领作用。中国医学科学院多年开发的系列干细胞相关技术获得包括国家科技进步一等奖等多项国家奖。血液病医院建立"天津市脐带血造血干细胞库"，是我国首批通过执业验收的脐血库之一，现已成为世界最大自体干细胞库之一。

　　肝癌是我国高发的，危害极大的恶性肿瘤。中国医学科学院肿瘤医院孙宗棠教授研究小组于 1970 年代基于抗原抗体特异识别原理，在国际上首创了可精确定量、方法稳定可靠的甲胎蛋白"放射火箭电泳"技术，为高发区人群"小肝癌"的发现奠定了基础，采用这一技术在启东人群中进行筛查而实现了肝癌的早诊早治。为此，孙宗棠、汤钊猷、朱源荣三位被授予 1979 年度负有国际盛名的 Willam B. Coley 肿瘤免疫奖。

1969 年吴英恺、刘力生等专家在石景山区首钢总公司建立了我国第一个慢性病防治网络，在此基础上吴锡桂教授等率先开展了慢性病监测、危险因素调查和综合干预工作。此后近 30 年，阜外医院三代科研人员与首钢人携手，查、防、治、研相结合，用高起点的流行病调查方法与国际水准接轨，坚持科研走出医院大门，与基层结合、为生产服务，有针对性地开展心血管病人群防治。1994 年，为表彰首钢在慢性病防治事业的突出贡献，世界卫生组织向全球推广慢性病防治领域的"首钢模式"。

中国医学科学院北京协和医院史轶蘩课题组通过对国内外最大系列（1041 例）垂体瘤病例的临床分析，在国际上首次提出垂体卒中后有完全和部分破坏两种结果的概念及治疗原则，建立整套先进的诊断方法，使我国垂体瘤诊断水平迈入国际先进行列。相关成果评为 1992 年国家科技进步一等奖。

中国医学科学院北京协和医院赵玉沛课题组多年来潜心专心致力于胰腺肿瘤综合诊治体系的建立和应用，制定多项国家级诊治指南，对行业内进行了规范和普及，通过多家胰腺疾病诊治中心覆盖全国，本课题组研究成果获得良好的社会效益，具有重要的国内、国际影响力。相关成果荣获 2016 年国家科技进步二等奖。

上世纪 80 年代初，在吴之康教授带领下，北京协和医院骨科在全国率先开展脊柱侧凸系统性治疗，将现代脊柱侧凸矫形理念和技术引入国内，并进行了国内首个脊柱侧凸流行病学调查，填补了我国在脊柱畸形研究领域的空白。邱贵兴教授课题组的"特发性脊柱侧凸系列研究及临床应用"获 2005 年度国家科技进步二等奖。

基础医学研究

中国医学科学院建院以来在我国的基础医学研究领域，取得了一系列开创性成果。

细胞遗传学是遗传学与细胞学相结合的一个遗传学分支学科。中国医学科学院基础医学研究所联合多家临床医院，在我国创建了细胞遗传学，开展了遗传病、复杂性状疾病的基因研究。1961 年，吴旻院士在苏联获得医学博士学位后回国，建立了我国第一个细胞遗传学研究组，开创了我国人体细胞遗传学和肿瘤细胞遗传学研究。他领导的研究小组系统开展并建立了人和小鼠等哺乳动物染色体研究技术，获得了中国人染色体的基本数据和模式图，成功用于遗传病的诊断，相关成果获 1985 年度国家科技进步二等奖。他们对中国人从儿童到成人的 8000 余个体细胞进行了相关参数的测量，得到了中国人体细胞染色体的基本数据和模式图，对我国人类和哺乳类动物细胞遗传学的建立和发展起了奠基和推动作用，对我国医疗事业的发展有重大的推动。1985 年，"人类和哺乳动物细胞遗传学在我国的创建、发展和主要成就"项目获国家科学技术进步二等奖。

1963 年，罗会元教授受张孝骞教授委派在中国医学科学院北京协和医院内科建立医学遗传组，在国内最早建立了医学遗传学学科体系，并在单基因病基因诊断和酶学诊断研究上取得系列成果，获 2000 年度国家科技进步二等奖。基础医学研究所吴冠芸教授开创了中国遗传病基因诊断研究，在地中海贫血（即珠蛋白生成障碍性贫血）产前诊断方面的研究成果获得我国遗传病基因诊断领域第一个国家级奖励。

沈岩和张学两个课题组先后发现了遗传学乳光牙本质、家族性反常性痤疮、Marie Unna 型遗传性稀毛症和红斑性肢痛症等单基因病的致病基因，鉴定了先天性全身多毛症等基因组病的 DNA 重排，在《科学

（Science)》和（Science）《Nature Genetics》等杂志上发表系列论文，产生了重大国际学术影响，相关成果获国家自然科学二等奖两项。

詹启敏、赫捷和王明荣三个课题组在食管鳞癌基因组学上研究的结果，展示了中国人食管鳞癌中最重要的突变基因与信号通路，发现了多个与患者的发病或预后显著相关的突变基因，具有潜在的诊断、分型和治疗应用价值，相关论文在《自然》和《Nature Genetics》上发表。林东昕和顾东风两个课题组通过全基因组关联研究发现一批食管癌等肿瘤和冠心病等心血管疾病的易感基因，在《Nature Genetics》等杂志发表系列论文，相关成果获国家自然科学二等奖。

中国医学科学院在"细胞遗传学创建及遗传病、复杂性状疾病的基因研究"领域取得的一系列研究成果极大推动了学科的研究与发展，发现了多种重要的遗传病致病基因，为强化产前诊断、提高人口素质做出了重要贡献。

中国医学科学院基础研究所强伯勤院士、吴旻院士、杨焕明教授为我国基因组研究做出了巨大贡献，正是他们的努力，才造就今天我国基因组研究在国际上的领先地位。

中国医学科学院基础研究所刘德培院士在分化与发育的基因表达调控、转基因动物与疾病模型、基因转移与基因治疗等方面的研究领域取得了一系列成果，比如在胎儿型珠蛋白基因重新开启表达与珠蛋白基因表达调控和地中海贫血基因治疗的基因位点，并建立了相关基因的转基因动物模型。

中国医学科学院基础研究所曹雪涛院士在免疫识别与免疫调节的基础研究、肿瘤等重大疾病的免疫治疗与基因治疗的应用研究领域取得了重大进展，其研究成果"免疫细胞分化发育与功能调控新机制研究"、"炎症消退和免疫稳态调控的新机制研究"分别入选 2014 年度和 2015 年度"中国高校十大科技进展"。

药物疫苗及医疗器械研发

建院以来，中国医学科学院在我国药物、疫苗的研发和医疗器械的研发中起到了举足轻重的作用。先后研制成功了丁苯酞、双环醇、联苯双酯、紫杉醇、人工麝香等多种新药；研制了新中国第一支青霉素，并相继将去甲万古霉素、乙酰螺旋霉素、大观霉素等多种抗生素推上临床；研制成功了脊灰疫苗、肠道病毒71型（EV71，国际首个）疫苗；研制成功了眼科超声诊断系统和医用胶原蛋白等。

丁苯酞（恩必普，dl-NBP）是中国医学科学院药物研究所研发的我国第一个具有自主知识产权的抗脑缺血一类新药，用于轻、中度急性缺血性脑卒中的治疗，目前已广泛应用于急性脑缺血的患者，年销售额已经超过10亿元，占国产一类新药重要的市场份额。如今，丁苯酞拥有近40项国内发明专利以及多项国际PCT（专利合作协定）专利，在世界几十个国家和地区受到保护。企业已与美国和韩国两家知名公司，签署了恩必普软胶囊在欧美和韩国市场的专利使用权转让协议，成为中国第一个以专利授权方式走出国门的化学药品。

联苯双酯和双环醇是药物研究所在天然产物五味子丙素研究中发明的重大新药。联苯双酯片及滴丸于20世纪80年代初先后上市，后者生物利用度更高，曾获国家发明奖等多个奖项。联苯双酯滴丸自上世纪90年代出口韩国、埃及等国后，创汇近千万美元。双环醇片于2001年上市，是我国首个问世的具有国际自主知识产权的一类化学新药，获国家科学技术进步二等奖。双环醇可以治疗慢性病毒性肝炎（乙肝、丙肝）、非酒精性脂肪性肝病、药物性肝损伤，总体研究达国际先进水平。通过产学研用协同创新成功实现产业化，作为独家产品其销售额达30亿元，份额稳居国内口服保肝用药首位。伴随着2004年双环醇在乌克兰的上市，这一国产抗炎保肝药物的国际化之旅正式开启；2015 年，双环醇在俄罗斯注册，至此，其已在 10 个国家正式获批进入临床，在 7 国注册上市，提供了保肝抗炎治疗的中国方案。

麝香系鹿科动物林麝脐下腺分泌物，属珍稀中药材。麝香药源紧缺，伪劣掺假品充斥市场，严重影响中成药质量和用药安全。1975 年，卫生部和中国药材公司委托中国医学科学院药物研究所牵头，组织了由山东济南中药厂和上海市中药研究所参加的联合攻关协作组，在国家科委"六五"攻关等项目的资助下，展开了系统的人工麝香研究。经过多年努力，该项目采用现代分析技术，首次系统地阐明了天然麝香的主要化学成分，分离出六大类、100 多种化合物并表征了结构；首次表达了天然麝香的功效，填补了天然麝香功效现代药理学资料空白，解决了人工麝香评价难题；发现了天然麝香中大分子多肽类主要药效物质及其代用品，解决了人工麝香研制面临的最大难点；项目基于"化学成分类同性、生物活性一致性、理化性质近似性、安全、低毒性"的仿生学思路，创新提出人工麝香组方策略，经临床前及临床试验，成功研制出与天然麝香功效与安全性相近的人工麝香，获国家 I 类新药证书。作为国家保密品种，自 1994 年推广以来，在全国 31 个省市 760 家企业应用，市场上销售的 433 种中成药中，有 431 种完全用人工麝香替代了天然麝香，替代率达到 99% 以上。2015 年获国家科技进步一等奖。

中国医学科学院医药生物技术研究所研制了新中国第一支青霉素，并相继将去甲万古霉素、乙酰螺旋霉素、大观霉素、克霉唑、美罗培南，以及吡哌酸、氟哌酸、环丙沙星、左氧氟沙星等喹诺酮类共几十种抗感染药物推上临床，约占国产抗菌药 50%，为我国医药卫生尤其是传染病防控做出了杰出贡献，使我国抗生素实现了从无到有，从仿制到创制，从进口到出口的历史性转变。此外，医药生物技术研究所启动了组合生物合成学研究，研制成功了基因工程抗生素阿米卡星，一类抗菌药可利霉素完成 III 期临床，标志我国组合生物合成技术实用化研究进入世界领先水平。由医药生物技术研究所构建的我国抗感染药物研发体系，完成了我国一半以上一类抗感染药物药效评价，包括绝大多数抗菌药，为我国抗感染药物研发提供技术支撑。

药用植物资源是大健康产业的基础，是国家基本药物制度顺利实施的重要保证，是重大新药创制及产业化的物质基础。中国医学科学院药用植物研究所肖培根院士领衔的研究团队取得了一系列研究成果，包括"创建了药用植物种质迁地和离体保护体系，突破了上千种珍贵药用植物种质资源迁地引种生长技术难题"、"创建了全新的中草药 DNA 条形码物种鉴定体系"等。徐锦堂教授针对我国 20 世纪 70 年代传统中药天麻野生资源匮乏，全国市场已三年断线供应的严峻局面，开展了天麻野生变家种的研究，取得了系列研究成果，帮助天麻产地农民增收致富，被誉为"天麻之父"。

1973 年中国医学科学院药物研究所与解放军第 187 医院合作开始研究海南粗榧及其有效成分的抗肿瘤作用，从植物资源、化学成分、有效成分合成、分析和药理诸方面开展了较为完整和系统的研究。随后国内一些临床单位在治疗急性非淋巴白血病时，已将三尖杉酯碱及高三尖杉酯碱作为联合化疗方案中的一个组成部分。相关成果被评为 1985 年度国家科技进步一等奖。

1984 年亚洲奥林匹克委员会理事会决定"1990 年在中国北京举办第十一届亚洲运动会"。按规定，主办国必需承担运动员的兴奋剂检测任务。在工作难度大、时间紧迫、又没有法定检测方法的情形下，医科院药物所周同惠教授迎难而上、毫不犹豫地接受了这项艰巨的国家任务，创建了中国兴奋剂检测中心，圆满完成了第十一届亚洲运动会的兴奋剂检测任务。相关技术达到国际先进水平，确立了中国的国际兴奋剂检测的重要地位。

近年来，中国医学科学院生物医学研究所李琦涵研究团队成功研制全球首个预防 EV71 病毒感染灭活疫苗。该疫苗的问世对于有效降低我国儿童手足口病的发病率，尤其是减少该病的重症及死亡病例，保护我国儿童生命健康具有重要意义。生物所廖国阳教授研究团队在全球率先提出采用 Sabin 减毒株制备脊灰灭活疫苗，并开始进行相关研究。2015 年 1 月 14 日，获得国家食品药品监管总局颁发的国家预防用生物制品 1 类新药证书和生产文号，成为全球首个 Sabin 株脊髓灰质炎灭活疫苗（单苗）。2015 年 7 月，中国医学科学院医学生物学研究所在昆明高新区"生物所疫苗产业基地"生产出首批 sIPV，实现中国孩子接种中国创新疫苗的目标。中国医学科学院药物研究所的蒋建东教授研究团队在"小檗碱的降脂降糖作用研究"方面取得了系列成果，将开辟代谢障碍性疾病防治新途径。

中国医学科学院生物医学工程所王延群教授课题组研制出了 BME-200 眼科超声诊断系统，荣获国家科技进步二等奖，该系统应用高频超声波对眼进行实时扫描成像，能清晰显示眼内组织结构，发现并诊断组织的占位性病变和病灶，替代了大量的国际同类进口产品，推广应用至全国各级医院，出口 60 多个国家和地区。工程所张其清教授在国内最早提出并发展了引导/诱导组织再生（GTR）的新理论和新技术，发明了以胶原为基本原料，制造可广泛用于临床医学各科的组织修复、具有引导/诱导组织再生效果的医用材料及其制造方法，申请了发明专利并获授权，组织实现了产业化并获产品注册证，引领了我国再生医学的发展。

科研基地平台建设

中国医学科学院建院以来科研基地平台建设形成新格局。目前院校获批 3 个国家临床医学研究中心、1 家国家医学图书馆、1 个国家医学智库，拥有 5 个国家重点实验室、31 个省部级重点实验室，数量在国内名列前茅。

中国医学科学院作为国家级医学中心，有 3 个国家临床医学研究中心获批建设。依托中国医学科学院阜外医院成立的国家心血管病中心是国家预防和治疗心血管疾病的研究、培训和教育的全国性领导机构和国家工作平台，负责协调和组织推进我国心血管病防治工作，以高血压和血脂异常防治为重点，开展心血管病人群综合防治，降低国民心血管病的发病和死亡，维护国民的心血管健康和提高国民生活质量。

依托中国医学科学院肿瘤医院成立的国家癌症中心负责协助国家卫生计生委制订全国癌症防治规划；建立全国癌症防治协作网络，组织开展肿瘤登记等信息收集工作；拟订诊治技术规范和有关标准；推广适宜有效的防治技术，探索癌症防治服务模式；开展全国癌症防控科学研究；开展有关培训、学术交流和国际合作。

依托中国医学科学院北京协和医院成立的转化医学中心将实施海内外高端人才的双聘、特聘制度，建立与国内外高水平机构间的交流互访和资源共享机制；同时发挥北京协和医院丰富的病例、临床专家队伍和先进的技术设备等资源优势，整合、共享中国医学科学院多家院所的优势资源，努力建成国家级、国际化的转化医学研究合作高端平台。

中国医学科学院/北京协和医学院图书馆，1957 年被国务院指定为"全国第一医学中心图书馆"，1990 年成为卫生部全国医学文献资源共享网络的国家中心馆和"WHO 储藏图书馆"，2000 年被指定为 NSTL 医学分中心，承担着国家医学图书馆的重要职能。

中国医学科学院正在建设医药卫生领域国家战略智库基地，坚持以有效支撑科技自主创新为目标，到"十三五"末，形成国际一流水平的医学数字知识资源保障体系和网络化的无缝服务机制，建成权威的医学信息研究产品体系和数字化科研信息支撑环境，建立国内领先水平的医药战略情报研究服务体系，打造具有国内领先位置和重要国际影响力的卫生政策分析与决策支持体系。

国家重点实验室是我国科技创新体系的重要组成部分，在促进重大科研成果的产生和杰出科学家的培育方面，发挥了不可替代的重要作用。中国医学科学院目前拥有 5 个国家重点实验室，分别是分子肿瘤学国家重点实验室、医学分子生物学国家重点实验室、实验血液学国家重点实验室、心血管疾病国家重点实验室、天然药物活性物质与功能国家重点实验室。重点实验室实行"开放、流动、联合、竞争"的运行机制，依托中国医学科学院各所院，在促进院校成果我国医学研究的国家队、提升院校的自主创新能力与核心竞争力方面起到了重要作用。

　　院校 31 个省部级重点实验室，是院校科技创新体系的重要组成部分，是院校创新性人才的培养基地，在院校学科建设、科技创新、人才培养和培育国家级科研基地中发挥着越来越重要的作用。院校省部级重点实验室在集聚优秀科研人才，引领院校科研方向、搭建成果推广与转化平台方面也做出了巨大贡献，为院校的科技发展提供了技术支撑。

　　另外，院校还建立了国家人口与健康数据共享平台，在灵长类动物基地、疾病动物模型平台、医学信息平台、药用微生物资源库、药用植物资源库、生物样本库、干细胞库等方面形成一批国家资源平台。

CAMS's Major Scientific and Technological Achievements since its Establishment

Liu Depei

Liu Depei, graduated from Peking Union Medical College in 1986 and was conferred a Ph. D. in biochemistry and molecular biology. From September 2001 to August 2011, he served as president of the Chinese Academy of Medical Sciences. His research focus is in gene expression regulation, gene therapy and cardiovascular diseases pathogenesis study. He is the PI of several key projects of the National Natural Science Foundation, the national 863 key projects, academic leader of the National Natural Science Foundation of "excellent innovation group", the chief scientist of 973 project in cardiovascular diseases. Former Member of the Academic Degrees Committee of the State Council. He is currently a member of the Standing Committee of the 12th National People's Congress, vice president of the Chinese Medical Association, director of the International Academy of Medical Sciences, director of the State Key Laboratory of Medical Molecular Biology.

Chinese Academy of Medical Sciences (CAMS), the sole academic and integrated research institution for medical science in China, was established in 1956. In 1957, when CAMS and Peking Union Medical College (PUMC) consolidated together, CAMS and PUMC shared the one administrative system. CAMS provided the most established and sound resources of faculty and expertise to support PUMC, while PUMC trained high-level professional talents for CAMS. The two is interdependent, mutual benefited and complemented, and thrived together. CAMS has 18 affiliated research institutes (and 5 branches), 7 clinical hospitals (including Tiantan Hospital in partnership with Beijing Municipality government), 7 affiliated schools, and 1 graduate school.

Since CAMS was established for more than 60 years, throughout its different historical periods, CAMS/PUMC has always been targeting on meeting the needs of the country, looking to the forefront of the world's science and technology, and the main agenda of the national economy, and focusing on the significant scientific and technological issues that has great impact on people's life and health. Through dedication, hardworking, pushing the boundaries, CAMS/PUMC has lived up to its mission and expectations, and has overcome great difficulties one after another and made several great hallmark achievements such as the development, production and application of the attenuated and inactivated poliomyelitis vaccine, the national control and elimination of leprosy, the complete cure of chorioepithelioma applying chemical therapy. Besides, CAMS won up to 7 first prize of National Scientific and Technological Progress Award. CAMS/PUMC has made significant contributions towards the prevention and control of major and catastrophic diseases, the protection of people's well-being, and the promotion of social and economic development. CAMS made an indelible contribution to the history of medicine in New China.

The summary and analysis of the main scientific and technological achievements of by CAMS/PUMC over the past 60 years is not only instrumental for enhancing the influence of CAMS/PUMC home and abroad, but also for encouraging the scientific and technological faculties dedicating to the research for medical science and technology to make more achievements and providing experiences and lessons to the administrative work of science and technology of CAMS/PUMC.

The prevention and control of major and catastrophic diseases

Since its establishment, CAMS, it has played an important role in the prevention and treatment of major epidemics and infectious diseases in China, performing a leading role in the development of clinical medicine in China.

The prevention and control of major infectious diseases

CAMS/PUMC has made great contributions to the eradication of poliomyelitis and leprosy. Poliomyelitis is one of the acute infectious diseases that could seriously threaten the health of children. most children with this disease would develop symptoms of lower limb muscle atrophy and muscular anomaly, resulting in permanent disability, which was commonly known as infantile paralysis. In 1955, the first poliomyelitis pandemic in China occurred in Nantong City, Jiangsu Province. Since then, the prevalence of poliomyelitis increased and there were reported cases in Shanghai, Jinan, Qingdao and other places one by one. Facing the epidemic, the newly established CAMS stepped in at this critical and difficult moment. In 1959, the Institute for Medical and Biological Research was established in Kunming and started the overall fight against poliomyelitis.

Professor Gu Fangzhou, who was the first director of poliomyelitis research laboratory in the Department of Virology at CAMS then, led the research team dedicating to the research into the etiology and prevention of "poliomyelitis" . In the extremely difficult environment and without frozen-chain transportation, the research team successfully developed China's first " oral poliomyelitis vaccine (OPV)", and proposed the immune solution and immune strategy that were different from other countries, which effectively controlled and blocked the transmission of the virus " poliomyelitis " and shortened the period of "poliomyelitis" eradication in China. In July 2000, the National Certification

Committee （NCC） for Poliomyelitis Eradication confirmed that China has successfully blocked the transmission of "poliomyelitis" within China and achieved the goal of "polio-free". This remarkable achievement benefits the society as well as the generations followed, protecting the physical and mental health of tens of millions of children in China and greatly improved the quality of the population.

Leprosy is one of the earliest infectious diseases ever recorded in the history throughout the word. It was recorded in the classics of Traditional Chinese Medicine "*Su Wen* (*Huang Di Nei Jing Su Wen*《黄帝内经·素问》)". In the long history of human development, a large number of people suffered from leprosy resulted in disability in limb, face and eye, due to lack of development in medicine in the past. Even today, many people are still intimidated by it.

After the founding of New China, the government paid high attention to leprosy. The Ministry of Health formed a vast network for the prevention and control of leprosy, led by Institute of Dermatology of CAMS, involving leprosy related organizations in the leprosy infected provinces （cities, districts）, carrying out initiatives to control and eradicate leprosy in different areas, including laboratory, clinic, rehabilitation, epidemiology, social medicine and field study, leading to remarkable results. In the 1980s, the Institute of Dermatology proposed the strategy of "early detection, combined with chemotherapy, chemical isolation, and home treatment". Through initiating the pilot project of WHO program of combined chemotherapy, the institute established and promoted the program of combined chemotherapy suitable for the situation in China. The findings of the research for leprosy prevention and control not only yields huge social and economic gain in China, but also become an example for the developing countries in realizing the stamping out of leprosy and basic eradication.

AIDS is a life-threatening infectious disease caused by the infection of human immunodeficiency virus (HIV). On June 3, 1985, Professor Wang Aixia of the department of Infectious Diseases of the PUMC Hospital reported the first case of the patient with AIDS found in China, starting the era in China's AIDS prevention and control. In the past few years, the "AIDS anti-viral treatment and immune reconstruction appropriate for the national conditions project" was carried out at the PUMC Hospital of CAMS, combining basic research with clinical transformation. It has made a series of innovative achievements, developing and optimizing the treatment strategy for AIDS that was not only suitable for the situation in China, but also effective, inexpensive and of low toxicity and side effects, which significantly reduced the case fatality rate; It was the first one to establish a comprehensive diagnosis and treatment system for AIDS, providing a scientific evidence to the reduction of the complications of important organs. In 2005, the hospital also took the lead in drafting *"Guidance to AIDS diagnosis and treatment"* -the first in China, which effectively regulated the HIV/AIDS diagnosis and treatment in China and curbed the epidemic of the disease.

In the past few years, CAMS also organized team to carry out the project of "research into the discovery, treatment and prevention of the pathogen of emerging and emergent infectious disease" and has made a series of remarkable achievements: establishing the world's first most systematic database of animal models for major infectious diseases. It fundamentally reversed the disadvantage of lacking of database of animal models for major infectious diseases in China. As the only one of its kind in China, it was also the most systematic one in the world, among which the HIV/AIDS model, influenza model, SARS model and MERS model were the first ones all over the world. CAMS created a technology system for the combinatorial screening of new pathogens, and it led to the solution to the international challenge: the integrated testing for identifying both the known pathogens and simultaneously the unknown ones. The technological system was used in a few major newly emerging infectious diseases in recent years, such as in the rapid screening and confirmation of pathogens of the H1N1 influenza in 2009, the epidemic of H7N9 Avian Influenza in 2013, and the human infection of H10N8 flu in Jiangxi Province in 2013 which was the first case in the world. It systematically expounded the infection pattern of respiratory virus in China's representative areas and discovered the spread of a number of important emerging viruses in China, providing a strong support for the national prevention and control of the epidemic of newly emerging and emergency of infectious diseases as well as maintaining the social stability.

The prevention and treatment of major and catastrophic non-communicable diseases

In the early 1960s, the choriocarcinoma was known as "the king of cancer", which greatly threatened women's health and was regarded as one of the most ferocious incurable diseases. The research team led by Professor Song Hongzhao of the PUMC Hospital successfully cured patients of choriocarcinoma with chemotherapy, so that the patients could preserve not only the uterus, but also the fertility. This achievement was purely a miracle of the world, and it was also China's contribution to the world. The achievement was of significant scientific and social value and won the 1978 National Science Conference Award and 1985 National Science and Technology Progress Award.

Prevention and treatment of malignant tumors is the biggest task in medical undertaking in China. In the 1960s and 1970s, led by Li Bing, president of the Cancer Hospital of CAMS, the hospital carried out the first cohort study in large scale, combining the field trip (Lin Xian, Henan Province), the laboratory and the clinical work together in the research of tumor prevention and treatment. The researchers of the Cancer Hospital, generations after generation, worked arduously to make a comprehensive study on the prevention and treatment of esophageal cancer and made extraordinary achievements. The Cancer Hospital of CAMS established the standardized model for the treatment and the key technical protocol for esophageal cancer, and published "*A Guide to the standardized diagnosis and treatment of esophageal cancer*"-the first one in China, the findings won the National Science and Technology Progress Award in 2013.

In the past 60 years, with the establishment and development of Fuwai Hospital of CAMS, in terms of level and the system of prevention and treatment of cardiovascular disease in China, the change was dramatic. Generations of medical workers of Fuwai Hospital have made great pioneering efforts in establishing the system of life saving and treatment of cardiovascular diseases.

In 1974, Professor Guo Jiajqiang completed the first case of coronary artery bypass surgery (CABS) at Fuwai Hospital, marking the beginning of coronary surgery in China. It was the trailblazer in applying surgical blood transportation to the construction of the vascularization for the treatment of coronary heart diseases. Subsequently, academician Gao Runlin of Fuwai Hospital was the first one in China practicing coronary thrombolytic for the treatment for acute myocardial infarction and the first one using the first generation of bare-metal stent for the treatment of coronary heart disease, which greatly reduced the in-patient mortality rate of the acute stage of myocardial infarction and that of the coronary restenosi. On this basis, academician Hu Shengshou took the lead in forming the platform for the treatment of coronary heart disease in China and widely promoted "the risk assessment model of using surgery on coronary heart disease of the Chinese". Academician Zhu Xiaodong led the development of China's first generation of bovine pericardial valves and performed China's first bioprosthetic valve replacement in July 1976, the first clinical use of bioprosthetic valves in China, playing a key role in promoting heart valve surgery in China.

Today, Fuwai Hospital of CAMS gradually becomes the national comprehensive center for the prevention and control of cardiovascular diseases, and constructs a complete treatment system of cardiovascular diseases, which fundamentally changed the overall picture of the treatment system and technology of cardiovascular diseases in China.

In China, Hematology Hospital of CAMS is the largest national research-oriented medical institution specializing in blood diseases, and it is the living proof demonstrating the diagnosis, treatment and research of blood diseases evolving from a weak beginning to a competitive stage now. In 1986, Professor Yan Wenwei successfully performed China's first autologous hematopoietic stem cell transplantation (ASCT). Since then, Professor Han Zhongchao and his colleagues invented the new technology of autologous peripheral blood stem cell transplantation (auto-PBSCT) for the treatment of lower limb ischemic diseases. The successful application and promotion of these two clinical treatment technologies have benefited many patients. In the past few years, Professor Cheng Tao led the implementation of several national important and large research projects such as "the regulatory mechanism study of the maintenance, the caducity and regeneration of the hematopoietic stem cell", many findings of which were published in the prestigious international magazines. It demonstrated that the China's basic medicine research of hematopoietic stem cell was keeping pace with the international society, and that it played a leading role in the research in areas of the reaction mechanism and its regeneration strategy of the hematopoietic stem cells under the condition of lesion or disease. The stem cell-related technology developed by CAMS in the past years won many national awards, including the first prize of National Science and Technology Progress Award. The Hematology Hospital of CAMS established "Tianjin hematopoietic stem cell bank of umbilical cord blood (UCB)", which was one of the first umbilical cord blood banks in China approved and has now become one of the largest autologous stem cell banks in the world.

Liver cancer is an extremely life threatening malignant tumor with high incidence. In the 1970s, based on the specific identification principle of antigen and antibody, the research team led by Professor Sun Zongtang of the Cancer Hospital of CAMS was the first in the world that invented the technology "radioactive rocket immunoelectrophoresis (RIEP)" of alpha-fetoprotein – a precise quantitative, stable, and reliable method, laying the foundation for the discovery of "small liver cancer" of people in high-incidence area. This technology was used in the screening cohort in Qidong, realizing the early diagnosis and early treatment of liver cancer. Because of this achievement, Sun Zongtang, Tang Zhaoyou, and Zhu Yuanrong were awarded the world-renowned Willam B. Coley Cancer Immunization Award in 1979.

In 1969, Wu Ying-k'ai, Liu Lisheng and other experts established China's first prevention and control network of chronic disease in Shougang-Capital Steel Corporation (CSC) in Shijinghsn District of Beijing, on the basis of which Professor Wu Xigui and others carried out the surveillance, risk factors investigation and integrated intervention of chronic diseases. Nearly 30 years later, three generations of researchers of Fuwai Hospital worked closely with CSC, combining screening, prevention, treatment, and research together, applying advanced epidemiological investigation method that was in line with the international standard, they insisted that the scientific research should go out of the hospital and outreach to the grass-roots, to serve the productivity, and carry out the targeted prevention and control service to the patients with cardiovascular diseases. In 1994, the World Health Organization (WHO) promoted the "Shougang model" in chronic diseases prevention and control to the whole world, honoring its outstanding contribution to the prevention and control for cardiovascular diseases.

By conducting the research into clinical analysis of pituitary tumors which was the largest disease cohort study (1041 cases) both in China and in the world, the research team led by Shi Yifan of PUMC Hospital was the first one which proposed the concept that there were two damages incurred after pituitary apoplexy-complete and partial, as well as the treatment principle. Also, the team developed a complete set of advanced diagnosis approach, so the diagnosis of pituitary tumors of our country ranked in the top group in the international society. The related achievements won the first prize of National Science and Technology Progress Award in 1992.

The research team led by Zhao Yupei of PUMC Hospital has devoted themselves to the establishment and application of comprehensive system for the diagnosis and treatment of the pancreatic cancer in the past few years. They developed a number of national guidelines to the diagnosis and treatment of the disease contributing to the standardization and dissemination of related practice, outreaching to the whole country through a number of pancreatic disease diagnosis and treatment centers. The findings of the research team have gained good social effect and made significant impact at home and abroad. The related findings won the second prize of National Science and Technology Progress Award in 2016.

In the early 1980s, led by Professor Wu Zhikang, a team from the Department of Orthopedics of PUMC Hospital took the lead in the systematic treatment of scoliosis in China, introducing the modern concept and technology of scoliosis correction into China, and carried out the first epidemic study on scoliosis in China, so that it filled the blanks in the field of spinal deformity research in China. The research - " A series study and clinical application of idiopathic scoliosis of the research group led by Qiu Guixing of PUMC Hospital won the second prize of National Science and Technology Progress Award in 2005.

The Research in basic medicine

Since its establishment, CAMS has made a series of innovative achievements in the field of basic medicine in China.

Cytogenetics is a sub area of genome study combining genome and cytology together. The Institute of Basic Medical Sciences of CAMS, together with a number of clinical hospitals created the cytogenetic in China and carried out the genetic research on genetic illnessand complicated diseases.

In 1961, upon obtaining his doctoral degree in medicine in the former Soviet Union, academician Wu Min returned to China and established China's first research team for cytogenetic study, initiating research on human cytogenetics and oncocytogenetics. The research team led by him performed and developed the research technology of mammal chromosome such as that of the human and mice, so that they obtained the basic data and model idiogram of the chromosomes of the Chinese, successfully used it in the diagnosis of genetic diseases. The related findings won the second prize of National Science and Technology Progress Awards in 1985. They measured the related parameters of more than 8,000 somatic cells of the Chinese people ranging from children to adults, so obtained the basic data and idiogram of the chromosomes of the Chinese people, laying the foundation and promoting the establishment and development of human cytogenetics and mammalian cytogenetics in China. It also greatly pushed forward the development of China's medical undertaking. In 1985, the project - "the creation, development and main achievements of human cytogenetics and mammalian cytogenetics in China" won the second prize of National Science and Technology Progress Awards.

In 1963, professor Zhang Xiaoqian appointed professor Luo Huiyuan to establish the medical genome research group in the Department of Internal Medicine of PUMC Hospital, so that PUMC created the first systematic medical genome discipline in China, yielding a series of achievements in the research on genetic diagnosis of single-gene disease and enzyme diagnosis, which won the second prize of National Science and Technology Progress Awards in 2000. Wu Guanyun, who was from the Institute of Basic Medical Sciences of CAMS, initiated the research on the genetic diagnosis of genetic diseases in China, and the research on the prenatal diagnosis of Cooley's anemia was the first one to win a national award in the field of gene diagnosis of genetic diseases.

The two research groups led by Shen Yan and Zhang Xue successively found the pathogenic genes of the following monogenic disease: the hereditary opalescent dentin, abnormal familial acne inversa, Erythromelalgia, Marie Unna hereditary hypotrichosis and erythromelalgia of Marie Unna type. Besides, they identified the re-arrangement of DNA of genome dieases like Congenital Generalized Hypertrichosis. What's more, they published a series of papers in magazines, such as *Science* and *Nature Genetics*, having a major international academic impact. The related achievements won two second prizes of National Natural Science Awards in 2000.

The findings on the genome of esophageal squamous cell carcinoma (ESCC) made by the three research groups led by Zhan Qimin, He Jie and Wang Mingrong respectively demonstrated the most important mutated genes and signal channels in China's ESCC, also they found a number of genes mutation significantly correlated with the patients' pathogenesis or prognosis, which has a potential applicable value in the diagnosis, genotyping and treatment. The relevant papers were published in *Nature* and *Nature Genetics*.

The two research teams led by Lin Dongxin and Gu Dongfeng, through the Genome-wide Association Study (GWAS), found a number of susceptible genes of esophageal cancer and that of the cardiovascular diseases such as coronary heart disease. They published a series of papers in *Nature Genetics* and other magazines. Their findings won the second prize of National Natural Science

Awards.

The research achievements one after another made by CAMS in the field of "genetic research on the creation of cytogenetics, genetic diseases and complex diseases" greatly promoted the research and development of the discipline, by identifying a variety of important pathogenic genes, which made significant contribution to the prenatal testing and improvement of the quality of the population.

Academician Qiang Boqin, academician Wu Min, and Professor Yang Huanming of the Institute of Basic Medical Sciences of CAMS made tremendous contributions to China's genome research. It was their efforts that the China's genome research was able to achieve its current leading role in the world.

Academician Liu Depei of the Institute of Basic Medical Sciences of CAMS has made a series of achievements in the field of regulation of gene expression in the period of differentiation and development, transgenic animals and disease models, gene transfer and gene therapy. For example, the gene locus of re-opening expression in the fetal globin gene, regulation of gene expression of globin gene, and gene therapy of Cooley's anemia. Besides, he established the transgenic animal model of the relevant genes.

Academician Cao Xuetao of the Institute of Basic Medical Sciences of CAMS has made great progress in the field of basic research on immunological recognition and immuno regulation, as well as in the field of application research on immune therapy and gene therapy of catastrophe diseases such as tumors. His research findings "Research on the mechanism of immune cells' differentiation, development, and function regulation", and "Research on the new mechanism of Homeostatic regulation of inflammation resolution and immunity" won the nomination of "Top Ten Scientific and Technological

Progress of Chinese Universities" in 2014 and 2015.

The research and development of drugs, vaccines, and medical technology

Since its establishment, CAMS has played a significant role in the development of research and development of drugs, vaccines, and medical equipments. CAMS has successfully developed a number of new drugs such as butyphthalide (NBP, bicyclol, Dimethyl diphenyl bicarboxylate (DDB), paclitaxel and artificial musk. Besides, it developed the first penicillin in new China and successively developed a number of antibiotics for clinical practice such as norvancomycin, acetylspiramycin and spectinomycin. In addition, it successfully developed the polio vaccines and EV71 vaccine, Ophthalmic ultrasound diagnostic system and medical collagen

Institute of Materia Medica of CAMS developed Butyphthalide (NBP) - the Class I drug for anti-cerebral ischemia that has an independent intellectual property right in China. The drug is used for the treatment of mild and moderate acute cerebral ischemic stroke. Now it has been widely used in patients with acute cerebral ischemic stroke. Its annual sales were more than 1 billion Chinese Yuan, accounting for a large market share of Class I new drugs produced in China. Today, butyphthalide (NBP) has nearly 40 domestic patents of invention and a number of patents of international PCT (Patent Cooperation Agreement). It is patented in dozens of countries and regions in the world. Agreements of the patent transfer of the drug have already been signed with two famous companies in the US and South Korea for the license of Butyphthalide (NBP) soft capsule in Europe, the United states and in South Korea. It was China's first chemical drug that went to the market abroad through patent licensing.

Dimethyl diphenyl bicarboxylate （DDB） and bicyclol are important new drugs invented by the Institute of Materia Medica of CAMS out of a natural products - Schisandra chinensis. DDB tablets and dropping pills were put into market in the early 1980s successively. The latter one had higher bio availability and won a number of awards including the National Invention Award. Since DDB dropping pill was exported to South Korea, Egypt and other countries since the 1990s, it has earned millions of US dollars. Bicyclol tablet was put into market in 2001 and was China's first Class I new drug in the market with independent intellectual property rights. It won the first prize of Beijing Science and Technology Award and the second prize of National Science and Technology Progress Award. Bicyclol could cure chronic viral hepatitis （hepatitis B and hepatitis C）, NAFLD （nonalcoholic fatty liver disease）, DILI （drug-induced liver injury）. The overall study of the bicyclol has reached the international advanced level. It has been successfully industrialized and internationalized through innovation in a coordinated effort involving industrialization, academic, research and application. The sales volume of the exclusive product - bicyclol tablet reached 3 billion Chinese Yuan, and its market share kept at the first place of the oral hepatoprotective medicine in China. Bicyclol was put into Ukraine's market in 2004, and this made-in-China drug with anti-inflammatory and hepatoprotective function started its journey to international market. In 2015 bicyclol was registered in Russia. By then it has been officially approved into clinical practice in 10 countries, providing a Chinese solution to the anti-inflammatory and hepatoprotective treatment.

Musk is the secretion of gland below the umbilicus from the cervine animal moschus berezovskii. It is valuable and rare resource for Chinese medicine. Musk is in short supply; therefore there are many fake, low-qualified or adulterated ones in the market, posing serious threat to the quality and safety of Traditional Chinese Medicine drugs. In 1975, the Ministry of Health and the Chinese Medicinal Material Company authorized the Institute of Materia Medica of CAMS to take the lead in organizing a collaborative joint research team including

Shandong Jinan TCM Factory and Shanghai TCM Research Institute. Supported by the projects such as National key scientific and technological project of the Sixth Five-Year Plan by the National Science and Technology Commission of the PRC and other programs, the team launched the systematic research into artificial musk. After several years of efforts, using modern analytical techniques, the team demonstrated the main chemical composition of natural musk for the first time, isolating six categories, more than 100 types of compounds and characterizing their structure. The research team first expressed the efficacy of natural musk, filling the blank in the modern pharmacological information of the efficacy of natural musk and solving the difficulty in evaluating the artificial musk. Besides, it found the main effective material and its substitute of macromolecular polypeptide in the natural musk, solving the biggest bottleneck in the development of the artificial musk. Following the idea in bionics of "homogeneity of chemical composition, consistency of biological activity, approximation of physical and chemical properties, safety, low toxicity", the project proposed the strategy of component plan of artificial musk. Through the pre-clinical and clinical trials, the team successfully developed the artificial musk with its efficacy and safety similar to those of the natural musk. It won the Certificate of the National Class I New Drug. It has been classified as a national confidential formula. Since its promotion effort started in 1994, it has been applied by 760 enterprises in 31 provinces and municipalities in China. Among the 433 kinds of Chinese patent medicine sold in the market, 431 kinds of them were completely made of artificial musk instead of natural musk, and the replacement rate has reached more than 99%. In 2015 it won the first prize of National Science and Technology Progress Awards.

The Institute of Medicinal Biotechnology of CAMS developed the first penicillin in new China and successively put dozens of antibiotic drugs into clinical practice, such as the norvancomycin, acetylspiramycin, spectinomycin, clotrimazole, meropenem as well as quinolone, norfloxacin, ciprofloxacin, levofloxacin tablets, accounting for 50% of home-made antibiotics, making outstanding contributions to the prevention and control of infections diseases in China and its health care. It made a historic transition in the evolution of China's antibiotics: starting from scratch, from generic to creation, from import to export. In addition, the Institute of Medicinal Biotechnology of CAMS has launched the research into combinatorial biosynthesis and successfully developed the gene engineered antibiotic amikacin, and its antimicrobial agent Kelimycin has completed phase III of clinical trial, marking that China's applied research in combinatorial biosynthesis technology was now among the leaders in the world. The R&D system of China's anti-bacterial drugs constructed by the Institute of Medicinal Biotechnology has completed more than half of the efficacy evaluation of China's anti-infection drugs, including on the majority of antimicrobial agents and providing expertise support for the R&D of China's anti-infection drugs.

The resource of medicinal plants was the basis of the health care industry, and very important in ensuring the sound implementation of the national essential drug system, as well as the material basis for the innovation and industrialization of new drugs with significant importance. The research team led by Academician Xiao Peigen of Institute of Medicinal Plants CAMS has made a series of research achievements, including "the creation of protective system for the Ex situ and ex vivo of germplasm of medicinal plants, and achieved the breakthrough in the technology of making the germplasm resources of thousands of precious medicinal plants moving and growing in an introduced foreign land", "the creation of a brand new species identification system with DNA bar code for Chinese herbal medicine" and so on. Facing the severe problem of the shortage in resources of the wild traditional Chinese herbal medicine and-Tianma with no supply in the market for consecutive three years in the 1970s in China, Academician Xu Jintang carried out the research on transforming Tianma from only wild growth to agricultural planting. He achieved a series of research findings and helped farmers living in the areas of origin of Tianma grow more and get rich, so that he was known as the "father of Tianma".

In 1973, the Institute of Medicinal Plants and No. 187 PLA Hospital began to collaborate on the study of the antitumor effect of Hainan cephalotaxus sinensis and its active ingredient. They carried out a relatively integrated and systematic study in aspects of the plant resources, chemical composition, synthesis of active ingredients, analysis and pharmacology. Subsequently some clinical institutes have incorporated harringtonine and homoharringtonine the component of the combined chemotherapy solution in the treatment of acute non-lymphoblastic leukemia. The related achievements won the first prize of National Science and Technology Progress Awards in 1985.

In 1984 the Olympic Council of Asia decided Beijing was the host city for the Eleventh Asian Games in 1990. According to regulations, the host country must undertake the task of doping testing of the athletes. The task was difficult, and time was pressing. There were no statutory test methods to follow. Facing all of these difficulties, Professor Zhou Tonghui of the Institute of Meteria Medica CAMS took the challenge and undertook this arduous task for the country without any hesitation. He established the China Doping Testing Center, and success-fully completed the task of doping testing of the Eleventh Asian Games. The technology reached the international advanced level, establishing China's important position in the international doping testing.

In the recent years, the research team led by Li Qihan from the Institute of Medical Biology has successfully developed the world's first inactivated vaccine against infection of EV71 virus. The invention of the vaccine was of great significance for the effective reduction of the incidence of hand-foot-and-mouth disease among Chinese children, especially for the reduction of the severe cases, fatality rate of this disease, and for the protection of the children's well-being in China. The research team led by Professor Liao Guoyang from the Institute of Medical Biology was the first in the world that proposed to use Sabin attenuated strain for the preparation of polio inactivated vaccine and began to carry out the related research. In January 14, 2015, they gained the Certificate of the National Class I New Drug and the production licensing code for prophylactic biological products issued by China Food and Drug Administration (CFDA), making the world's first Sabin strain polio inactivated vaccine-sIP (monospore seedlings). In July 2015, the Institute of Medical Biology CAMS producedthe first batch of sIPV in Kunmig's High-tech Zone "vaccine industrial base of the Institute of Medical Biology", achieving the goal to vaccinate Chinese children with China's innovative vaccines. Inaddition the research team led by professor Jiang Jiandong of the Institute of Meteria Medica has made a series of achievements in the research of "berberine effect in the reduction in blood lipid and blood sugar", which would provide a new approach to the prevention and treatment for metabolic diseases.

The project team led by Professor Wang Yanqun from the Institute of Biomedical Engineering CAMS developed the BME-200 Ophthalmic Ultrasound Diagnostic System and won the second prize of National Science and Technology Progress Award. The system used high-frequency ultrasound to perform the real-time scanning imaging of the eye, which could clearly show the intraocular tissue structure, detect and diagnose the occupied lesions and focus lesions of tissues, replacing a large number of imported products of the same kind of technology. It has been promoted and applied to hospitals at all levels in China and exported to more than 60 countries and regions. Professor Zhang Qixing from the Institute of Biomedical Engineering CAMS firstly proposed and developed the new theory and new technologyof Guiding/Inducing Tissue Regeneration (GTR) in China. He invented medical materials and their manufacturing methods made of collagen as the basic raw material which can be widely used in tissue repair in all disciplines of clinical medicine with GTR effect. He applied for the patent of invention and was approved. He made the industrialization of the invention and was granted the registration certificate of the product, leading the development of China's regenerative medicine.

The construction of the platform base for scientific research

Over the past 60 years' development since the establishment of CAMS, the scientific research base now manifested a new look. At present, CAMS/PUMC has been approved three national clinical medical research centers, five key national laboratories and 31 key laboratories at provincial and ministerial level, the number of which ranks at the top in the whole country.

As the medical center at national level, CAMS had three national clinical medical research centers being approved for construction.

Based on the Fuwai Hospital of CAMS, a national center of cardiovascular diseases was established, which was the leading institute and national working platform for the research, training and education of prevention and treatment of cardiovascular diseases in China. The center coordinated and organized the efforts to promote the prevention and treatment of cardiovascular diseases in China. Focusing on the prevention and treatment of hypertension and dyslipidemia, the center carried out the comprehensive prevention and treatment of cardiovascular diseases in the population, reducing the mortality and the morbidity of cardiovascular diseases of the Chinese people, safeguarding the health of heart and vascular, and improving the quality of life of the Chinese people.

Based at the Cancer Hospital of CAMS, a national cancer center was established, assisting the National Health and Family Planning Commission in formulating a plan for national cancer prevention and control. The center established a national collaborative network for cancer prevention and control, and organized the information collecting initiative such as registration of tumor and etc. The center is working on drafting the technical norms for diagnosis and treatment as well as relevant standards, promoting the appropriate effective technology of prevention and treatment, exploring the delivery model of cancer prevention and treatment, carrying out the national scientific research on cancer prevention and control, providing training, promoting academic exchanges and international cooperation, and undertaking other tasks assigned by the National Health and Family Planning Commission.

Based at the PUMC Hospital, the center for translational medicine was established. PUMC center for translational medicine adopted the recruitment methods of "dual-appointment of high-level talents from home and abroad" and "special appointment for experts"; jestablished a mechanism of exchanges and resource sharing with leading institutions at home and abroad. Meanwhile, the center made full use of its advantages - bundant cases, clinical expert team and advanced technology, integrating and sharing the advantages and resources of the affiliates of CAMS, so as to build an advanced platform for the research and cooperation of translational medicine, not only in China, but also in the world.

In addition, CAMS/PUMCalso established a sharing platform of national database for population and health, and has established a number of national platforms of resources in the areas of primate animal base, platform for animal model of diseases, platform of medical information, resource platform for medicinal microorganism, resource platform of medicinal plants, platform of biological samples, and platform of stem cells.

The CAMS/PUMC Library was designated as the "No. 1 National Medical Center Library" by the State Council in 1957, and became the National Center Library of the Ministry of Health's Resource Sharing Network for National Medical Literature as well as the "WHO storage library" in 1990. In 2000, it was designated as the medical branch center of NSTL, performing the important function of a national medical library.

The CAMS is building a national strategic think tank in domain of medicine and health, insisting on the goal of effectively supporting the independent innovation of science and technology, so as to form the world-class supporting system for digital medical knowledge resources and the seamless networking service mechanism by the end of "the 13th 5-year plan"; and to establish the authoritative system of the medical information research outcome and the supporting environment of digitalized scientific research information; to build the cutting-edge system of medical and pharmaceutical strategic informatics research in China; to create an system of health policy analysis and decision making - leader in China and of important international influence.

The key national laboratories comprise an important component in China's scientific and technological innovation system. They played an irreplaceable important role in promoting the production of significant scientific research achievements and the training of outstanding scientists. Five key national laboratories has been approved at CAMS, namely the Key National Laboratory of Molecular Oncology, the Key National Laboratory of Medical Molecular Biology, the Key National Laboratory of Experimental Hematology, the Key National Laboratory of Cardiovascular Diseases, and the Key National Laboratory of Active Substances and Function of Natural Medicine. Implementing the operating mechanism featuring "openness, mobilizing, collaborating, competition", as well as relying on the affiliated of CAMS, the key national laboratories have played important role in promoting the building up of the national team, facilitating the output of CAMS/PUMC, and promoting CAMS/PUMC independent innovation capacity and core competence in China's medical research.

CAMS/PUMC's 31 provincial and ministerial key laboratories are an important part of the scientific and technological innovation system of CAMS/PUMC and CAMS/PUMC's training base of innovative talents, playing an increasingly important role in CAMS/PUMC's discipline construction, scientific and technological innovation, personnel training as well as in nurturing the national scientific research base. CAMS/PUMC's provincial and ministerial key laboratories have also made great contributions in gathering outstanding scientific research personnel, in leading the direction of CAMS/PUMC's scientific research, and in building the platform of the outcome promotion and transformation, providing technical support for CAMS/PUMC's development of science and technology.

协和的创造力和影响力——纪念协和建校 100 周年

巴德年

　　巴德年，中国工程院院士，美国国家医学院外籍院士，免疫学家。1992 年 12 月至 2001 年 9 月，出任中国医学科学院院长、中国协和医科大学校长。之前曾任中国驻日本大使馆教育参赞等职务。目前担任的社会职务有：第九届全国政协委员、中华医学会副会长、中国免疫学会理事长、中国生物医学工程学会名誉理事长、国务院学位委员会委员、中国工程院管理学部常务委员，并承担多种国家级杂志的主编、常委等工作。

协和百年，人才辈出，硕果累累。值得纪念，值得总结，更值得期待和展望。

协和造就出中国最好的医师、医学教授、医学科学家和医学界高级管理专家

　　众所周知，中国最好的医院是北京协和医院，最著名的医师、医学教授、医学科学家好多出自协和系统（协和医大/医科院，时而略曰协和）这所学术殿堂。张孝骞、林巧稚、胡正祥、刘士豪、诸福棠、李宗恩、钟惠澜、董承琅、罗宗贤、黄家驷、吴阶平、李洪迥、吴英恺、许应魁、冯应琨、张庆松、朱贵卿、文士域、王桂生、邓家栋、曾宪九、周华康、宋鸿钊、黄宛、尚德延、胡懋华、王世真、张乃铮、史轶蘩、方圻、朱预、刘彤华、葛秦生、郎景和、邱贵兴；陶寿淇、蔡如升、刘玉清、郭加强、刘立生、朱晓东、高润霖；吴桓兴、黄国俊、宋少章、谷铣之、吴旻、哈宪文、屠规益、陆士新、孙燕、程书钧、宋儒耀、吴宪、刘思职、冯德培、张锡钧、沈其震、吴襄、汤飞凡、谢少文、白希

清、黄祯祥、冯兰洲、侯宝璋、杨简、张鋆、梁植权、薛社普、何观清、顾方舟、朱既明、王琳芳、佘铭鹏、罗会元、梁晓天、黄亮、周同惠、刘耕陶、肖培根、甄永苏、于德泉、韩锐等。

抗战胜利到新中国成立初期，完成学业的协和学子，如卢世璧、罗慰慈、张之南、连利娟、潘国宗、朱元珏、蒋朱明、戴玉华及陈元方等，他们经历过战乱、各种政治运动，也经历过协和历史性变迁。他们服从组织，艰苦奋斗，在成为一代名医的同时，为协和传承、为国家医学发展起到了承前启后和桥梁纽带作用。

党和政府高度重视协和的人才成长，特别是在钱信忠部长的力主下，把当时从苏联留学回国的最优秀人员留在协和系统。如吴旻、华光、侯云德、钟守先、毕增祺、徐乐天、李泽坚等。

在"文革"前周总理力主，选拔一批优秀学者赴英国留学，包括陆召麟、朱晓东、曾毅、刘士廉、章静波等。

"文革"刚结束，肿瘤医院的李冰院长，以超人的眼力和魄力，识才用才，把下放农村的优秀科技人才抢先请回肿瘤医院，强化研究所。其中包括吴旻、李铭新、张友会、孙宗棠、陆世新、程书钧等。

改革开放学成回国一批批优秀人才，如强伯勤、修瑞娟、陈德昌、宋增璇、陈璋、詹启敏、赫捷、金奇、秦川、李太生、赵春华等。

外校毕业协和成长，成为医学界优秀代表者，如汪忠镐、劳远琇、王爱霞、张承芬、郭玉璞、王直中、罗爱伦、刘晓程等。

"文革"十年，大学停办，人才流失，协和同样也面临青黄不接、人才断层的严重局面。但天无绝人之路，特别是，对协和系统而言，有着得天独厚的人才资源和取之不尽、用之不竭的发展潜力。自 1993 年起，连续八年，采取不拘一格降人才，培养、晋升、提拔、重用相结合，自己培养与国外引进相结合。一大批睿智、能干、正派又有奋斗精神的年轻的学术骨干、学术带头人茁壮成长，不仅为协和解决了人才断层问题，更为国家的医药卫生行业和各医学学科输送了今天的和明天的学术领袖（许多已成为中华医学会，中国医师协会的会长，副会长，或专业委员会的主任或后任主任）。其典型代表是：赵玉沛、钱家鸣、金征宇、刘大为、姜玉新、黄宇光、沈铿、王任直、王宝玺、陈杰、崔丽英、张奉春、江骥、吴清玉、胡盛寿、刘应龙、孙立忠、刘进、杨跃进、顾东风、赵平、石元凯、刘德培、沈岩、何维、张学、王晓良、庚石山、邵荣光、褚嘉佑、李奇涵等。

引进的优秀人才很多，包括杨焕明、林东昕、韩忠朝、蒋建东、惠汝太、王恒、蒋澄宇、程涛、王建祥等。

从协和到北医，成为北医的学术领袖的有：胡传揆（1927 届）、吴朝仁（1928 届）、王叔咸（1930 届）、马万森（1935 届）、刘家琦（1937 届）、陈景云（1937 届）、冯传汉（1940 届）、严仁英（1940 届）、王光超（1940 届）、吴阶平（1942 届），以及朱洪荫、关颂韬、孟继懋等。

从协和到上医，成为上医的学术领袖的有：荣独山（1929 届）、徐苏恩（1932 届）、林飞卿（1932 届）、李鸿儒（1934 届）、范日新（1934 届），以及沈克非、陈翠贞、颜福庆、林兆耆、戴自英、张昌绍、徐丰彦、崔之义等。

从协和到天津，成为天津医学史上最光辉最著名的医师有：施锡恩（1929 届）、朱宪彝（1930 届）、卞万年（1930 届）、金显宅（1931 届）、范权（1931 届）、方先之（1933 届）、司徒展（1933 届）、赵以成（1934 届）、俞蔼峰（1939 届）等。

从协和到中山，成为中山的学术领袖的有：汤泽光（1929 届）、秦光煜（1930 届）、钟世藩（1930 届，钟南山的父亲）、陈国桢（1933 届）、周寿恺（1933 届）、卢观全（1937 届）等。

从协和到四川，成为四川的学术领袖的有：陈志潜（1929 届）、原华西大学医学院院长曹钟梁（曹泽毅的父亲）（1935 – 1937 协和进修）。

从协和到军科院、301、北京医院、中日友好医院的一批批的学术带头人，也为这些顶尖的医疗机构的建设和发展奠定了基础。做出重大贡献的：刘永、周金黄、俞焕文、蒋豫图、李耕田、陆维善、叶慧芳、吴蔚然、杨友凤等。

朱章赓、刘瑞恒、林可胜和沈克非都曾在国民政府任过卫生部部长或副部长，朱章赓还曾任中央卫生实验院院长并为世界卫生组织（WHO）筹建人之一。刘瑞恒创立中央医院、中央卫生实验院，兼任两院院长，并任禁烟委员会委员长。林可胜 1947 年担任国防医学院院长。1948 年兼任中华民国卫生部部长。

陈敏章 1987 年国家卫生部部长，王陇德、彭玉、刘谦曾任或任卫生部副部长。陈文杰和陆如山都曾担任过 WHO 的副总干事。刘德培曾任中国工程院副院长，沈岩任国家自然科学基金委员会副主任。

25 年间的协和职业生涯，陶冶了我，锤炼了我，甚至一直加工到"切削"、"打磨"、"熏蒸"、"热处理"，让人饱尝了酸甜苦辣，但使人坚定了信念，铸就了修养，提高了本事。不知过了多久，我终于悟出个道理，其实所有协和人都和我相似，在协和这座"熔炉"，这个"加工厂"，这所"大学校"里，情愿或不情愿地接受协和的洗礼，自觉不自觉地传承协和的文化。令人欣喜的是协和的人才薪火相传，协和的人才五湖四海，协和的人才兴旺发达。

依我的体会，能吸引一流学生并培养成一流人才的大学就是一流大学。当然要选用有思想有作为有担当的一流校长，要在育人上下大力气，动真功夫，不是教会而是让学生学会、悟懂、践行"做人做事做学问"的基本道理和一辈子用得上的真本事。要用慢工，要做细活，要长以计宜，还要因材施教。协和的三基三严，不仅是要求学生的，首先是要求校长的。恕我直言，当今的985大学也好，C9大学也好，进步很快，但性子太急，虚工太多，特色趋淡，攀比过多。2007年上海医学院80年校庆的时候我做过一个讲话，我列举了上医校友的成功人士的一个名单，说明上医是"有大师，出大师，育大师"的一流大学。现在，我又列举了一个协和人的名单，不难看出协和更是一所有更多大师、出更多大师、育更多大师的更一流的大学。

协和创造并成就了中国的高等护理教育

协和的高等护理教育，1919年筹建，1920年9月就正式招生。其校训是：勤、慎、警、护。当时的校名定为：北京协和医学院护士学校，并同时在美国纽约州立大学及中华护士会注册。这所学校截止1952年，共毕业28个班，263人，其中近60人工作在国外，绝大多数成为中国护理学界的先驱。其中林斯馨、徐霭诸、聂毓禅、林菊英、王琇英、王懿、陈琪、梅祖懿等都曾担任过中华护士（学）会的会长，副会长。田粹励总干事为学会工作15年（1934～1949），维护了学会尊严，坚持了护士毕业会考。王琇英是中国第一人获得南丁格尔奖章。

值得一提的是从1940年到1953年，协和护校第四任校长聂毓禅，在抗战期间历尽艰辛，长途跋涉，"长征"到四川，保存了协和护校并坚持办学。真可谓抗战英雄，护理教育的模范。

改革开放以后，中国又恢复了高等护理教育。但办学不规范，学制不统一。特别是护理本科5年制，授予医学学士学位。课程也几乎是医学课，或医学省略版。严重的问题是，毕业生不安心护理工作，人才流失。中国协和医科大学在美国中华医学基金会（CMB）支持下，得到国家教委的认同和批准。1996年在中国第一个将护理系升格为护理学院，将护理本科 5 年制改为 4 年制，授予护理学院合格毕业生理学学士学位。并聘请国内外十余位护理教育学专家，制定了专本衔接的护理学教学大纲、教育计划及一整套护理学教材。此举得到了业内的普遍认同，特别是得到了国家教委的高度赞许和大力支持，被列为面向 21 世纪的教育教学改革项目，向全国推广。

在这一系列的改革、建设、发展护理教育工作中，当时的护理学院院长沈宁带领护理学院的广大教师，做出了重大贡献。着眼未来，储备人才，大学选送刘华平赴美完成护理学硕士课程又完成博士课程及护理学博士论文，获得护理学博士学位。十几年过去了，如今的刘华平不仅是协和的护理学学术带头人，必将成为中国的今天和明天的护理学学术领袖。

协和创造了中国的现代医学、药学

创造是一种引领，是一种示范，是一种带动。现代医学和药学在中国的产生和发展过程中，协和的作用举足轻重。

远在协和建校初期，协和关于北京猿人的研究闻名世界，而北京猿人的头盖骨就保存在协和的解剖教研室。抗战时期，日本侵略军占领协和，头盖骨丢失，造成人类文明史上巨大损失。

1922－1923 年间，协和的药理学家陈克恢教授从中药麻黄中提取出化学单体麻黄素，开创了真正的中草药现代化的先河。20 世纪 30 年代协和的生物化学家吴宪教授发明血糖测量法，又与刘思职教授一起提出了蛋白质变性学说。刘思职教授用化学反应与数学计算的方法，提出抗体是二价的，即一个抗体分子结合两个抗原分子。张锡钧教授关于乙酰胆碱的研究，李宗恩教授与钟惠澜教授关于黑热病的研究，刘士豪教授与朱宪彝教授关于钙磷代谢的研究，诸福棠教授关于胎盘球蛋白预防麻疹的研究都闻名国内外。四十年代吴英恺教授成功完成中国第一例食管癌根治术，并效果良好。

解放后，在传染病防治，特别是消灭麻风和脊髓灰质炎方面做出了巨大贡献。协和校友汤飞凡在世界上首次发现沙眼病毒（沙眼衣原体）。特别值得强调的是，由顾方舟教授带领的脊髓灰质炎疫苗研究，开发，生产一条龙团队，在环境极其艰苦、当时没有冷链运输的情况下，他们发明的脊髓灰质炎糖丸疫苗解决这个严重疾病的预防问题。中国人就是靠服用中国人发明的这个"糖丸"，在中国消灭了这个病。在这里，我必须强调一句，能解决问题的技术就是高技术，能彻底解决实际问题的技术就是最高技术。在 20 世纪 60 年代初期，针对严重危害妇女健康又称"癌中之王"的绒毛膜上皮癌，协和医院妇产科宋鸿钊教授领衔的研究团队，用化学疗法成功地治愈了绒毛膜上皮癌的患者，不仅可保留子宫，而且可保留生育能力，实乃世界之奇迹，是中国对世界医学的一大贡献。60 年代由华光教授主持的关于东莨菪碱的研究，为治疗中毒性休克开辟了新途径，也为微循环研究奠定了基础。各种抗生素的研究，开发与生产解决了国家医疗与防病治病的需求。肿瘤的防治是我国医学界的最大课题，60、70 年代在李冰院长力主之下，中国医学科学院肿瘤医院在肿瘤防治研究方面，开展了现场、实验室、临床三结合的最早的大规模人群队列研究，以河南林县为现场，长期坚持，特别是对食管癌的早期发现早期诊断早期治疗起到了样板作用。而 70 年代由全国肿瘤防治办公室牵头完成的中国肿瘤发病回顾调查图谱，也是一部很有科学价值的宝贵文献。

1978 年全国科技大会之后，迎来了科学的春天。协和系统广大科技人员爆发出极大的积极性和创造力，成绩显著。甲肝疫苗研制成功，人工麝香、联苯双酯、双环醇、紫杉醇、丁苯酞等多种新药陆续上市，研发成功国内首个利用合成生物学技术研发的药物可利霉素，取得巨大的经济效益和社会效益。高难度先天心脏病、冠心病各类手术接连成功，开展了多项具有重大国际影响力的心血管病防治大规模多中心临床研究，心脑血管疾病防治水平显著提高。国内共发现人类单基因遗传病 60 余种，其中四分之一是协和系统发现的。世界上首次从胎盘分离干细胞获得成功，间充质干细胞治疗小腿供血障碍性坏死等疾病已取得良好效果。小檗碱的降脂降糖作用的发现，将开辟代谢障碍性疾病防治新途径。肿瘤防治长期随访大样本队列研究，为了解我国肿瘤病因、掌握肿瘤发病流行规律和建立完善防治策略提供了有力支撑。在食管癌等重要肿瘤基因组学研究方面取得多项突破，完成多项抗癌新药的临床试验研究，连续获得国家科技进步一等奖。建立完善了疫苗研发体系，世界首个预防小儿手足口病的 EV71 疫苗和脊髓灰质炎病毒灭活 Sabin 株疫苗已批准上市。"海南粗榧抗癌有效成分的研究""兴奋剂检测方法的研究与实施""食管癌规范化治疗关键技术的研究及应用推广""人工麝香研制及其产业化"等多项成果协和均作为第一完成单位获得国家科技进步一等奖。"免疫细胞分化发育与功能调控新机制研究"、"炎症消退和免疫稳态调控的新机制研究"分别入选 2014 年度和 2015 年度中国高校十大科技进展。

突出国家队作用，建设高端医学科研平台。协和筹建医学领域首个国家实验室，转化医学国家重大科技基础设施（北京协和医院）和 3 个国家临床医学研究中心获批建设。建立了国家人口与健康数据共享平台，在灵长类动物基地、疾病动物模型平台、医学信息平台、药用微生物资源库、药用植物资源库、生物样本库、干细胞库等方面形成一批国家资源平台。圆满完成 SARS、手足口病、甲型 H1N1 流感、人感染 H5N1、H7N9 和 H10N8 等禽流感，输入性脊髓灰质炎应急防控以及援助非洲抗击埃博拉等多项重大应急科技支撑任务。

以下几个数字，也许会在一定程度上说明协和系统在国家医药卫生科技创新中的作用和贡献：国家重点实验室 5 个；获国家级科技成果一等奖 11 项；在协和系统工作的两院院士入选 55 位（其中已故 21 位），协和校友（有协和"血缘"的）不在协和系统工作的两院院士 25 位；外国科学院院士 10 位。

国家医药卫生事业发展战略是国家医药发展的旗帜，是蓝图。协和在相关战略的制定、实施、评估、验收起到了核心作用。从健康中国2020 到医药卫生 863、973、国家重大专项等都体现出协和人的智慧和力量。其实，协和系统是新火花闪烁、新火花碰撞、新思想诞生、新行动开始的地方。想当年，想搞基因组的人是院校的杨焕明，支持他并一直支持他搞基因组的是吴旻，是当时的第一副院校长强伯勤，是本院校长。后来才有了那个了不起的"1%"，南方基因，北方基因，华大基因。在奥巴马提出"精准医学"之前两年，协和就向国家申请"精细化科学化诊疗体系建立"的项目，并通过了专家论证。奥巴马的国情咨询报告刚一出炉，协和/医科院"关于中国精准医学发展战略及其实施方案"向国务院做了报告，才有了今天的"精准医学"的热与火。同样，协和历来主张基础与临床相结合，当"转化医学"的概念刚一问世，中国第一家国家批准的转化医学中心在协和揭牌。刘德培、沈岩、赵玉沛、詹启敏、何维等都具有战略科学家的素质和作为。当然更具潜力、更有才华的国家医学科学战略科学家即将发挥更大作用。

"三基""三严"是协和的传统作风，坚持创新是协和的科学精神，科学至上，学术民主，独立思考，拒绝平庸，团队合作，共同构筑了协和文化的基本内涵。这种"协东西之德，和天地之道"的文化，已百年传承，已变成人们行为规范，已是协和人共同维护和不断完善的精神家园。可想而知，在这样美好家园里怎能不人才辈出，硕果累累。

协和培养和造就了中国最知名医学院校的大学校长

协和不仅是培养学生，训练医师，是医学家的摇篮，也是医学院校大学校长的"养成所"，医学教育家的"培训班"。

马文昭，北京协和医学堂毕业，协和解剖学教授，北医解剖学教授，组织胚胎学专家，1946～1947 年任北京大学医学院院长。

颜福庆，1926 年任北京协和医学院副院长，1927 年被国民政府任命为第四中山大学医学院（即上海医学院，上海医科大学）第一任院长。

胡传揆（1927 届），皮肤科专家，1948 年～1981 年任北京医学院

（北京医科大学）院长（校长），长达 33 年，是百年北医三分之一时间的掌门人和历史见证者。

朱宪彝（1930 届），内分泌学专家，1951 年～1984 年任天津医学院（天津医科大学）院长（校长）。

李宗恩，热带病学专家，曾任北京协和医院院长，抗战开始 1937 年被国民政府任命为国立贵阳医学院院长，抗战胜利后回协和，任北京协和医学院院长。

王季午（1934 届），传染病学专家，李宗恩的学生，1947 年任浙江大学医学院院长，1952 年院系调整后任浙江医学院（浙江医科大学）副校长，校长至 1984 年。

吴阶平（1942 届），泌尿外科专家，1960 年～1970 年北京第二医学院副院长、院长，1970 年～1983 年协和医科大学／中国医科院副院校长，1983 年～1985 年协和医大校长、医科院院长。

我本人 1992 年～2001 年任协和医大校长／医科院院长，实际上是在协和在医科院受熏陶，受训练，受锻造。在 2002 年以后我到浙江大学医学院任院长时，浙大要求我把浙大医学院办成"南方协和"，我在协和形成的理念、练就的修养，乃至习得的方法和工作的套路真正派上了用场。我不敢说协和的模式、协和的理念和套路，对办好中国的医学教育是放之四海而皆准的，但至少在浙江大学医学院是成功的。浙大医学院在不到十年的时间里，由一个排位居于十多位的省属校，逐年上升，异军突起，现已稳居中国医学院校的最先进的第一方阵。

作为协和系统培养，熏陶出来的詹启敏院士刚刚成为北大医学部掌门人，不仅用他歌声"征服"了北医广大师生，更以他的能力和人格将把北医越办越好。

国家科技创新大会，向全国人民发出了向科技强国进军的伟大号召，刚好是百年协和总结经验、展望未来、向新目标进发的大好时机。协和要响应习主席的伟大号召，创建一流大学，创建一流的医学学科，将中国医学科学院早日成为中国的"NIH"，具有创造力影响力的协和医大要培养出更多的医学骨干和医学领袖。在创新驱动发展、实践中国梦的今天，在人口与健康领域，中国医学科学院和协和医大一定会充分发挥"国家队"和"火车头"的作用，为中华民族的传承、健康和繁荣做出新的更大贡献。

参考书目

1. 邓家栋：中国协和医科大学校史，北京科学技术出版社，1987。

2. 玛丽．布朗．布洛克：油王洛克菲勒在中国，商务印书馆，2014。

3. 巴德年：改革开放与协和医大，中国协和医科大学校报，1999.1。

4. 巴德年：人文心、科学脑、世界观、勤劳手——我的医学教育观及其实践，《科学时报》2010年3月3日，头版。

5. 巴德年：在CMB 100周年纪念大会上的讲话，中国协和医科大学校报，2014.10。

6. 巴德年：在上医80周年纪念大会上的讲话（录音整理稿），2007.9。

7. 王荣金：北京协和医院（1921—1991），协和70周年纪念画册，（内部印刷，发行）。

Creativity and Influence of Peking Union Medical College

The Commemoration of 100th Anniversary of Peking Union Medical College（PUMC）

Ba Denian

Ba Denian, immunologist, academician of Chinese Academy of Engineering, and a foreign member of National Academy of Medicine (US) . From December 1992 to September 2001, he served as president of the Chinese Academy of Medical Sciences and pumc Medical College. Previously served as the educational counselor of the Chinese Embassy in Japan. Current positions include: the Ninth CPPCC National Committee members, vice president of the Chinese Medical Association, the director of Chinese Society of Immunology, honorary chairman of the Chinese Society of biomedical engineering, member of the State Council Academic Degrees Committee, the executive member of the Management Committee of the Chinese Academy of Engineering, executive and editor of a variety of national science journals.

PUMC has produced generations and generations of excellent scholars and made fruitful achievements in the past century; thus, the history of PUMC deserves a careful retrospective review and commemoration; however, we expect even greater achievement in the future of PUMC.

PUMC produces the best doctors, medical professors, scientists, and medical executives in China

Well known by the public, the best hospital in China is Peking Union Medical College Hospital. The most famous physicians, medical professors, and medical scientists① were nurtured and developed in PUMC system (short for PUMC/Chinese Academy of Medical Sciences), a significant academic institute.

From the end of Sino-Japanese War to the early era of People's Republic of China, PUMC graduates②experienced the turbulence of the wars, various political movements, and witnessed the historical transitions of PUMC. These excellent doctors unconditionally submitted to the organization and worked arduously to become distinctive physicians for that era. At the same time, they

---

① Some of the most prominent representatives are: Zhang Xiaoqian, Lin Qiaozhi (Lim Chiao-chih), Hu Zhengxiang (Hu Cheng-hsiang), Liu Shihao (Liu Shih-hao), Zhu Futang (Chu Fu-t'ang), Li zdong'en (Lee Chung-en), Zhong Huilan (William H. L. Chung), Dong Chenglang, Luo Zongxiang (Luo Tsung-hsien), Huang Jiasi (Huang Chia-ssu), Wu Jieping (Wu Chieh-p'ing), Li Hongjiong (Li Hung-chiung), Wu Yingkai (Wu Ying-k'ai), Xu Yingkui, Feng Yingkun (Feng Ying-k'un), Zhang Qingsong (Chang Ch'ing-sung), Zhu Guiqing, Wen Shiyu, Wang Guisheng, Deng Jiadong, Zeng Xianjiu (Tseng Hsien-chiu), Zhou Huakang, Song Hongzhao, Huang Wan, Shang Deyan, Hu Maohua, Wang Shizhen, Zhang Naizheng, Shi Yifan, Fang Qi, Zhu Yu, Liu Tonghua, Ge Qinsheng Lang Jinghe, Qiu Guixing, Tao Shouqi, Cai Rusheng, Liu Yuqing, Guo Jiaqiang, Liu Lisheng, Zhu Xiaodong, Gao Runlin, Wu Huanxing, Huang Guojun, Song Shaozhang, Gu Xianzhi, Wu Min, Ha Xianwen, Tu Guiyi, Lu Shixin, Sun Yan, Cheng Shujun, Song Ruyao, Wu Xian, Liu Sizhi, Feng Depei, Zhang Xijun (Chang His-chun), Shen Qizhen, Wu Xiang, Tang Feifan, Xie Shaowen (Samuel H. Zia), Bai Xiqing, Huang Zhenxiang, Feng Lanzhou, Hou Baozhang, Yang Jian, Zhang Yun, Liang Zhiquan, Xue Shepu, He Guanqing, Gu Fangzhou, Zhu Jiming, Wang Linfang, She Mingpeng, Luo Huiyuan, Liang Xiaotian, Huang Liang, Zhou Tonghui, Liu Gengtao, Xiao Peigen, Zhen Yongsu, Yu Dequan, Han Rui and so on.

② Such as Lu Shibi, Luo Weici, Zhang Zhinan, Lian Lijuan, Pan Guozong, Zhu Yuanjue, Dai Yuhua, and Chen Yuanfang

played a role of bridges and ties in carrying on the great heritage of PUMC and the development of medical science in China.

After the wars, the Chinese Communist Party and Chinese Government put a new premium on the development and growth the talent pool in PUMC. Excellent scholars joined PUMC by following means:

● Initiated and advocated by Qian Xinzhong, the minster of Ministry of Health, a group of excellent scholars such as Wu Min, Hua Guang, Hou Yunde, Zhong Shouxian, Bi Zengqi, Xu Letian, Li Zejian were invited to work at pumc System after studying in the Soviet Union.

● Before the Cultural Revolution, Premier Zhou Enlai strongly advocated for selecting and sending a group of excellent scholars, including Lu Zhaolin, Zhu Xiaodong, Zeng Yi, Liu Shilian, Zhang Jingbo to study in the United Kingdom.

● Right after the end of the Cultural Revolution, Li Bing, the president of Cancer Hospital, affiliate of PUMC, with his exceptional insight and courage, pioneered a search for brilliant talent in science and technology fields among the young people who had been sent to the countryside for "life experience" during the Cultural Revolution. These young intellectuals, including Wu Min, Li Mingxin, Zhang Youhui, Sun Zongtang, Lu Shixin, Cheng Shujun were invited to join the Cancer Hospital to strengthen the capacity of the research institute.

● Owing to Chinese reform and opening-up policy, many excellent scholars returned to China and joined the PUMC after completing their studies abroad. Among these scholars were Qiang Boqin, Xiu Ruijuan, Chen Dechang, Song Zengxuan, Chen Zhang, Zhan Qimin, He Jie, Jin Qi, Qin Chuan, Li Taisheng, Zhao Chunhua.

● Excellent graduates from other medical schools joined the PUMC workforce where they grew and developed, and ultimately became excellent representatives of medical practitioners and leaders in China, such as Wang Zhonggao, Lao Yuanxiu, Wang Aixia, Zhang Chengfen, Guo Yupu, Wang Zhizhong, Jiang Zhuming, Luo Ailun, Liu Xiaocheng and others.

Unfortunately, brain drain occurred in China during the ten-year Cultural Revolution as universities were closed. PUMC also faced the serious issues of generation gap with personnel, who while competent, were either aged or novice. The good thing is that heaven never seals off all the exits, especially for pumc System. We had distinctive advantages in human resources and inexhaustible potentials for development. Starting from 1993, for the following eight consecutive years, pumc did not limit itself to one mode of faculty recruitment and development, but rather adopted multiple approaches to attract and develop talent, including providing training and academic opportunities in a combination of domestic and overseas training programs, as well as offering positional promotions such as placing an outstanding recruit in a key position. As a result, a large number of young academic elites and leaders who were wise, competent, full of integrity and hard-working, matured and thrived at PUMC. By doing so, this corps of recruits not only addressed the faulty age of the personnel, but also supplied the healthcare professions and disciplines with academic leaders to meet the current and future needs. In fact, many have become the presidents or vice presidents of Chinese Medical Association or Chinese Medical Doctor Association, or chairs or candidates for chairs of various professional societies[3].

---

[3] The outstanding representatives are Zhao Yupei, Qian Jiaming, Jin Zhengyu, Liu Dawei, Jiang Yuxin, Huang Yuguang, Shen Keng, Wang Renzhi, Wang Baoxi, Chen Jie, Cui Liying, Zhang Fengchun, Jiang Ji, Wu Qingyu, Hu Shengshou, Liu Yinglong, Sun Lizhong, Liu Jin, Yang Yuejin, Gu Dongfeng, Zhao Ping, Shi Yuankai, Liu Depei, Shen Yan, He Wei, Zhang Xue, Wang Xiaoliang, Yu Shishan, Shao Rongguang, Chu Jiayou, Li Qihan, and others.

Many young stalwarts came to PUMC from abroad, doctors such as Yang Huanming, Lin Dongxin, Han Zhongchao, Jiang Jiandong, Hui Rutai, Wang Heng, Jiang Chengyu, Cheng Tao, Wang Jianxiang and others.

Furthermore, PUMC graduates became academic leaders at Beijing Medical University (now known as Peking University Health Sciences Center): With their year of graduation they are Hu Chuankui (Hu Ch'uan-k'uei, 1927), Wu Chaoren (Wu Ch'ao-jen, 1928), Wang Shuxian (Wang Shu-Hsin, 1930), Ma Wansen (Ma Wan-sen, 1935), Liu Jiaqi (Liu Gia-chi, 1937), Chen Jingyun (Ch'en Ching-yun, 1937), Feng Chuanhan (Feng Ch'uan-han, 1940), Yan Renying (Yen Jen-ying, 1940), Wang Guangchao (Wang Kuang-ch'ao, 1940), Wu Jieping (Wu Chieh-p'ing, 1942), as well as Zhu Hongyin, Guan Songtao (Kwan Sung-tao), Meng Jimao and others.

Some PUMC graduates assumed leadership positions at Shanghai Medical College: Rong Dushan (Jung Tu-shan, 1929), Xu Su'en (Hsu Su-en, 1932), Lin Feiqing (Lin Fei-ch'ing, 1932), Li Hongru (Li Hung-ju, 1934), Fan Rixin (Fan Jih-hsin, 1934), as well as Shen Kefei, Chen Cuizhen, Yan Fuqing (F. C. Yen), Lin Zhaoqi, Dai Ziying, Zhang Changshao, Xu Fengyan, Cui Zhiyi and others.

Other PUMC graduates became the most brilliant and prestigious doctors in Tianjin medical history: Shi Xien (Shih His-en, 1929), Zhu Xianyi (Chu Hsien-I, 1930), Bian Wannian (Bien Wan-nien, 1930), Jin Xianzhai (Kimn Hyen-taik, 1931), Fan Quan (Fan Ch'uan, 1931), Fang Xianzhi (Fang Hsien-chih, 1933), Situ Zhan (Szutu Chan, 1931), Zhao Yicheng (Chao Yi-ch'eng, 1934), Yu Aifeng (Yu Ai-feng, 1939) and others.

Still others, PUMC graduates became the academic leaders at Sun Yat-sen Medical College in Guanzhou including: Tang Zeguang (T'angTze-kuang,

1929), Qin Kuangyu (Ch'in Kuang-yu, 1930), Zhong Shifan (Chung Shih-fan, 1930, father of Zhong Nanshan), Chen Guozhen (Ch'en Kuo-chen, 1933), Zhou Shoukai (Chou Shou-k'ai, 1933), Lu Guanquan (Lu Kwan-ch'uan, 1937).

Furthermore, PUMC graduates became the academic leaders in Sichuan: Chen Zhiqian (Ch'en Chih-ch'en, 1929), Cao Zhongliang (father of Cao Zeyi, former Dean of West China University Medical College, a fellow at PUMC, 1935 – 1937).

In addition, PUMC graduates became the academic leaders in the Academy of Military Medical Sciences, Chinese PLA General Hospital, Peking Hospital, Sino-Japanese Friendship Hospital: Liu Yong, Zhou Jinhuang (Edward C. H. Chou, 1938), Yu Huanwen, Jiang Yutu (Chiang Yu-t'u, 1939), Li Gengtian Lu Weishan, Ye Huifang, Wu Weiran, Yang Youfeng and others. They paved the way for the founding and development of these top medical institutions and made significant contributions.

PUMC alumni also became key government ministers. Zhu Zhanggeng (Chu Chang-keng), Liu Ruiheng (Liu J. Heng), Lin Kesheng (Lim Kho-seng), and Shen Kefei used to serve as a Minister or Deputy Minister for the Ministry of Health in the Nationalist Government. Chu Chang-keng also served as the director of Institute of Health and was one of those involved in the preparatory work to found World Health Organization (WHO). Liu J. Heng founded Central Hospital and National Institute of Health and served as a president for both organizations and chaired the Anti-tobacco Committee. Lim Kho-seng served as the dean of National Defense Medical College in 1947 and also the first Minister for the Chinese Ministry of Health in 1948.

Chen Minzhang served as Minister of Health in 1987 while Wang Longde,

Peng Yu, Liu Qian were/are the Deputy Ministers. Chen Wenjie and Lu Rushan used to serve as Deputy Director-General of WHO. Liu Depei served as the Vice President of Chinese Academy of Engineering and Shen Yan is the Vice Director of National Natural Science Foundation of China.

On a personal note, my 25-year work experience at PUMC molded my temperament and shaped me, as if I went through a refinery process of "casting", "grinding", "steaming" and "heat treatment". All the bitterness and sweetness that I tasted there cemented my belief, cultivated my characteristics and improved my competence. I do not know how long it took before I could realize a truth that all people in PUMC were actually just like me — whether willingly or unwillingly, we received some sort of baptism at PUMC which is like a "furnace", the "processing factory". Thanks to that refining whether consciously or unconsciously, we pass on the great heritage of PUMC's culture and traditions. The most exciting thing is that the talents at PUMC never ceased to flourish and replenish from generation to generation, and now hasspread all over the world.

To my understanding, top universities are the ones that can attract top students and cultivate the finest minds. To that point, presidents for the top universities must be the visionary and accountable leaders. They spare no effort in nurturing people. Instead of teaching the students, leading academics encourage students acquire knowledge, learn to understand and practice the fundamental principles of "being an authentic person, doing the right things and exploring wider knowledge", as well as skills they need for a life time. Furthermore, the presidents of top universities advocate for long-term planning of individualized teaching with a belief that "soft fire makes sweet malt". The requirements of "three basics and three stricts" (basic theory, knowledge, and skills; strict attitude, requirements, and methods) specific to PUMC are not only for students, but also for the president to meet first. To be frank, the common problems for the "985 universities" or the "C9 universities" are that they are progressing too fast with no patience; they are featureless, with too much empty work, and too many meaningless comparisons with other universities.

In 2007, I delivered a speech at the 80th anniversary of Shanghai Medical College. I made a list of successful alumni of Shanghai Medical College, which showed that this college is one of the top universities producing and cultivating masters in their fields. Now I just presented a similar list above for PUMC. It was not difficult to tell that PUMC is the best among the top medical universities producing and cultivating even more masters.

PUMC created and dispersed higher education for nurses in China

Higher education programs for nurses in China began in 1919 at PUMC, which started to enrollsuch students in September 1920. The school's motto was "diligence, prudence, vigilance, and caring". At first it was called School of Nursing of Peking Union Medical College, and registered with the State University of New York, in the United States and the nurses' Assouation of China (NAC, later changed to Chinese Nursing Association). From that beginning until 1952, the School of Nursing graduated 263 students in 28 classes. Among those graduates, 60 worked abroad and most of the graduates became pioneers in Chinese nursing society. For example, Lin Sixin (Lin Sz-sing, 1926), Xu Aizhu (Hsu Ai-chu, 1930), Nie Yuchan (Vera Nieh, 1927), Lin Juying (Lin Chu-yin, 1941), Wang Xiuying (Wang Hsiu-ying, 1931), Wang Yi, Chen Qi (Ch'en Ch'I, 1931) and Mei Zuyi (Mei Tsu-yi, 1941) served as the Presidents or Vice Presidents of Chinese Nursing Association. Director-General Tian Cuili served the association for 15 years (1934 – 1949). She protected the dignity of the nursing association and advocated for a standardized national nursing graduation exam. Wang Xiuying was the first Chinese nurse to win the Florence Nightingale medal in the nation. It is worth mentioning that Ms Nie Yuchan, the fourth dean of PUMC School of Nursing, led a "long march" to Sichuan where despite the many hardship during the Sino-Japanese War, she maintained and kept running the school of nursing from 1940 to 1953. She deserves the name "heroine" for her role in nursing education during the war.

After reform and the "opening up", higher education for nurses was re-launched in China. At that time, however, the nursing schools were running with no uniform standards and programs. The bachelor program in nursing was five years with a degree in medicine. The nursing courses followed the same or a shorter version of the medical school curriculum. Another drawback was that many of the students did not enter clinical work after graduation, which caused a brain drain. In 1996, supported by China Medical Board and approved by the National Education Commission, PUMC was the first university to upgrade the department of nursing to a collegiate level (School of Nursing, PUMC) and change its bachelor degree program of nursing from five years to four years, conferring the B. S. degree in nursing. At the same time, the school of nursing invited several domestic and foreign nursing experts to develop the nursing curriculum, syllabus, teaching plan and series of the textbooks for upgrading the associate program to the bachelor program. This was widely recognized in the nursing society and received high commendation and great support from the National Education Commissionof China. It was listed as the most significant education and pedagogy reform project leading to the 21st century and was disseminated throughout the nation. During the transitional period of reform, capacity building and development, the Dean at that time, Shen Ning, led the faculty for nurses at PUMC School of Nursing and made significant contributions to Chinese higher education for nurses.

Looking to the future and the need to develop the talent pool, the school of nursing sent Liu Huaping to the U. S. for studies in higher education and there she received her doctorate of nursing diploma. More than a decade has passed,

Liu Huaping not only became an academic leader at PUMC but is a current and future academic leader in Chinese nursing.

PUMC created modern medicine and pharmacology in China

Innovation is to stand at the fore front, to exemplify and to lead. In this regard, PUMC played a pivotal role in the creation and development of modern medicine and pharmacology in China. Dating back to the early years of PUMC, its research on Peking Man was known worldwide and the skull of Peking Man was stored in the anatomy laboratory of PUMC. Unfortunately, the skull was lost during the Sino-Japanese War when the Japanese occupied PUMC, a huge loss to the history of human civilization. Around 1922, when Chen Kehui (Chen Ko-Kuei), a pharmacologist of PUMC, extracted the chemical compound ephedrine from Ephedra herb, that marked the beginning of true modernization of herbal medicine. In the 1930s, biochemist Wu Xian (Wu Hsien) at PUMC invented quantitative measurement of blood glucose, and along with Professor Liu Sizhi, proposed protein denaturation theory. Professor Liu applied a mathematical model to calculate chemical reactions and proposed that antibodies are bivalent, which means a singular antibody molecule binds with two antigen molecules. The list of outstanding work by PUMC scientists goes on: Professor Zhang Xijun's (Chang His-chun) study on acetylcholine, Professor Li Zongen (Lee Chung-en) and Professor Zhong Huilan's (William H. L. Chuang) study on kala azar disease, Professor Liu Shihao (Liu Shih-hao) and Professor Zhu Xianyi's (Chu Hsien-i) study on calcium phosphate metabolism, Professor Zhu Futang's (Chu Fu-t'ang) study on placental globulin in the prevention of measles as well as Professor Wu Yingkai (Wu Ying-k'ai) successful first surgery to eradicate esophageal carcinoma in the 1940s are all well-known.

Furthermore, after the Liberation, PUMC made great contributions to the prevention and treatment of infectious diseases, particularly, in the eradication of leprosy and poliomyelitis. PUMC alumni, Tang Feifan discovered trachoma virus （Chlamydia trachomatis） for the first time. The team led by Professor Gu Fangzhou worked very hard with very few resources to create the oral poliomyelitis vaccine in candy form that would keep without refrigerated transport. Giant steps toward the eradication of poliomyelitis in China was achieved by taking this oral vaccine invented by Dr. Gu's team.

Here, I must stress that we need advanced technology to solve practical problems. In early1960s, chorionic epithelioma, known as " King of the cancers" threatened women's health. Professor Song Hongzhao （Soong Hung-chao, 1943）, a gynecologist at PUMC hospital, led a research team to successfully treat patients with chorionic epithelioma using chemotherapy. This regimen not only saved patients, but also their fertility. That was a true miracle in the world and a remarkable contribution to medicine made by China. About that same time, Professor Hua Guang conducted a study of scopolamine and initiated a new approach to treat toxic shock and laid the groundwork for microcirculation. Research, development and production of antibiotics of various kinds addressed the needs of the nation's healthcare and disease prevention and treatment. Li Bing, the first president of Cancer Hospital strongly advocated for prevention and treatment of cancer, China's largest medical project. Cancer hospital conducted the earliest large-scale cohort study, combining field study, laboratory work and clinical medicine for better cancer treatment. A team from PUMC traveled to Linxian County in Henan Province to study esophageal cancer. Their long-term efforts resulted in significant findings for early detection, diagnosis and treatment of esophageal cancer. In the 1970s, initiated by National Cancer Prevention and Control Office, an atlas of the prevalence of cancer in China, based on the findings of this retrospective study was completed and published. This atlas is a precious document with high scientific value.

In 1978, China embraced the spring of science after the National Science and Technology Conference was held, which brought into full play the initiatives and creativity of leading scientists. Remarkable achievements were displayed: A vaccine for Hepatitis A, Artificial musk, biphenyl ester, bicyclol, taxol, butylphthalide and other new drugs were gradually put onto market. PUMC was the first to use synthetic biology techniques to develop kelimycin, which has great economic and social benefits. Tough and complicated surgeries on heart diseases were successfully performed. Large-scale multicenter clinical research on prevention and treatment of cardiovascular diseases was conducted with significant international influence. The level of cerebrovascular disease prevention and treatment improved significantly. More than sixty human monogenic inherited diseases were discovered in China, one fourth of which were discovered by scientists at PUMC. The university was the first in the world to successfully isolate stem cells from the placenta. Good clinical outcomes were achieved in the treatment of ischemic necrosis in the leg by using mesenchymal stem cells. The discovery of effects of berberine on lowering lipid and glucose initiated new treatment regimen for metabolic disorders. Long-term follow-up cohort study of mega sampling on prevention and treatment of cancers provides strong evidence for cancer etiology, cancer incidence and prevalence pattern, and the improvement of cancer prevention and treatment strategies in China. Additionally, a number of breakthroughs were achieved in key genomics research on esophageal carcinoma. Many clinical trials of new anti-cancer drugs were completed and continuously won the first-place National Prize for Progress in Science and Technology. A vaccine research and development system was established and developed. The first EV71 vaccine used in prevention of hand-foot-mouth disease for children and inactivated poliovirus Sabin strain vaccines have been approved for sale. Many research projects, led primarily by PUMC have won the first-place National Prize for Progress in Science and Technology, such as research on effective anticancer components of Hainan Cephalotaxus; study and implementation of artificial musk; PUMC's project on new mechanism research of immune cell differentiation; development and functional regulation and research on new mechanism for inflammation resolution and immune homeostasis regulation were nominated as top ten projects in China's College and University Science and Technology Advancement Award in 2014 and 2015 respectively.

PUMC highlights its role as the national team in medical science and constructs high-end medical research platforms. For instance, PUMC has built up the first national key laboratory in medicine, national key science and technology infrastructure for translational medicine (PUMC Hospital) and was approved to construct three other national clinical medical research centers. A national demographic and health information sharing platform has been established at PUMC and a series of national resources platform were formed, such as primate animal base, animal models of disease platform, medical information platform, microbiology sampling database, and stem cell database. PUMC also successfully accomplished a number of major scientific support tasks for emergency prevention and control of disease, such as SARS, hand-foot-mouth disease, (influenza) H1N1, human infection of bird flu such as H5N1, H7N9, and H10N8, emergency control of imported polio and assisted in the fight against Ebola in Africa.

The following numbers might illustrate PUMC's role and contribution to science and technology innovation in the medical and health sector in China. PUMC owns five key national laboratories; has been awarded the first-place prize for National Scientific Achievements for 11 projects. Fifty-five faculty of PUMC and its affiliates were elected as Academician of the Chinese Academy of Sciences or Chinese Academy of Engineering (21 of them passed away), an additional 25 PUMC alumni who do not work at PUMC were elected as Academician of Chinese Academy of Sciences or Chinese Academy of Engineering. Ten PUMC faculty were recognized as fellows of Academy of Sciences in other countries.

China's national healthcare development strategy serves as a blueprint and flagship for the advancement of medicine and health in China. PUMC plays a pivotal role in the planning, implementation, evaluation, and approving of relevant strategies. From Healthy China 2020, to Medical and Health in national projects of 863 and 973, PUMC has demonstrated its wisdom and power in these National Key and Specialized Mega projects. In fact, PUMC is the place where fresh sparks erupt and collide, where new ideas are conceived, and new actions initiated. Looking back, when Yang Huanming, faculty member of PUMC wanted to do research on genome, it was Wu Min, Qiang Boqin and I who gave him strong support, so that the exceptional "1%" of the genome project-southern genes, northern genes and BGI-were later created. Two years before President Barack Obama advocated for Precision Medicine Initiative, PUMC had already initiated a national project to establish precise and scientific diagnosis and treatment system which was approved by experts. Once President Obama delivered his address, PUMC submitted a report to the State Council on Chinese precision medicine developmental strategies and implementation plan, which led to the popularity of precision medicine today. Similarly, PUMC has always advocated for combining basic science with clinical medicine. The first nationally approved translational medicine center in China was launched at PUMC Hospital as soon as the concept of translational medicine first emerged. Liu Depei, Shen Yan, Zhao Yupei, Zhan Qimin, and He Wei all possess the qualities and vision of strategic scientists. Of course, those strategic medical scientists who are more capable will emerge and play a bigger role in China.

The "three basics" and "three rigorousness" is the heritage of PUMC, while innovation is the scientific spirit of PUMC. As for science-academic democracy, independent thinking, pursuit of excellence, and teamwork form the fundamental essence of PUMC's culture. This culture of *pumc of virtue from the east and west and harmony of the universe* has been a heritage for a century and now has become the norm for PUMC. It is the spiritual heaven that all people from PUMC strive to maintain and improve upon. Without doubt, generations of intellectuals will keep coming out of this heaven and will continue to make fruitful achievements.

PUMC cultivated and created presidents for the most prestigious medical universities in China

PUMC is not only a school to train students and physicians and a cradle for medical scientists, but it is also an institute to create presidents for medical universities, and a "training class" for medical educators.

• Ma Wenzhao (Eiko Ma), a PUMC graduate, Associate Professor of Anatomy of PUMC and later tenure Professor of Anatomy of Beijing Medical University (currently the PKUHSC), a renowned embryologist, served as the President of Beijing Medical University from 1946 to 1947.

• Yan Fuqing (F. C. Yen), served as Associate Dean of PUMC in 1926 and was appointed by the Nationalist Government as the first Dean of Medical College of the Forth Sun Yat-sen University (later became the Shanghai Medical College and Shanghai Medical University).

• Hu Chuankui (Hu Ch'uan-k'uei, 1927), a renowned dermatologist, served as the Dean of Beijing Medical College and the President of Beijing Medical University for 33 years (1948 – 1981). He headed Beijing Medical College for one third of its 100 years of history and was its historical witness.

• Zhu Xianyi (Chu Hsien-I, 1930), a renowned endocrinologist, served as the Dean of Tianjin Medical College and the President of Tianjin Medical University from 1951 to 1984.

• Li Zongen (Lee Chung-en), specialized in tropical medicine, served as the President of Peking Union Medical College Hospital. He was appointed by the National Government as the Dean of National Guiyang Medical College at the beginning of the war in 1937. He returned to PUMC and served as the President of PUMC after the Sino-Japanese war.

● Wang Jiwu (Wang Chi-wu, 1934), specialized in infectious diseases, student and disciple of Lee Chung-en, served as Dean of the School of Medicine, Zhejiang University in 1947. He served as the Vice-President and President of Zhejiang Medical College (Zhejiang Medical University) after the merging of the school from 1952 to1984.

● Wu Jieping (Wu Chieh-p'ing, 1942), a renowned urologist served as Vice-President and President of Beijing Second Medical College from 1960 to 1970; Vice-President of PUMC/CAMS from 1970 to 1983; President of PUMC/CAMS from 1983 to 1985.

● I formed my own philosophy, cultivated my characteristics, and learned a disciplined approach to work during the time I was president for PUMC and CAMS from 1992 to 2001. What I gained became very useful when I was the Dean for School of Medicine, Zhejiang University and was requested to make the medical school a "PUMC" in southern China. I cannot claim that PUMC's model, concept and approach will work in all Chinese medical education institutions, but at least, it was successful in Zhejiang University. The medical school of Zhejiang University, a provincial college originally not ranked in the top ten, moves forward annually. Within a decade it has become a new force that has risen suddenly to make its way to enjoy a firm position among the top medical schools in China.

● Academician Zhan Qinmin, trained and edified in PUMC, has just recently been appointed Director of Peking University Health Sciences Center. He captured the hearts of students and faculty with his beautiful songs. We also believe that he will make Peking University Health Sciences Center a better institution with his talents and character.

The National Science and Technology Innovation Conference applauded people in the nation for making a powerful country with strong science and technology. This is perfect timing for PUMC to reach new goals as we celebrate our 100th anniversary, reflect on our past and look forward to the future. In response to President Xi's great call to create top universities and top medical disciplines and to turn CAMS into the "NIH of China" as early as possible, innovative and influential PUMC must cultivate more medical elites and leaders. To realize China's dreams through innovation-driven development today, CAMS/PUMC will fully execute its role as "the national team" and "locomotive" in the field of population and health, engage itself in making greater contributions to carry on the great national heritage and to promote the wellbeing and prosperity of the Chinese nation.

Bibliography

1. Ba D. N. （2014）. Speech on 100th anniversary commemoration of CMB. Peking Union Medical College Newsletter.

2. Ba D. N. （2010）. Liberal Heart, Scientific Mind, World Perspectives, Hardworking Hand, My Medical Education Perspective and Practice. Science Times.

3. Ba D. N. （2007）. Speech on 80th anniversary commemoration of Shanghai Medical School.

4. Ba D. N. （1999）. Economic Reform and Peking Union Medical College. Peking Union Medical College Newsletter.

5. Bullock, M. B. （2014）. The Oil Prince's Legacy: Rockefeller Philanthropy in China. The Commercial Press.

6. Deng, J. D. （1987）. History of Peking Union Medical College. Beijing Science and Technology Press.

7. Wang, J. R. Peking Union Medical College Hospital （1921 – 1991）, 70th Anniversary commemoration album of PUMC. 990530

让我们共同迎接挑战——写在协和百年之际

柯杨

柯杨，北京大学常务副校长，美国国家医学院外籍院士。2004 年至 2006 年任北京大学医学部（PUHSC）任常务副主任。全国政协第十一，十二届全国委员，国务院学位委员会委员，中华医学会副会长，中国学位和研究生教育委员会常务委员会委员。她的主要研究领域是上消化道恶性肿瘤的环境因素和遗传因素。

今年是协和医学院一百周年纪念。一百年前的此时，一批带着救世情怀、怜悯之心的美国人来到中国，建立了著名的北京协和医学院。彼时，正是美国的医学教育刚刚调整到更加严格规范的世纪之初，并在本土的医学院形成了标杆。与上世纪初中国几个西医院校的成立相呼应，协和的成立，使当时中国的北方地区也有了一家标准的西医院校。

长期以来，协和以其高质量的教学、严格的临床培训、优秀的教师及尖子学生形成了国内医学教育的象牙塔，也影响了一批国内优秀医学院的成长。

作为兄弟院校，北医就曾在不同历史阶段吸收了几批著名教师，引进了协和精神。例如，北医早期的住院医培训就是效仿的协和模式。

在祝贺协和百年辉煌的日子里，作为医学教育的同行，我愿在此分享北医在过去十几年中通过教育实践、改革与思考，对医学教育面临的机遇、挑战的认识，以资共勉。

回顾医学教育发展，以美国为代表的医学教育引领世界近百年。上世纪初，从弗莱克斯纳（Flexner）在系统评估了医学教育之后，提出学科规范，学制固定，注重质量，学术引导的教育改革，因此而推动了正规医学教育的普及。百年后的今天，当我们再次反思，可以不无惊奇的发现，医学教育仍然是当今迅速发展的世界中受到挑战最多的、需要调整改革最多的高等教育。如果归纳之，如下五条似乎更为显著：

首先，医学教育的综合性在当代变得更加明确和突出。这种综合性体现在专业的多样性、各专业知识体系的综合性和对个人素质要求的综合性上。医学教育包括临床医学、口腔医学、公共卫生、护理、药学、检验、影像、康复、麻醉、眼视光等医技类学科以及与医学相关的社会科学类学科和法医学等其他类学科。这有别于既往和国外目前医学教育所指的单纯临床医生的培养。随着科学技术的发展、社会服务类型和水平的提高、医疗体制的理顺，尤其是人们对健康的需求日益高涨，等等这些因素都导致社会对各类懂医的相关人才从数量上和类型上的需求越来越大。而"大医学"背景下培养临床医生和上述各类相关的医学人才是发展趋势，是全球医学教育改革的重要内容之一。2011 年发表在《柳叶刀》杂志上的全球医学教育独立委员会的分析报告客观地分析了医学教育存在的问题，指出对于健康问题，医疗只是整个链条中的末端，而预防、基层医疗、慢病康复及管理将成为保证人群健康和最终解决医疗高额成本的关键。除了传统的专业化培养，打破专业界限培养复合型人才及各类各层懂医的专业人员，通过护理、公共卫生（卫生经济学者、卫生监督人员、健康教育者、食品与营养师、懂医的各类政府官员等）、临床、全科医生整合的团队，回归基层工作方式是实现这一目标的重要一环。这将是医学教育改革的"第三次革命"。在我国，历史上大多数医学教育包含了医学相关的各个学院，如基础医学、护理、临床医学院（附属医院）、公共卫生、药学等等，专业齐全，因此才能称作"医科大学"。在诸多优秀医科大学并入综合大学的今天，坚持在"大医学"背景下培养临床医生及其医学相关人才恰恰符合新时代社会对人才的需求。而医学内部的学科交叉整合也是医学教育改革发展的大趋势。

医学综合性的另一个体现是知识结构。就临床医学生培养而言，医学教育思想方法涉及多学科。在我国，医学生是由理科分类的高中生报考，大家自然容易将医学片面定位为理科。但它既不是单纯的理科也不是工科，还需要有很重要的社会科学思想方法以及人文精神的培养和教育。所以，医学是综合性非常强的专业。医学生需要综合思维，不但需要具备工科解构认识对象、发现问题、解决问题的能力，同时也需要理科所具备的无限细分深入到分子研究功能的素质，更需要社会科学中流行病和统计学等对病因和疗效等复杂问题的研究技能，以及社文"四课"和伦理、医史、交流学、心理等人文精神的素养。加之医学对动手能力的要求，加之医学的职业精神，这些综合素质最终构成了医学生的"岗位胜任力"。

其二，社会体制转型、科技进步、全球化、网络信息化等深刻改变着人们的生活和思想理念，进而对医学教育产生深刻影响。因为医学教育职业性的特征，她不可能独立于、孤立于社会。结合我们中国的现状更是如此——一方面我们正在经历的社会转型，改变了人们的价值理念、生活条件、生活习惯、健康期望以及诚信互信。这些不但直接影响着人群的健康，改变了疾病谱，也决定了新型的医患关系和医学生对待职业的态度。在我国社会转型时期，我们正在经历的社会转型包含了医疗体制这一重大社会体制的重构，从计划经济转向中国特色模式，既保持公益性又融入市场规律。而这一历程在时间和难度上远远超出人们的预期。在这一艰难过渡阶段，公共卫生的加强，基层医疗的恢复，三级医疗的质量与安全，医院的生存方式等等，不但决定了体制本身，也影响着医学及健康相关职业岗位对优秀人才的吸引力。与此同时，年轻人经历了信仰危机、社会诚信危机、职业的多元性选择、物质利益的诱惑……当今的医学生正经历前所未有的焦虑。这些都要求我们对医学生加强"全人教育"和职业精神的引导，做出综合努力，助其综合能力的提高。唯有这样的努力才能让医学生更加坚定、自信与成熟。总之，今日的医学生再也不是当年选择了学医就坚定不移、两耳不闻窗外事，一心只读"圣贤书"了。医学教育再也不能像过去那样，单纯的传授医学知识与技能，而不关心医学生的心灵成长。我们不能等待社会的进步和体制的完善，必须做出教育的改变和应对。

其三，随着医学技术的快速发展，医疗的能力大为提高，对人类的期望寿命的提高做出了很大贡献，但也带来"技术至上"的弊端。我们应该看到，由于技术进步带来的科技进步体现在医疗技术上的极致，大大强化了我们的医疗能力。但进步让百姓受益的同时，提高了诊疗成本，提高了人们对"治愈"的期望值；分科过细肢解了人的整体性；机器的使用隔离了人与人之间的交流，淡化了医学不可或缺的人文关怀；新材料新方法的涌现促进了过度诊疗。同时医疗能力的提高并不覆盖所有疾病，并不覆盖疾病及健康维护的全过程。占疾病 70% 以上的慢性复杂性疾病仍然要依靠强有力的预防和长期监控和康复……这些变化强烈呼唤医疗模式的改变，医学教育需要主动通过人才培养促进之。其中培养适应中国的现实的全科医生，是教育必须"超前"并配合医疗体制相应改革的重要任务。除了一些重要专业人才的补充，如护理人才、医学社工、临床药师、康复师等等，专科医生的人文精神和综合能力也需要受到足够的重视与基础性的加强。

其四，伴随科技发展，教育手段和获取知识的方式发生改变，面对爆炸式增长同时又有融合的医学知识，不可能靠传统教育方式完成。医学基础知识的爆炸，信息化知识传播的出现，需要我们的医学教育彻底改变书本为中心、教师为中心、一言堂灌输式的陈旧落后的方式，更加突出问题引领，实践感悟的教育手段。医学人一辈子终生学习的能力，也早已成为不可或缺的要求。这些都需要医学教育通过改革灌输式、书本知识传授式、教师讲授为中心、背考试内容及基础和临床脱离式的陈旧教育模式，使现状得到根本性的改变。

其五，医学教育的阶段性、持续性、实践性，使总的学制较长，既有在校的知识传授，又有医院的实践，身份的转换和过渡较复杂。各国的医学教育既有共性，又有特性。在我国，学制和医学教育改革经历了复杂过程：学制上，从最初的相对短学制的"欧洲模式"，又引入了"改良"的长学制的"北美模式",使原本较整齐划一的学制出现了分化,在时间切口上出现差别甚至混乱。在学历上,临床医学从只有本科学历、发展出研究生教育。在学位上,从只有科学学位,发展出专业学位,使临床专业的"住院医培训"更规范,同时解决了临床专业学生获得名副其实的高学历之学位问题。在行业管理上,从原本的医疗行业主管,转变为医、教共管。本科教育和研究生教育归教育部,涉及实践的教育(研究生教育和继续教育)归卫生部,而且后者在实践教育的规范性上和准入上逐渐规范严格。所有这些变革、变迁、调整、发展、进步的过渡,都需要教育者的理解,主动进取与被动适应和调整。

面对问题与挑战,我国医学教育工作者都在做出自己的应对,尤其借鉴国际同行的经验开展各种方式、内容的改革。其中包括研讨问题,更包括自我改革全方位加强全人教育、理顺学制、强化各类实践、改革课程体系、建立急需新学科、走国际化道路……北大医学教育近十年也做出了自己的努力,改革取得了一些成绩,但仍然只是开端,需要不断探索并与国内外同行交流互助。改革永远在路上,因为我们处在快速发展变革的时代,教育既有万变不变之内核,更有与时俱进不断顺应改革之需求。医学教育更是如此。

Rising Up to Our Shared Challenges
Remarks at the Centenary of Peking Union Medical College

Ke Yang

Ke Yang, Executive Vice-president of Peking University (PKU), a foreign member of National Academy of Medicine (US). She served as Executive Vice President of Peking University Health Science Center (PUHSC) from 2004 to 2016. a member of the 11th and 12th CPPCC national committee, member of the Academic Degree Committee of State Council, Vice-president of China Medical Association, and member of the Standing Committee of Chinese Committee for Academic Degree and Postgraduate Education. Her major research area is on the environmental and genetic factors of upper digestive tract malignant tumor.

This year marks the centenary of the Peking Union Medical College (PUMC). A hundred years ago, a group of Americans came to China in their benevolence and built the PUMC in accordance with the latest and more rigorous benchmarks that had just taken shape in the American medical education. The establishment of the PUMC coincided with several other Chinese schools of Western medicine, and completed the jigsaw puzzle as the piece from North China.

Since then, the PUMC with its high-caliber teaching and training, outstanding faculty and excellent students, has been a lighthouse for medical Education in China, admired by its fellow institutions at home.

As a sister university, the Peking University Health Science Center (PUHSC) for one has in its history recruited groups of PUMCers into its faculty, bringing in some of the practices observed in the PUMC. The residency program of the PUHSC, for instance, was initially modeled after the PUMC.

As we celebrate the 100 years of the PUMC, I would also like to talk about the opportunities and challenges in medical education in general, based on the practices, reforms and explorations at PUHSC over the last two decades.

Medical education in the past 100 years has been largely under the influence of the American model, a model that came into being following Dr. Abraham Flexner's systematic evaluation of medical education in the early 20th century. His efforts led to an educational reform that standardized disciplines, fixed length of training, shifted emphasis on quality and introduced mechanisms for academic supervision, making medical education what we have come to know today.

This system, however, is far from perfect. A hundred years after the Flexner Report, medical education is still one of the most challenging branches of higher education, where reform is most needed.

First, medical education is becoming more comprehensive. This comprehensiveness is shown in the diversity of its disciplines, the richness of each discipline and the components of competency.

In its broad sense, medical education goes beyond clinical medicine, dentistry, public health, nursing, pharmacology, laboratory, imaging, rehabilitation, anesthesia and ophthalmology, to include disciplines such as health-related social sciences and even forensic medicine. In practice, however, the term only refers to the training of clinical doctors. With the development of technologies, diversification and improvement of social services, reform of healthcare system, and in particular the rise of demand for health, an increasing number of health professionals with diversified disciplines will be needed. Training clinical doctors and other health professionals with a holistic approach to medicine will be the future and thus addressing a major issue that educational reforms around the world.

In its 2011 report published on *The Lancet*, the Commission on the Education of Health Professionals for the 21st Century looked into problems in current medical education and indicated that medicine is merely a last link in the chain to maintain health, and that the solution to population health and excessive medical costs lies in prevention, primary health care and management of chronic diseases. Therefore on top of traditional training, we must break the boundary between specialties in producing trans-disciplinary personnel, build an integrated team of nurses, public health specialists (health economists, health inspectors, health promoters, nutritionists and health officials), clinical doctors and GPs, and shift our focus to primary care. This will be the theme of the third revolution in medical education.

In China, higher education institutions of medicine used to be called universities because they each consisted of a complete cluster of medicine-related schools, such as schools of basic medicine, nursing, clinical medicine, public health and pharmacology. Most of these institutions have now merged into other comprehensive universities, but their holistic approach to the training of clinical doctors and other health professionals is everything but obsolete. Integration of medical disciplines will continue to build momentum in the unfolding reform.

The comprehensiveness of medicine also leads to the requirement of an equally comprehensive structure of knowledge on the part of the professionals. Training of clinical doctors alone involves multiple disciplines. In China, medical schools enroll students of science from high school, which gives people an impression that medicine is all about science. In fact, it is more than science or engineering; it requires trainings of social sciences and humanities, too. Accordingly, students need to have a comprehensive way of thinking. They should be able to de-structure the object, identify the problem and solve it like an engineer, dig deep into molecules to explain physiological functions like a scientist, investigate cause of disease and efficacy of treatment with epidemiological and statistic methodologies like a researcher, and learn about ethics, history of medicine, communication and psychology as a properly educated person. Adding to this list are operational skills and medical professionalism, and all of these constitute the competency of a medical student.

Second, people's lifestyles and mindsets are going through great changes brought about by social transformation, technological advancement, globalization and informatization, which has far-reaching implications on medical education as well because medicine is not practiced in a vacuum.

This is especially true to what we see in China. The Chinese society is evolving rapidly, which gives rise to changes in people's values, living standards, lifestyles, health expectancy, and mutual trust. These factors have direct impacts on population health and disease spectrum; more importantly, they are re-shaping physician-patient relations and medical students' attitudes toward their career.

One aspect of China's social transformation comes in the form of its healthcare reform, a transition from an old model geared for a planned economy to a new one that pursues public welfare in a market economy and keep its public welfare as well. This process turns out to be much more difficult and time-consuming than anybody could initially anticipate. How we manage to enhance capacity of public health interventions, build capacity in primary health care, improve quality and safety of the tertiary system, and design sustainability strategy for health providers will be the key elements to both the system that emerges from the reform and the attractiveness of health-related career to a new generation.

On the other hand, medical students are experiencing greater anxiety amid conflicts of values, collapse of trust, diversified career paths and temptation of materialism. This is an urgent call for holistic education and professionalism cultivation which will help students grow into mature, confident and committed human beings. The days were gone when stepping into medical school meant a life devoted to the career, and so were the days when medical education meant nothing more than training of skills. We cannot sit back and wait for society and its institutions to perfect themselves; we must push for change from the educational front.

Third, although progress in medical technologies has expanded the limits of health care and contributed to a higher life expectancy, it has also led to an excessive and lopsided emphasis on technology itself. While the significance of technology should never be underestimated, we must be fully aware of the problems that come with it. For instance, deployment of new technologies pushes up medical costs, raises unrealistic expectations of a cure and encourages excessive medical treatment; medical specialties sub-dividing into smaller fields makes it difficult to maintain a holistic view; and use of machinery reduces communication between doctors and patients, making the practice less humanistic. Besides, despite the advancement in treatment, control of complex chronic diseases which make up over 70% of the disease burden still hinges on prevention and long-term management. All of these again call for a transformation of healthcare model, and medical education should act as a contributor to this change. The training of GPs for instance is what we can do now to match the trend of reform in the future. Similarly, we should train more nurses, social workers, clinical pharmacists, rehabilitation therapists and other much needed professionals. At the same time, we must make education of humanities an important part in the training of specialist doctors to improve their competency.

Fourth, technological development has changed the ways of teaching and learning, and conventional pedagogy is no longer valid when facing the explosion and integration of medical knowledge. We should therefore abandon the lecture-based method that revolves around textbooks, teachers and tests, adopt an alternative that is problem-and practice-oriented, and help students become lifetime learners.

Fifth, medical education is a widespread yet continuous spectrum of practice-based stages. Students are trained both in medical schools and in hospitals, which gives them mixed roles and identities.

The system of medical education in China has its unique characteristics which came into being after rounds of complex reforms. 1) Lengths of training. In the beginning, China followed the so-called European model with a relatively short length of student training. This model was later abandoned by some institutions in favor of the North American model which required longer training period. This created a mixture of training programs varying in lengths. 2) Degrees. Academic degrees used to be the only type of degrees that medical students could expect after finishing their training. This was changed when professional degrees were introduced. This positive change helped standardize residency training and gave graduates of clinical programs a certificate that they truly deserved. 3) Administration. The Chinese Ministry of Health used to be the only government authorities of medical education. It now, however, has ceded administration of undergraduate education and non-practice-based graduate education to the Ministry of Education. By focusing on practice-based education（graduate education and continuing education）, the MOH managed to establish more rigorous standards on training of students and accreditation of sites. As educationists, we should study the rationale behind these changes, adapt to them and push for new progress.

To address these challenges, Chinese educationists have put in tremendous efforts. We have, in particular, learned from our international peers and carried out reforms on both what we teach and how we teach it. These reforms did not stop at solving isolated problems, but went on to reshape the system by emphasizing holistic education, pursuing uniformity in the length of training, intensifying practices, redesigning curriculum, establishing disciplines, and tuning to international standards. This is also what has been happening at the PUHSC over the last decade. We have seen fruits coming out of such efforts; yet still, we have before us a long way to go. Being in rapidly evolving society means reform will always be an ongoing effort. So is educational reform, and so is medical education.